Thirty Days to Natural Blood Pressure Control

The "No Pressure" Solution

Publisher:

COMPASSHEALTH CONSULTING, INC.

FORESTHILL, CALIFORNIA

www.compasshealth.net

Copyright © 2016 by CompassHealth Consulting, Inc.

Published in the United States of America

All Rights Reserved

Edited by Clifford Goldstein

Cover by Akira007/ Akiragraphicz and Heather R. Steinke

Graphics by Naomi Schumacher, Sherle Curtice, and RRGraph

Layout by Indie Publishing Group

Publisher's Notice

The authors greatly appreciate the time you're investing to improve your health by reading this book. Please help extend the influence of this important topic by leaving a review where you bought the book, or telling your friends about it. Thank you.

The information in this book is designed for educational purposes only. It is not intended to be a substitute for informed medical advice or care. You should not use the information provided to diagnose or treat any health problems or illnesses without first consulting your primary health care giver.

ISBN: 978-1-942730-02-6

DEDICATION

To our families, for their years of patience and support in the midst of long clinical hours and countless hours teaching, writing, and otherwise communicating the good news about non-drug therapies for illness.

To our patients, for sharing their lives and stories with us.

CONTENTS

ABOUT THE AUTHORS

David DeRose, MD, MPH

Heard on more than 140 radio stations, syndicated radio show host and practicing physician, Dr. David DeRose for three decades has been helping people address, with natural therapies, disease processes. DeRose brings solid credentials as a board-certified specialist in both Internal Medicine and Preventive Medicine, in addition to holding a Master in Public Health degree, with an emphasis in Health Promotion and Health Education.

Dr. DeRose's commitment to educating the masses on optimal health strategies has taken him far beyond the radio booth and medical clinic. He has taught at the college level, held numerous seminars for health professionals and lay audiences alike, and has been featured in TV and video health series. DeRose's research has been published in peer-reviewed medical journals, including *The Journal of the American Medical Association*, *The Annals of Epidemiology*, and *Preventive Medicine*.

Greg Steinke, MD, MPH

As a Lifestyle Medicine Specialist, Dr. Greg Steinke has had the opportunity to help many patients reverse their blood pressure naturally. Steinke is board-certified in Family Medicine and Preventive Medicine, holding a Master in Public Health degree, with an emphasis in Public Health Nutrition. In addition to his clinic and hospital practice, Steinke regularly conducts community-based lifestyle education programs designed to reverse and improve chronic diseases such as heart disease, high blood pressure, high cholesterol, diabetes, depression, and tobacco addiction.

He was part of the inaugural graduating class in the first Lifestyle Medicine program in America. His training, at Loma Linda University in California, especially prepared him to help those motivated to leave a life of sickness, medications, and helplessness for, instead, a life of vigor and vitality and with less medication. He believes people can take charge of their health and leave nearly every trace of their prior state of ill health behind.

Trudie Li, MSN, FNP

Trudie Li is a family nurse practitioner passionate about engaging others in the pursuit of a healthier lifestyle. A graduate of Loma Linda University, Trudie worked in China at Sir Run Run Shaw Hospital as Loma Linda's nursing representative. It was during the SARS epidemic there that Trudie's commitment to public health was solidified while working with the local Center for Disease Control. Since then, Trudie has regularly assisted with staff development and health education at lifestyle centers in China. Her stateside experience revolves around incorporating lifestyle education into medical-surgical nursing and family practice. Her enthusiasm is renewed with each patient's commitment to evidence-based lifestyle choices.

THE STORIES IN THIS BOOK

As health care professionals, we've been grateful to care for thousands of people with high blood pressure. The stories and the lives they represent hold great value to us and we wish to hold them in honor as we retell them. Therefore, the names and identifying details have been changed to maintain anonymity.

About this Book's Voice

Other than our introductory notes, we've written this book using a single voice. Although our collective clinical experience and research is represented on these pages, when relating first-hand experiences with our patients or sharing bits of our own journeys, we have chosen to use the first person pronoun "I," without indicating who is telling the story. Among the reasons for this choice are: First, it adds an additional element of confidentiality to the stories. Although we always change the names and circumstances of our patients, blurring the practitioner's identity adds an additional level of anonymity. Second, we are authoring this book as a team, and none of our clinical experiences or life journeys carry more weight than do another's. It would be counterproductive to set readers up to give more credence to sections written by one of the authors rather than another. Third, each of us as authors is on a journey with you, our readers. We're all trying to improve our health by bringing our lives more into harmony with the laws of our being. In view of this, in the body of the book, we reserve the use of the second person to our common journey—readers and authors together—to that state of better health.

FOREWORD

If as many lives were claimed by a natural disaster, we would not be so complacent. But because the villain is hypertension, and because it resides in so many of our homes, we're in danger of tolerating its presence.

However, when it comes to loss of life, hypertension (the medical term for high blood pressure) wreaks far more havoc worldwide than do all natural disasters combined. Globally, the World Health Organization estimates that 9.4 million people die annually from only the cardiovascular complications of hypertension.[1] Compare that to data linking less than 80,000 deaths annually to natural disasters.[2] In other words, high blood pressure claims more than 100 times as many lives as the effects of all natural disasters combined. The tragedy is augmented when we realize hypertension's complications are largely preventable with essentially side-effect-free natural strategies!

This book is not a hypothetical treatise relating merely good suggestions to help your blood pressure. It is a book based on evidence, solid medical research studies, as well as the changed lives witnessed by the health care providers authoring this book. It is a book that provides practical strategies to help you get your blood pressure (BP) under control, once and for all, without depending on costly, side-effect-ridden medications.

Yes, hypertension is far more deadly than any tsunami, earthquake or tornado on record. But there are typically no sirens, urgent news reports, or alarms commanding our attention. Furthermore, unlike such natural disasters, we can actually stop most of high blood pressure's root causes. The reality is this: many individuals can get their blood pressure under control in 30 days or less. Even if your BP is more sluggish to respond, the roadmap provided in this book is calculated to lead you to a new life with less medications and far better blood pressure readings.

Join us on this life-changing 30-day journey. Your life will never be the same.

David DeRose, MD, MPH

Greg Steinke, MD, MPH

Trudie Li, MSN, FNP

Thirty Days to Natural Blood Pressure Control

The "No Pressure" Solution

By David DeRose, MD, MPH; Greg Steinke, MD, MPH; and Trudie Li, MSN, FNP

1

THE PERSONAL AND GLOBAL TOLL OF HIGH BLOOD PRESSURE

THE NIGHT SKY WAS clear, the air crisp and clean. Once I got out of my car at the lecture venue, the only noise interrupting that night's stillness was the repetitive sound of my feet hitting the pavement until an older model Chevy pickup began reversing out of its parking space. My eyes met the eyes of the pickup driver. It was Norman, my patient.

I was excited Norman was here, apparently to sign up for our heart healthy program. He sure needed it. However, I was confused. He was leaving, not coming. As Norman continued backing up, he rolled down his window and broke the news, "Doc, I really do appreciate the opportunity. But I've got a lot of work to do on the other side of the state. Can't attend this time. Maybe next time." Though concerned, what could I say?

Norman and his wife, Judy, had been successful Wisconsin farmers. However, tired of the cold winters, they recently sold their farm and moved to our community with its more temperate climate. Judy thought it would be easier for Norman to get healthy, free from the demands of farm life. His blood pressure was poorly controlled, which she knew only added to the risks of his diabetes and high cholesterol.

Not many days before that brief parking lot meeting, Norman was in my medical office complaining of shortness of breath. I offered him a variety of treatment options but he wouldn't commit. I ordered some heart tests, but he hadn't had them done.

As Norman drove off, I had an uneasy feeling. He needed to take his health seriously. He was too nonchalant. He wasn't interested in the treatments I had offered. He wasn't interested in living healthier. "Doc, come on," he said, trying to reassure me. "Other than a little shortness of breath, I feel fine."

A few days later, I received a call. Norman had been admitted to the hospital with a catastrophic, life-threatening stroke. He was on life-support. He couldn't move his limbs. He was confused. The hospitalist told me he was doubtful Norman would ever leave the hospital. He didn't. Norman hung on for two weeks in the ICU before breathing his last.

I was deeply saddened. The warning signs were there. I had attempted to impress Norman with their gravity. However, his apathy indicated he thought that I was the one with the problem: excessive concern regarding a healthy patient!

Now I was faced with one of those times when every compassionate health practitioner hates to be right. Norman was dead; his life had ended far too soon. Judy was a widow. It was all so unnecessary.

Blood pressure. Within appropriate limits, we need it to stay alive. However, high blood pressure is a beacon of warning. Refuse to respond at your own risk. Please, don't follow in Norman's footsteps.

What Might Have Been

Ed was a successful accountant in his mid-fifties. He had worked hard for many years and had finally come to the place where he could start slowing down. Unfortunately, Ed had neglected his health for several decades. He had gained weight, overworked, neglected exercise, ate far too many snacks, and typically ate excessively even at mealtime. Ed's blood pressure had risen to dangerous levels. Headaches had become routine. He took several medications to address his blood pressure; they were, however, inadequately controlling his problems.

With such a medical and lifestyle history, Ed joined our four-week lifestyle education program. Unlike Norman, he was concerned and motivated. And our team rapidly took advantage of that receptivity and helped Ed understand the principles needed to reverse his blood pressure naturally. He carefully followed those recommendations.

A few days into the program, Ed came to me astonished. He was experiencing episodic dizziness. His blood pressure had dropped into the 110's-120's systolic and 70's-80's diastolic. He had reduced some of his medication on his own, but this clearly wasn't enough.

I had the joy of helping Ed eliminate several of his blood pressure medications. Only then did the dizziness resolve. Getting off his blood pressure medication was just one of his rewards for intentional healthy living. Ed also lost weight, improved his cholesterol, stabilized his blood sugars, and improved his energy level. His sense of wellbeing was enhanced, and his mood brightened considerably. Although not everyone improves his or her blood pressure that quickly, Ed was astonished at his own improvements as he studiously implemented natural lifestyle principles.

The stories of Norman and Ed remind us that elevated blood pressure works insidiously, undermining the very foundations of health. Addressing our blood pressure naturally, we can reap amazing benefits. Greet a high blood pressure diagnosis with nonchalance or ambivalence, and we're asking for trouble. To borrow a phrase from case law, high blood pressure is genuinely of "clear and present danger." Let's look carefully at data that supports this undeniable conclusion.

The Scope of High Blood Pressure

In order to assess fully the damage done by hypertension, we must first understand the scope of the problem. After all, a given medical condition might have severe individual consequences but make relatively little societal impact if few people are affected. Where does high blood pressure rank as far as numbers involved?

In the United States, high blood pressure's scope is staggering. About 67 million American adults have hypertension, with roughly an equal number having a less severe elevated blood pressure condition known as *prehypertension* (blood pressures higher than normal but not yet high enough to be labeled hypertension).[3] Added together, over 120 million American adults, almost 1 in 3, have elevated blood pressures. Some states fare better than others as depicted in Figure 1.1.[4]

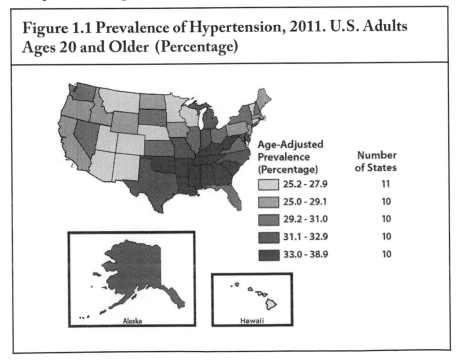

Figure 1.1 Prevalence of Hypertension, 2011. U.S. Adults Ages 20 and Older (Percentage)

Age-Adjusted Prevalence (Percentage)	Number of States
25.2 - 27.9	11
25.0 - 29.1	10
29.2 - 31.0	10
31.1 - 32.9	10
33.0 - 38.9	10

If you reside in the Southeastern U.S.—watch out! Your risk of hypertension is very high. But if you are a resident of Minnesota, Colorado or another less heavily affected state, don't feel smug. Yes, compared to the Southeast and a host of other regions, a smaller percentage of your state's residents are dealing with hypertension. However, notice the numbers affected. Even in places like Minnesota and Colorado, over one-quarter of the adult population has high blood pressure. On the other hand, that figure approaches a whopping 40% in the hardest hit states.

Furthermore, hypertension is not merely an American problem. The World Health Organization found that globally some 40% of all adults are affected, and those ranks are swelling.[5] Figure 1.2 illustrates the expanding reach of high blood pressure over time.

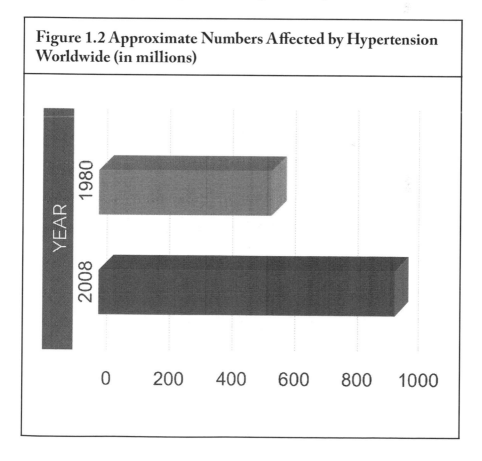

Figure 1.2 Approximate Numbers Affected by Hypertension Worldwide (in millions)

However, the plot thickens when we look in the mirror. Whether or not you think your appearance testifies to the fact, each of us is getting older. And with increasing age comes a staggering increase in high blood pressure risk. This has been well documented in U.S. data.[6,7] Figure 1.3 highlights this sobering reality.

Figure 1.3 Greater Likelihood of High Blood Pressure as U.S. Adults Age

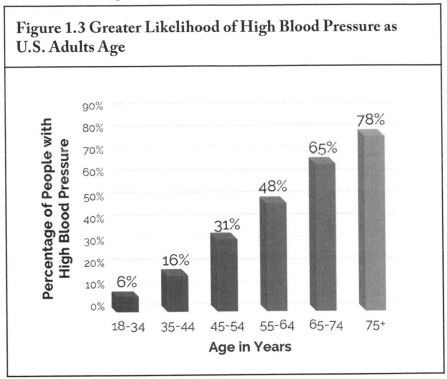

The bottom line is this: If you live long enough, high blood pressure is almost sure to come knocking. However, don't be discouraged. There is good news. The principles in this book are not only for hypertensives; i.e., those with high blood pressure; they are also for *normotensives*; i.e., those currently running normal blood pressures. Indeed, the simple natural strategies herein are powerful enough to keep many of you from ever being diagnosed with the condition.

Health Implications of High Blood Pressure

OK, high blood pressure—hypertension—is extremely common, but don't millions of people have the condition and suffer no ill effects? Yes and no. Although many individuals with hypertension may feel fine, those higher blood pressures are taking a toll on a host of bodily processes.

Look at it this way: Imagine an 8-year-old girl walked up to you and punched you in the arm. Would you be rendered permanently disabled? Not likely. The average child that age might be able to inflict some pain, but we wouldn't expect her to incapacitate you. However, what if that same 8-year-old just kept pummeling your arm? Severe damage could ultimately be inflicted.

The same is true of modestly elevated blood pressures. In this setting, a head of pressure is pounding away at your blood vessels, your heart, your brain, and your kidneys (as well as virtually every other tissue in your body). Like the blows from that 8-year-old, the pounding causes no distress initially. However, over time, the effects of those relatively small repeated traumas accumulate, thus risking serious or life-threatening complications. Now don't take that illustration too far. If your blood pressure ("BP" in medical lingo) is *very* high, a more appropriate analogy might envision a professional boxer dealing the blows. In that scenario, the high blood pressure itself might cause significant distress, perhaps in the form of severe headaches, a stroke, or worse.

Whether the complications of high blood pressure visit you in the short or in the long run is largely due to how high your blood pressure goes, and how susceptible your body is to hypertension's effects. But make no mistake: High blood pressure is dangerous even when the elevations are only modest.

Specific Complications of High Blood Pressure

Richard never gave much thought to his blood pressure. Sure, his numbers were very high, but in his mid-40s, he was healthy and strong.

On the rare occasions when he checked his pressure, it was not uncommon to see readings like 210/120. When in medical settings for other reasons, Richard noted that his BP numbers always got the attention of health professionals. So over the years he had tried a variety of their prescription medications. However, they all made him feel "lousy." "Why take a drug," he reasoned, "if I feel good and don't have any problems?"

For many years it seemed as if Richard's life story was going to end up "happily ever after." That was until he began noticing fluid retention, nausea, and weakness. When Richard finally sought medical attention, he received the shocking news that his kidneys were shutting down due to end stage kidney disease. He was counseled to prepare for dialysis. What happened? Unbeknownst to Richard, hypertension had for years been performing its relentless work of pounding away at his kidneys until those vital filtering organs were destroyed.

If you can't relate to Richard's story today, you may one day follow in his footsteps. As we've already seen, most of us are destined to have high blood pressure. And, along with those elevated pressures, come hypertension's complications. In addition to kidney failure, complications include stroke, heart attack, blindness and arterial aneurysms. See Figure 1.4.

Let's look at the cost of this devastating disease. Heart attacks and strokes claim hundreds of thousands of lives worldwide each year. And hypertension ranks among the most important of preventable risk factors for both conditions.

As if avoiding heart attacks and strokes weren't enough to motivate us, consider the effect of high blood pressure on the risk of aneurysms, a condition that weakens and stretches out blood vessel walls, often with devastating consequences. As an artery expands, it gets progressively weaker, finally setting the stage for a catastrophic rupture. For example, if you have an aneurysm and rupture of the major vessel that runs through your belly, the abdominal aorta, you face an 88% chance of sudden death.[8]

Figure 1.4 Selected Complications of High Blood Pressure

"Target" Organ	Complications
BRAIN	✓ Stroke ✓ Dementia ✓ Hypertensive encephalopathy (confusion, lethargy, seizures, coma)
HEART	✓ Heart attack ✓ Heart enlargement ✓ Increased risk of heart rhythm problems
BLOOD VESSELS	✓ Aneurysms ✓ Atherosclerosis (narrowed, hardened arteries)
KIDNEY	✓ Kidney damage ✓ Kidney failure and dialysis
EYES	✓ Retinal damage ✓ Blindness
PROSTATE (MEN)	✓ Slow, weak urine stream ✓ Trouble voiding

Some are surprised to learn of the millions of cases of eye and kidney damage linked to high blood pressure. Along with diabetes, hypertension contributes to a majority of cases of blindness and kidney failure in Western nations like the United States.

Another surprising linkage exists between high blood pressure and symptoms related to prostate gland enlargement. The higher a man's blood pressure, the greater his risk of troublesome prostate symptoms.[9] Although this may sound like nothing more than a nuisance, men who have had surgeries for such symptoms realize this may be far from the case. Even the relatively "simple" transurethral resection of the prostate (where a "roto-rooter" inserted through the penis removes excess prostate tissue) can lead to problems like bleeding, sexual dysfunction, narrowing of the urethra (the tube that drains the bladder), urinary retention, and urinary incontinence.

Perhaps the most devastating effects of high blood pressure impact the brain. While having a stroke may be the most immediately devastating and feared complication, hypertension also appears to accelerate brain aging.[10] High blood pressure among middle-aged adults has been linked to future cognitive decline and dementia, with high systolic numbers seeming to inflict the most damage.[11] High blood pressure leads to deficits in numerous brain functions: memory, reaction time, attention, focus, reasoning, task flexibility, problem solving, planning, execution, and cognitive processing speed.[12] And, if that's not bad enough, if you already have some degree of cognitive decline, hypertension accelerates that decline over time.[13]

The Benefits of Treating High Blood Pressure

Hypertension is extremely damaging. However, effectively treating it can significantly lessen its toll on your body. In fact, the authors of the monumental JNC7, a comprehensive set of high blood pressure guidelines for doctors, articulated that the benefits of treating high blood pressure are "a universal finding." They asserted emphatically: "lowering arterial pressure can remarkably reduce cardiovascular morbidity and mortality rates as well as slow the progression of renal disease, retinopathy, and all-cause deaths."[14] Expressed more simply, these experts were attesting to the huge benefits of controlling high blood pressure: decreasing the pain, suffering and death from things like heart attack, stroke, cognitive decline and dementia ("cardiovascular morbidity and mortality"); as well as helping prevent damage to the kidneys (renal disease) and eyes (retinopathy). A graphical expression of the evidence relating to stroke appears in Figure 1.5.[15]

The graph is eloquent, and dramatic. It shows us that people less than 60 years of age who adequately treat their high blood pressure are 50% less likely to have a stroke. That's a big improvement. Among people over 60 years of age, adequate blood pressure treatment rendered them 35% less likely to have a stroke. That's still a lot.

If you don't want to have a stroke, get your blood pressure under control, whatever your age.

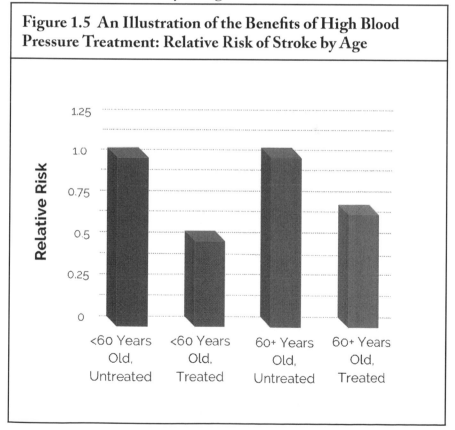

Figure 1.5 An Illustration of the Benefits of High Blood Pressure Treatment: Relative Risk of Stroke by Age

How Are We Doing at Addressing Blood Pressure?

With such a serious range of complications, you might assume that society would be doing all it could to curb this killer. However, despite the millions affected, and the potentially life-threatening and life-impairing consequences of high blood pressure, many people—like Richard—seem incredibly cavalier about the condition. Current data indicate that only about 50% of individuals residing in the U.S. with high blood pressure have their numbers under reasonable control. (See Figure 1.6.[16]) And from the vantage point of the World Health Organization, the U.S. represents a best-case example.

There's no question our nation has made a lot of progress, especially when you consider that only ten percent of individuals with hypertension had their BP controlled in the late 1970s. However, in every class I ever took, 50% was still a failing grade. Yes, it's a whole lot better than 10%, but clearly quite dismal when it comes to performance on such an important front.

Figure 1.6 U.S. Trends in Awareness, Treatment, and Control of High Blood Pressure

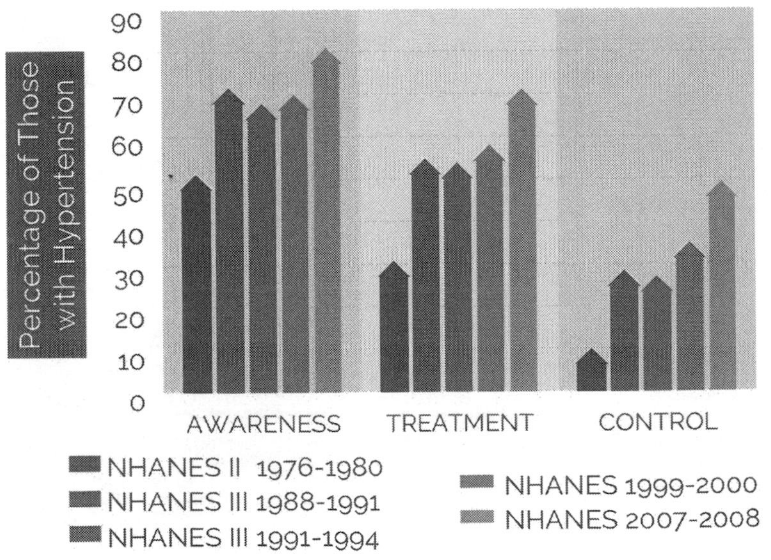
Percentage of Those with Hypertension
90
80
70
60
50
40
30
20
10
0
AWARENESS
TREATMENT
CONTROL
NHANES II 1976-1980
NHANES III 1988-1991
NHANES III 1991-1994
NHANES 1999-2000
NHANES 2007-2008

Why—with all we know about high blood pressure, and the medical community's focus on this condition—are we still doing so poorly?

Part of the answer likely is reflected in one of hypertension's common nicknames: *the silent killer*. That moniker is apt. Most people feel perfectly fine as they walk around with the elevated blood pressures that are insidiously undermining their health. However, another part of the answer likely resides with just how we, in the medical community, typically treat high blood pressure. In Chapter 3 we'll look at this possibility in some detail. But before going there, I want to tell you some of the "best" news about a diagnosis of "hypertension."

Harnessing Hypertension

Clearly, hypertension is a serious, often silent health hazard. However, through years of working with patients I've seen how even a sobering diagnosis can help a person more than hurt them. Years ago, this truth was riveted in my mind by two strikingly similar patients who were living with a different chronic condition—diabetes.

I met Sue and Phyllis years ago while I was working at a residential lifestyle change facility. If these two ladies had not come through our program at the same time, I don't know whether I would so vividly remember their remarkably similar medical histories.

Both Sue and Phyllis were in their seventies, and both had been diagnosed with type one diabetes decades earlier. In spite of that chronic condition, both were in good health. Even more remarkably, each had outlived all of her relatives.

I was impressed with the similarity of their stories, a similarity of life paths that caused my mind to fill in details to which I was never privy.

I could envision Sue as a teenager flanked by family members celebrating a relative's birthday. The soft drinks were flowing; ice cream and cake were there in abundance. Sue partook in few of the delicacies. Hushed words were spoken: "Poor Sue. It's a surprise she's not depressed." "It's sad such a nice girl can't join in the fun."

My mind saw similar story lines playing out in Phyllis's life. Friends and family members socialize, eat, and talk in the living room. A young Phyllis excuses herself to take a walk on a cold winter's day. "I'm sorry," she says, "my blood sugar's running high and I've got to get some more activity." Again, whispered tones witness to the pity that they feel for a young woman who seems to have been robbed of the innocence of her youth.

Then my mind returns to the present. The chronic disease that Sue and Phyllis no doubt thought was a curse was, really, the very thing that motivated them to live differently than did their cousins and siblings. They had, in a sense, harnessed their diabetes. A silent health robber had become an agent of change. That which threatened to compromise health ended up enhancing it instead.

The same is true of high blood pressure. Whether or not you've been labeled with the "hypertension" diagnosis, whether or not high blood pressure runs in the family, if you get serious about preventing or treating this condition through natural means, you're likely to end up a winner in the long run.

2

BLOOD PRESSURE ESSENTIALS

What Exactly is Blood Pressure?

BLOOD PRESSURE CAN BE defined simply as the force transmitted throughout your arteries after blood leaves your heart. It's likely you know at least some basic cardiovascular physiology (i.e., the science of how the heart and blood vessels function). But let me make it simple.

Oxygen-poor blood returns to the heart via the veins. These low-pressure vessels ultimately direct blood to the right side of the heart, into a chamber called the right atrium (see Figure 2.1). This "used" blood has already made its circuit through the body. During that journey, it surrendered its oxygen to the body's tissues, picked up carbon dioxide, and has now returned to the heart, where it will be first pumped to the lungs (to become re-oxygenated), and then ultimately pumped back out to the rest of the body.

If you were to follow a single blood cell after its arrival to the right atrium, you would see it pumped from there to the right ventricle, and then ultimately to the lungs through what are called the pulmonary arteries. Once in the lungs, this blood cell releases its carbon dioxide and picks up a fresh supply of oxygen. It makes the short return path to the heart via the pulmonary veins, arriving back in the heart's left atrium. From there it is pumped to the most muscular and strongest of all the heart's pumping chambers, the left ventricle.

Figure 2.1 Diagram of the Heart[17]

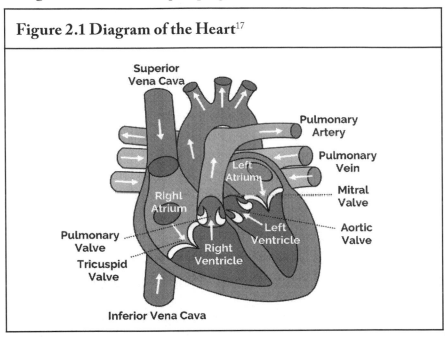

Although in special medical situations we may measure the pressure on the right side of the heart (such as the pulmonary artery pressure), when it comes to typical "high blood pressure," the pressures we are concerned about involve the left side of the heart. (If you are wondering, there is a medical condition called "pulmonary hypertension" that deals exclusively with elevated pressures in the pulmonary arteries and ultimately in the lungs.) So, the hypertension we're exploring in this book is concerned with the pressures in the arteries supplying your body as a whole, pressures that reflect the pumping force of the left ventricle.

Understanding the Numbers

You're now prepared to better appreciate what is being measured by the two numbers that describe human blood pressure. The upper value is called the *systolic* pressure. The lower number is referred to as the *diastolic* pressure. Systolic pressure, as illustrated in Figure 2.2, indicates the highest pressure that your arteries see during each pumping cycle.

I say "pumping cycle" because the heart does take a break, not for minutes or hours at a time. But the heart does rest, and does so for roughly twice as long as it pumps.

The pumping cycle or cardiac cycle represents one full circuit of pumping and resting. Think of it this way: if your heart rate is 60, then your heart is pumping once per second. If your heart is normal, that pumping action will take place within 1/3 of a second. Afterward, your heart will rest for 2/3 of a second.

When your heart pumps, that head of pressure generated by your heart is called the systolic pressure (systole refers to the pumping phase). By convention, we record the systolic pressure as the upper number in the blood pressure reading. In the example in Figure 2.2 that pressure is 120.

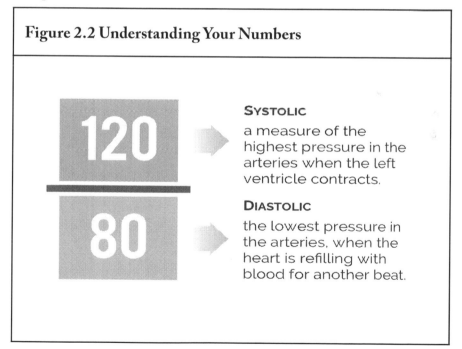

Figure 2.2 Understanding Your Numbers

120

SYSTOLIC
a measure of the highest pressure in the arteries when the left ventricle contracts.

80

DIASTOLIC
the lowest pressure in the arteries, when the heart is refilling with blood for another beat.

When the pumping ceases, your heart (technically your left ventricle) moves into the phase of rest or diastole. At this point, the pressure in your arteries quickly falls until it reaches its lowest point, called the diastolic pressure. Figure 2.2 lists a diastolic pressure of 80.

So How Do We Decide How High is Actually Too High?

High blood pressure is, then, pressure in your arteries *elevated to such an extent that it causes problems for organs and tissues "downstream."* Think of your arteries as constituting a high pressure plumbing system. In this analogy, your arteries are acting as pipes, carrying "water" to destinations throughout your home. If pressure in your pipes becomes too high, it will damage your toilets, showers, hot water heaters, and other appliances attached to those pipes.

What, then, would be an ideal pressure? One sufficient to adequately supply all your appliances—but no higher. The same is true of blood pressure in your body. Your heart needs to generate an adequate head of pressure, but more than that causes cumulative harm to the organs at the receiving end of that pressure.

Systolic or Diastolic: Is One More Important than Another?

By now you realize your blood vessels are actually seeing pressures that bounce between the upper systolic level and the lower diastolic one. Because the heart rests for twice as long as it pumps, the diastolic phase influences your average pressure twice as much as the systolic phase. Consequently, doctors calculate something called Mean Arterial Pressure (i.e., the average pressure) with the following equation:

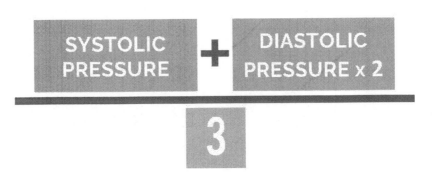

This greater influence of the diastolic pressure led physicians in the past to believe the diastolic number was the more important of the two. However, we now realize that, if too high, either number is damaging.

This stroke of illumination was relatively late in coming. In describing the history of hypertension control through 2003, Dr. Claude Lenfant and colleagues summarized the data this way:

"Almost immediately after the NHBPEP [National High Blood Pressure Education Program] began, hypertension awareness, treatment, and control rates began to improve. Death rates from coronary heart disease and stroke declined shortly thereafter. The decline is real, seen in both genders, and in blacks and whites. The improvements continued until the early 1990s, when blood pressure control rates did not improve further and the decline in stroke and coronary heart disease mortality rates appeared to have waned and certainly were not what the program was accustomed to seeing. The sails were no longer set correctly; the ship was losing momentum. The question was why?

It was because clinical trials focused primarily on diastolic blood pressure, and the JNC [Joint National Committee] and NHBPEP educational messages were on treating the diastolic number, which clinicians were doing quite well. However, data from the NHLBI [the National Heart, Lung, and Blood Institute—a division of the National Institutes of Health] Framingham Study and other studies suggested that systolic blood pressure was stronger than diastolic pressure as a predictor of cardiovascular disease in people over the age of 50."[18]

The clear message in the 21st century is this: both systolic and

21

diastolic numbers are important. We want to optimize both values to minimize our risk of damage. What then are those magic values?

Definitions of High Blood Pressure

One of the most frustrating things about the practice of medicine is that, although it is a science with life or death consequences, it is inexact. Because health professionals continue to accumulate medical knowledge, their understanding of what is normal changes over time.

Consider the case of diabetes. Several decades ago, you could consistently run fasting blood sugars in the 130s and still avoid the "diabetes" label. Why? Because the cut off for diabetes was then set at 140 mg/dl. However, today a blood sugar reading consistently above 125 mg/dl merits the diabetes designation.

Why the change? It was because health professionals and researchers realized that many people who were told they did not have diabetes were nevertheless suffering from diabetic complications. In other words, what was being labeled a normal blood sugar was actually too high.

The same is true with blood pressure. There was a time when doctors told patients that a systolic number of 100 plus your age was normal. In other words, an 80-year old whose blood pressure ran 175/85 would likely be told her numbers were just fine.

As it was with high blood sugar (diabetes), so it is with hypertension. Doctors realized that lenient cut-offs were not doing their patients any favors. Individuals who were told they had normal blood pressures were having complications from hypertension.

In order to keep up with the growing knowledge base of the medical profession, the coordinating committee for United States' National High Blood Pressure Education Program regularly convenes an expert group to make recommendations on blood pressure guidelines and treatment. Roughly every four to five years this group, known as the Joint National Committee on Prevention, Detection, Evaluation, and Treatment of High Blood Pressure (JNC), releases a summary report.[19]

In 2003, the Joint National Committee released their 7th report (often referred to as JNC7). Their recommendations continued a trend toward further lowering the cut-offs for normal blood pressure. Those guidelines are shown in Figure 2.3.

Figure 2.3 Goal Blood Pressures Recommended by JNC7

CLASSIFICATION	SBP	DBP
General guideline if no diabetes (DM) or chronic kidney disease (CKD)	<140	and <90
General guideline if DM or CKD present	<130	and <80

In December 2013, after considerable delay, JNC8 was released. The report had some air of intrigue surrounding it. Like all the preceding panels, the JNC8 panel was originally commissioned by the NHLBI. However, NHLBI pulled out of the guideline development process midway through 2013, preferring to have medical specialty organizations coordinate the process. Nonetheless, some six months later, the existing JNC8 panel members published their recommendations.Consequently, when it was released, JNC8 was not an official NHLBI-sanctioned report.[20]

This background seemed to add to the buzz the report generated in medical circles. JNC8 presented a dramatic change in emphasis. In the panel's assessment, the preceding decade had demonstrated that getting blood pressures to "optimal" levels with medications was actually counterproductive. Specifically, they concluded that lowering the BP below 140-150/90 was not warranted. So, when JNC8 rolled off the press, a new balance was added: don't be too aggressive when it comes to drug therapy of high blood pressure. The JNC8 guidelines are summarized in Figure 2.4.

Figure 2.4 Goal Blood Pressures Recommended by JNC8

CLASSIFICATION	SBP	DBP
If 60 years of age or older and no diabetes (DM) or chronic kidney disease (CKD)	<150	and <90
If 18 - 59 years old, or ≥60 years old with DM or CKD	<130	and <80

The easing of blood pressure goals articulated by the JNC8 panel is of great importance. To provide one glimpse of the kind of data that likely influenced their decision, consider Figure 2.5.[21] Researchers Sleight, Redon and colleagues were presenting to the medical community a striking reality. Even when examining medications from two of the very best tolerated high blood pressure drug classes, angiotensin receptor blockers (ARBs) and angiotensin converting enzyme inhibitors (ACEIs), more medication is not necessarily better. True, the risk of cardiovascular events fell by well over 50% when subjects decreased their systolic blood pressure from 161 to 130 using these medications. However, if the average study participant used more of those drugs to get his blood pressure down from 130 to 112 systolic, he would experience a striking *increase* in cardiovascular risk.

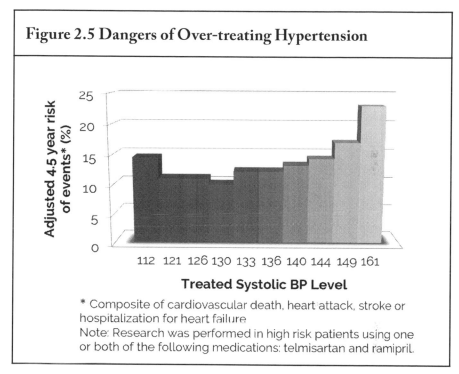

Figure 2.5 Dangers of Over-treating Hypertension

* Composite of cardiovascular death, heart attack, stroke or hospitalization for heart failure
Note: Research was performed in high risk patients using one or both of the following medications: telmisartan and ramipril.

JNC8 didn't have the last word, of course. Controversy continues. How aggressively should we treat blood pressure with medications? Even the experts continue to argue the question. One of the more recent salvos in that medical battle occurred with the publication of the National Heart, Lung, and Blood Institute (NHLBI)-sponsored Systolic Blood Pressure Intervention Trial (SPRINT).

SPRINT recruited over 9000 individuals from 102 centers throughout the U.S. Participants had to be at least 50 years old with both high blood pressure and at least one other cardiovascular disease risk factor. Over the course of just over three years, study participants who received standard hypertension care demonstrated an average systolic blood pressure reading of 134.6 mm Hg. Those randomly assigned to more intensive treatment showed an average systolic of 121.5 mm Hg.[22,23] Most importantly, the SPRINT researchers found the lower blood pressure group reaped an impressive 25% decrease in cardiovascular disease events and a 27% decreased risk of dying from any cause.

However, we've already seen in Figure 2.5 that some individuals appear to be worse off if they get their blood pressure down to these levels through the use of drug therapies. Other data indicates that lowering blood pressure below 120 systolic *with medications* can be risky.

For example, such overly aggressive BP lowering increases the risk of two vision-robbing conditions. Individuals who use drugs to lower their pressure below 120 systolic are at greater risk of open-angle glaucoma (a cause of elevated internal eye pressure) and ischemic optic neuropathy (damage to the nerve that carries vision signals from the eye to the brain). This increased risk appears to result from excessively low blood pressures in the night-time hours, a problem that may be worst with evening doses of high blood pressure meds.[24]

So, what should *my* goal blood pressure be? I'll tell you where I stand: unless your doctor has given you specific reasons to target a lower number, in general, medications should be used to lower blood pressures into the range of 140-150 systolic and 90 diastolic only. I make this recommendation very guardedly—especially since the emerging evidence suggests that many individuals would likely benefit from a systolic goal closer to 120. However, this is really the state of the science. As a case in point, consider an invited editorial accompanying the *New England Journal of Medicine* article that communicated the SPRINT data.[25] There University of Sydney researchers Vlado Perkovic and Anthony Rodgers opined: "Clearly, our current concept of hypertension is insufficient to determine who benefits from blood-pressure lowering or how far to lower blood pressure."

In short, this is the point: all the data convincingly argues that getting your blood pressure lower than 120 systolic *without medication* is beneficial, regardless of who you are. Expressed another way: if you are not on high blood pressure drugs, there are continuous, graded benefits from getting your blood pressure down to probably 110/75, if not lower. This is illustrated in Figure 2.6.[26]

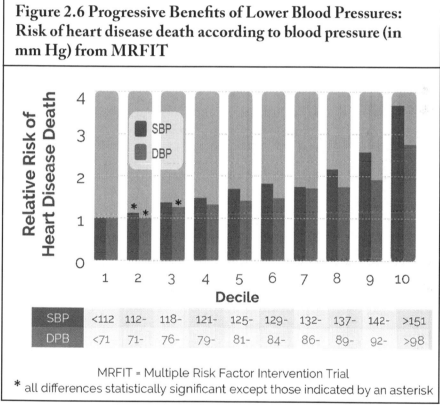

Figure 2.6 Progressive Benefits of Lower Blood Pressures: Risk of heart disease death according to blood pressure (in mm Hg) from MRFIT

	Decile									
	1	2	3	4	5	6	7	8	9	10
SBP	<112	112-	118-	121-	125-	129-	132-	137-	142-	>151
DPB	<71	71-	76-	79-	81-	84-	86-	89-	92-	>98

MRFIT = Multiple Risk Factor Intervention Trial
* all differences statistically significant except those indicated by an asterisk

Figure 2.6 reminds us of an important fact: Within acceptable physiologic limits, the lower you can get your blood pressure using natural means, the better. I say "physiologic limits" for obvious reasons. For example, certain medical conditions can lead to dangerously low blood pressure. In their most extreme form, these conditions are referred to as "shock." Whether it is due to blood loss ("hypovolemic shock"), overwhelming infection ("septic shock"), recent heart attack with heart failure ("cardiogenic shock"), or other causes—these extreme low blood pressure situations are often life threatening. No one will tell you a blood pressure of 60/30 is desirable.

In conclusion, if your blood pressure is "low" due to a healthy lifestyle, this is desirable because, to some extent, any elevation above your physiologically lowest attainable blood pressure may be increasing your risk of long-term problems. However, unless specifically instructed otherwise, don't try to get your blood pressure below 140/90 while on medications.

Once in that ballpark, further blood–pressure-lowering efforts should utilize lifestyle changes alone. When you see blood pressure improvements, work with your healthcare provider to carefully wean medications to avoid potential complications.

Indeed, the latest round of research makes an eloquent case—often not heard in research circles—for finding non-drug ways to get your BP even lower than the current JNC8 guidelines. And that's what this book is all about.

A Difficult Juncture

The medical community's efforts to control blood pressure have reached an extremely difficult juncture. First, some patients, with years of medication-fostered "well controlled" blood pressures, have been subjected to what we only now realize was overly aggressive blood pressure lowering. Second, in the context of such messages expressing concerns about excessively-exuberant medication regimens, a majority of the population with hypertension still *do not* have their blood pressure under control. The public health difficulty is obvious. How do you encourage some people to get serious about taking blood pressure medications when messages are circulating about the overmedication of hypertension?

Plus, we've seen that the data indicates a final problem with our current approaches. Namely, individuals can reap optimal benefits by getting their blood pressure far lower than the current JNC8 guidelines, provided they do so *without medications*. It is almost as if once health professionals put a patient on hypertension medications, they preclude those individuals from benefitting from the lowest attainable BP readings.

The solution no doubt lies with non-drug strategies for blood pressure reduction. Such an approach can help us on all three fronts:

- If you have hypertension and your blood pressure is currently under good control with medications, you could well decrease your dependence on those drugs.

- If you have uncontrolled high blood pressure, you stand a reasonable chance of bringing that blood pressure under control without the use of more medications.

- If you have blood pressure requiring no drug treatment according to current guidelines (generally below 140/90), you probably can lower your risk of cardiovascular and related diseases by bringing your BPs into a more optimal range.

Now, some health professionals would argue that the dangers of excessive blood pressure lowering are not due to the side-effects of blood pressure pills, but rather to changes in a person's physiology after all those years of higher pressure. Although there may be some truth in this, if you can get your blood pressure down to 118/72 without medications (no matter how high your blood pressure was in the past), no doctor is going to put you on drugs to raise your pressure to 140/90. In other words, medical professionals can argue about *why* lower blood pressures are harmful in medicated hypertensives. Nonetheless, the evidence points to the benefits of naturally lowering blood pressure as low as possible (within those physiological limits) using natural strategies.

The data indicate that we, as a world population, need to get our blood pressures lower in order to have optimal long term health. What obstacles are preventing us from making progress? In the next chapter we turn our attention to what may be the greatest problem when it comes to blood pressure control, as well as a surprising road map toward a solution.

3

THE GREATEST CAUSE OF OUR BLOOD PRESSURE FAILURES?

WHEN GIVING PUBLIC LECTURES on high blood pressure, I often display a slide that contrasts the short-term side effects of high blood pressure treatment with the untreated hypertensive state. I first project a list like the one that appears in Figure 3.1, detailing common problems with typical antihypertensive medications.

Figure 3.1 Common Symptoms of Blood Pressure Medications

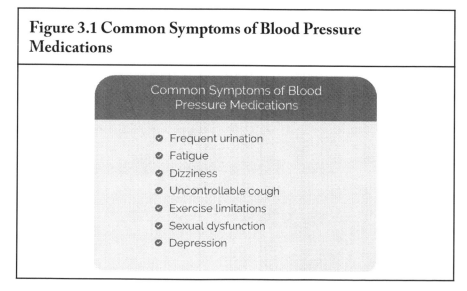

Common Symptoms of Blood Pressure Medications

- Frequent urination
- Fatigue
- Dizziness
- Uncontrollable cough
- Exercise limitations
- Sexual dysfunction
- Depression

No audience finds that list particularly appealing. Then, after those side-effects sink in, on the same slide, I project a list of the common short-term side-effects of high blood pressure itself. Based on what we've already been learning, that second list shouldn't surprise you. Figure 3.2 shows it alongside the initial list.

Figure 3.2 Short-term Symptoms of Treated and Untreated High Blood Pressure

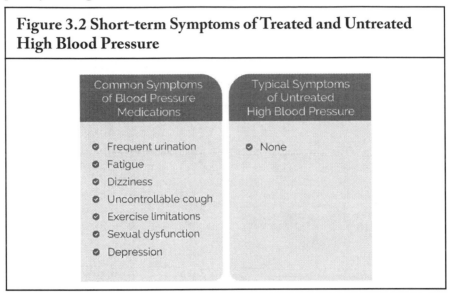

Common Symptoms of Blood Pressure Medications	Typical Symptoms of Untreated High Blood Pressure
● Frequent urination	● None
● Fatigue	
● Dizziness	
● Uncontrollable cough	
● Exercise limitations	
● Sexual dysfunction	
● Depression	

What's the point of that exercise? Although every expert group testifies to the power of natural approaches when it comes to blood pressure lowering, the typical emphasis in most of the world is this: you have high blood pressure; therefore you need to take medication(s).

Listen to how one prestigious publication expressed it: "Although counseling about lifestyle factors plays a role, prescribing antihypertensive medications remains the cornerstone of the medical management of hypertension."[27]

Stephanie, a 47-year-old, came into our office, apparently attracted by our reputation for using natural therapies. About six months earlier, while feeling fine, she was incidentally found to have high blood pressure.

Stephanie had quite a saga. She had been placed on six different high blood pressure drugs in succession, only to have the same response to each one. Stephanie's quality of life decreased with each of the medications, only to rebound when she stopped the drug. We had the privilege of sharing with Stephanie the principles in this book, and explaining how she could likely get her blood pressure under control without having to resort to another pill.

This is not an isolated incident. Consider the very provocative data conveyed in Figure 3.3.[28] That graphic depicts data involving some of the world's most popular classes of high blood pressure medications. Note that these studies are generally looking in terms of months—typically less than a year.

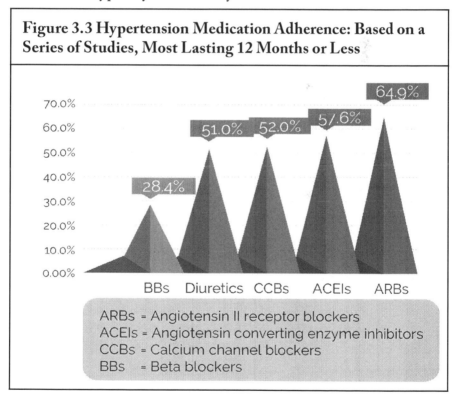

Figure 3.3 Hypertension Medication Adherence: Based on a Series of Studies, Most Lasting 12 Months or Less

ARBs = Angiotensin II receptor blockers
ACEIs = Angiotensin converting enzyme inhibitors
CCBs = Calcium channel blockers
BBs = Beta blockers

Let's walk through the graphic to ensure we don't miss the message. If you start at the bottom of the graphic you see "BB" for beta blockers. The figure indicates that if you were started on a beta blocker for high blood pressure, odds are less than one in three

(28.4%) you would still be on that drug a year later. When it comes to water pills (diuretics), and calcium channel blockers (CCBs) there's only about a 50-50 chance you will stick with those drugs for a year. Even when it comes to the best tolerated of medications, the ARBs and ACEIs, less than 2 of 3 individuals stick with (or "adhere" to) the therapy for a mere 12 months!

Why such dismal data? If you're like Stephanie, feeling perfectly fine, would you be happy to take a medication that made you feel worse? I've already reviewed the long term risks of high blood pressure. But "risk" is not *inevitability*. Short term quality-of-life tends to trump worries about a distant stroke or heart attack. (Granted, that equation may change significantly if you are lying in the emergency room with crushing chest pain or right-sided paralysis).

Scientists studying health behavior have known for decades that humans typically choose things that will make them look, feel, or function better, rather than things that may help to stave off some distant complication, even if that complication is death!

The Real Cause of Poor Blood Pressure Control Rates?

It is hard not to walk away from the average physician's office, or from the medical literature, with at least a serious question: Isn't it likely that the less than optimal rates of blood pressure control worldwide relate to patients' lack of acceptance of medication therapy, the conventional approach to high blood pressure?

Figure 3.2 holds, perhaps, the most important key for the less than optimal compliance when it comes to blood pressure therapies. Many individuals are not willing to sacrifice quality of life to decrease risk down the road, especially if they have not had any medical or family history to suggest that they are personally at risk from elevated blood pressures.

Isn't it ironic that many people are more stressed out—and "pressured"—by the medication treatments for high blood pressure than by the hypertension itself? Wouldn't it be wonderful if there was a "no pressure" solution to blood pressure? A solution that could lower those BP readings without causing collateral damage to one's quality of life?

Lessons from an Unsatisfying Shower

Hours before, they had been working outside my home. The laborers had been addressing some rather serious neighborhood plumbing problems. It was no small job. Heavy equipment had been on the scene. Pipes were dug up and replaced.

It was evening when I stepped into the shower. But there was a serious problem: "no pressure." Yes, I think those were the exact words I used when shouting to my wife: "Honey, there's no pressure coming out of this showerhead." However, there *was* water coming out of the fixture.

What was I trying to communicate? I was simply relating that there was insufficient pressure coming out of the showerhead to remove the dirt from my body.

However, what's bad for cleaning your body is good for sustaining your health. In other words, "no pressure" from your showerhead is undesirable, but "no pressure" in your arteries is beneficial.

Now, I'm not talking about a "no pressure" scenario where your blood pressure drops to 0/0. (Actually, such a state, if it persists, is called "death.") Instead, I'm recommending a "no pressure" scenario where there is no unnecessary elevation to your BP, where your blood pressure will do no more damage to your organs than that sputtering shower did to the dirt on my body! But more importantly, it's a "no pressure" solution where there is no added pressure or stress from the *treatments* used for your higher than optimal BP numbers.

In fact, the very words, "no pressure," constitute a powerful acronym that brings into focus ten natural strategies for blood pressure control. These are illustrated in Figure 3.4.

Figure 3.4 The "NO PRESSURE" Mnemonic

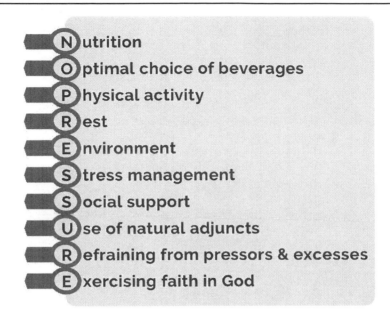

N utrition
O ptimal choice of beverages
P hysical activity
R est
E nvironment
S tress management
S ocial support
U se of natural adjuncts
R efraining from pressors & excesses
E xercising faith in God

There's some risk in putting up a comprehensive list like this from the outset. Although some of you may already be getting excited about a comprehensive non-drug approach, others may have a different reaction, thinking that: "blood pressure medications sound less quality-of-life-impairing than implementing all those ten factors." Others of you may have gravitated to a single element and are hung up on that. For example, "This won't work, I hate to exercise." Or, "'Faith in God!' What does that have to do with blood pressure? I'm an atheist!"

Let me assure you of several things:

1. There is solid scientific evidence supporting each of these ten areas.

2. This is not a one-size-fits-all program. If you can implement only seven (or fewer) of the ten components, you can still reap significant benefits from the program.

3. The struggle to motivate ourselves to achieve results in each phase of the *No Pressure* treatment protocol is real. Studies show that incorporating spiritual principles can enhance your likelihood of success, even if you're an atheist.

Other Hidden Dangers in Lifestyle Approaches

Most of the *No Pressure* strategies focus on lifestyle habits. Whether our dietary practices, how much we exercise, our approach to stress, or our sleeping habits, all come under the realm of our personal choices. There are at least two dangers here. The first is that some of you may feel this book blames you for your high blood pressure. Not true. Secondly, others may be tempted to play the blame game themselves. Don't fall into the trap of telling your friends and loved ones: "If you had just followed the *No Pressure* program, you wouldn't have high blood pressure."

Let me give you the bottom line: Although we'll be looking at lifestyle and other natural therapies, the presence of hypertension *does not* necessarily mean a person is following a poor lifestyle. With that out of the way, let's look at a vital question.

Why Do I Have High Blood Pressure to Begin With?

Although lifestyle factors clearly have a bearing on blood pressure, you can find plenty of examples of people who do "everything wrong" and have good BP numbers. Similarly, many individuals living generally healthy lives seem cursed with hypertension. What is going on?

First, let me talk to those in the latter category. Please, don't shelve this book thinking you've already secured all the benefits possible from non-drug therapies. (For example, you may find you are doing well with the early *No Pressure* components like nutrition, beverage choices, and physical activity, only to find some significant areas for improvement when we get to the latter components.) *I'll give you a host of strategies in this book. It is extremely unlikely you are already following all of them.*

So, why do some of us seem predisposed to high blood pressure? If you were sitting in on a medical school class on the topic, your teacher would probably begin by listing the two major categories of high blood pressure: primary and secondary.

Secondary hypertension refers to a high blood pressure state that is being caused by some other, usually treatable, condition. It accounts for approximately 10% of all cases of hypertension in the United States.

On the other hand, primary hypertension refers to individuals with elevated BPs in the absence of a causative disease or process. The vast majority of individuals with high blood pressure, approximately 90%, have the "primary" variety. (Sometimes primary hypertension is called "essential" hypertension. This doesn't refer to having a need for the condition, but is *essential* in that it seems inherent, occurring apart from any other pathologic state.)

Although primary hypertension is the diagnosis most likely affecting those with elevated blood pressures, it is clearly wise to look first at secondary hypertension. *If* your high blood pressure is due to a treatable condition, you'll likely want to prioritize treatment of the condition, perhaps even before finishing this book.

Figure 3.5 provides a partial listing of some of the causes of secondary hypertension.

Might you have secondary hypertension? The answer often lies with a thorough medical evaluation. If you're already seeing a doctor but don't feel you've had such a comprehensive assessment, consider a second opinion. However, some of the conditions listed in Figure 3.5 may offer "red flags" that call attention to themselves.

For example, you might be tipped off to the presence of sleep apnea syndrome by excessive daytime sleepiness (e.g., falling asleep at inappropriate times such as while eating, having a conversation, or reading a stimulating book like this one, etc.). The same condition might be noted by a partner or friend who actually observes you while sleeping. The syndrome is witnessed when a person during sleep stops breathing ("apnea" literally refers to not breathing). Those apneic episodes are often preceded by snoring. In most cases, sleep apnea can be easily treated with a nighttime breathing device called CPAP (an abbreviation for "continuous positive airway pressure"). Treatment of sleep apnea may be all that is needed to fully normalize blood pressure.

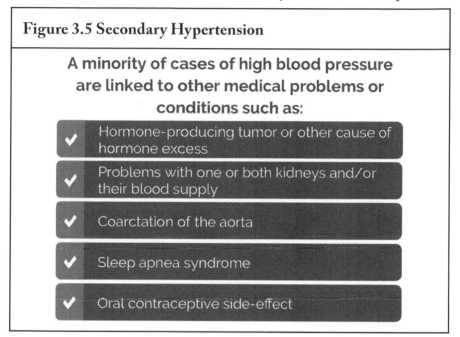

Figure 3.5 Secondary Hypertension

A minority of cases of high blood pressure are linked to other medical problems or conditions such as:

- ✔ Hormone-producing tumor or other cause of hormone excess
- ✔ Problems with one or both kidneys and/or their blood supply
- ✔ Coarctation of the aorta
- ✔ Sleep apnea syndrome
- ✔ Oral contraceptive side-effect

Another example is provided by hormone-producing tumors. Depending on the type of hormone involved, a person may obtain clues that something is not right. For example, excess production of growth hormone may not only raise blood pressure, it may also cause a coarsening of one's hands and face. Excess cortisol can cause fat accumulation around the midsection and upper back. It can also make an individual's face become more rounded ("moon-shaped") in addition to elevating BP. Hormone-producing tumors are usually benign, so making a correct diagnosis, then removing the growth, may be a cure not only for high blood pressure but also for other related hormonal problems. Again, all of these secondary forms of hypertension boil down to getting a precise diagnosis.

One last example is warranted. Figure 3.5 also lists kidney

problems. Many lay people are surprised to learn the kidney is a very important organ when it comes to blood pressure control. The tissues of the kidney, particularly a region called the juxtoglomerular (JG) apparatus, are especially sensitive to blood pressure. If the JG tissues sense that blood pressure is low, they will release a hormone called renin that helps to raise blood pressure. This can be especially useful if you are in shock from blood loss, for example.

However, let's imagine another scenario. Your blood pressure, measured in your left arm is running consistently at 170/100 or higher. It just so happens that the artery going to your left kidney, called the left renal artery, is over 80% blocked. See Figure 3.6. Would you like to guess what blood pressure your left kidney is registering? Due to the large amount of blockage decreasing its blood supply, that kidney might be seeing a pressure as low as 75/40. The JG apparatus is programmed to interpret such low blood pressure as a life-threatening situation, so it has been working overtime pumping out large amounts of renin. What do you think all that renin is doing? Perpetuating your high blood pressure.

In certain causes of renal artery blockage (especially a condition called *fibromuscular dysplasia*—common in women between the ages of 25 and 50), removing the blockage with angioplasty (the balloon procedure used to open up blocked arteries), may be sufficient to normalize the blood pressure. However, as illustrated in Figure 3.6, atherosclerosis (fatty buildup in the arteries) is the most common cause of blocked kidney blood vessels. Angioplasty is generally not recommended in those situations.

Why Would I Have Primary or Essential Hypertension?

We've already seen that most individuals who have high blood pressure—probably some nine out of ten —have "primary" or "essential" hypertension. With this condition there is no easily identifiable cause. Why, then, does it develop?

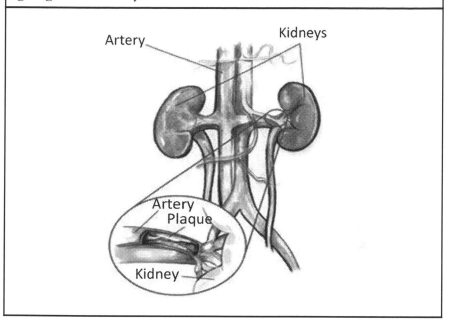

Figure 3.6 Renal Artery Stenosis (Narrowing of an artery going to the kidney)

Imagine you're joining me on a trip to some of the nephrology wards of today's research hospitals. Those halls are the domain of kidney specialists (nephrologists) who have made some remarkable discoveries when it comes to primary hypertension. Some of the most provocative lessons come from the area of kidney transplantation.

Imagine you are a woman in your 40s who has always had excellent blood pressure. However, two years ago, you were diagnosed with systemic lupus erythematosus (SLE), often simply referred to as "lupus." Despite the best of care, the condition followed a particularly devastating course, robbing you of your kidney function. After some 12 months of dialysis, your lupus is finally under control and you receive word that a 25-year-old man just died in an auto accident. You are the first person on the transplant list who is a suitable match, so you'll be receiving one of his kidneys.

Fast forward another 12 months. You are feeling great. Your

lupus has stayed in remission. Your new kidney is functioning marvelously. There is only one thing troubling you: your blood pressure. Before your lupus, your blood pressure ran a steady 105/60; after the transplant it quickly rose to 195/105. You're now taking three high blood pressure medications, and your pressure is still running 150/85. Your nephrologist just obtained some interesting information that your donor's parents volunteered. Their son's blood pressure before his fatal accident was always high. He never took medication for a blood pressure that ran typically around 195/105.

While sitting in the nephrologist's office a few weeks later, you begin visiting with another recent transplant recipient. John, a 62-year-old man, lost his kidneys due to diabetes and high blood pressure. He had the good fortune of receiving a kidney from his oldest son, Richard. John explains how blood pressures of 220/120 were not unusual for him even in his 30s. He was on as many as five blood pressure drugs even before his kidneys "gave out." But your ears really perk up when John tells you his blood pressure is now normal—without any medications. In fact, he observes, "My pressure now runs around 120/70—just like my son Richard."

That hypothetical scenario highlights a real phenomenon observed in the context of kidney transplantation. Namely, once you are the recipient of a transplanted kidney, your blood pressure will tend to be similar to that of your donor.

Observations from transplant surgeries, as well as other nephrology studies, have led to a fascinating understanding: Our likelihood of having hypertension is often determined by our kidneys. However, the plot thickens when you realize that our kidneys are especially influenced by circumstances surrounding our birth.

A landmark German autopsy study analyzed kidneys from ten middle-aged hypertensive individuals (35 to 59 years old) and compared them with kidneys from ten normotensive individuals who were otherwise similar in other respects (age, height, weight, and gender). The researchers found, on average, those with high blood pressure had only about half as many *glomeruli* (the filtering portion of the kidney's functional units) than those with normal blood pressure: 702,379 vs. 1,429,200 per kidney.[29]

What would cause deficient numbers of nephrons and glomeruli? Nothing that can be attributed to your personal lifestyle choices. However, research has revealed that nephrons are formed when we're developing in our mother's womb, between the 28th and 36th weeks of pregnancy. If your mother was stressed during that developmental window in your pregnancy, your kidney development might have been impaired and, thus, you could well have been born with fewer nephrons than optimal.[30]

Of course, genetic factors and other influences can affect whether or not we are at risk for high blood pressure. I'm not saying the only mechanism by which one could be programmed toward hypertension in utero has to do with faulty development of glomeruli. Maternal stress during pregnancy can have other long term effects on the fetus, all of which might predispose the infant to higher blood pressures later in life.[31] Consider the following.

We've already seen how hormonal abnormalities can affect blood pressure. If a mother is under significantly increased mental or physical stress during pregnancy (presumably greater than the normal demands of pregnancy), her body can ramp up levels of "glucocorticoid" stress hormones like cortisol. These hormones can then pass through the placenta to her baby. Such a hormonal milieu may have long-term effects, predisposing to high blood pressure years later.

Furthermore, maternal stress during gestation can set the stage for something called "uteroplacental insufficiency," where the fetus receives inadequate blood flow from his or her mother. This condition predisposes to low birth weight, which in turn can result in impaired blood vessel development. This can have profound implications when it comes to blood pressure years later. If the lining of arteries is not properly developed, "endothelial dysfunction" may ensue, leaving those vessels impaired in their ability to relax. Impaired arterial relaxation (think *stiffer arteries*) necessitates higher blood pressures in order to move blood through those relatively inelastic conduits.

To summarize, when it comes to "primary" or "essential" hypertension, an underlying genetic or intrauterine predisposition is later augmented by lifestyle and/or other environmental factors. Those triggering factors may be few or many. For some, several factors must be superimposed on a tendency toward hypertension before overt high blood pressure occurs; for others, it may take a single triggering factor.

Two important messages emerge. First, we can be predisposed to hypertension independent of lifestyle choices. Second, lifestyle factors can still play a powerful role in helping us control our blood pressure, or avoid hypertension altogether. Therefore, if you have essential hypertension, you would be well advised to heed this book's recommended program as elucidated in the *No Pressure* acronym.

4

A 30-DAY BLUEPRINT FOR BLOOD PRESSURE CONTROL

THROUGHOUT THE UPCOMING CHAPTERS we'll be walking step-by-step through the *No Pressure* mnemonic. However, let's begin with some general observations.

The Envisioned Outcome

To increase your likelihood of success, every plan needs a mental picture of the outcome. Ask yourself the question, "What is my life going to look like when I finish this book?" Your expected outcome probably is, "I will have normal blood pressure." Realize, however, as you make the lifestyle changes listed on the ensuing pages, you probably will accomplish far more than just improving your blood pressure. You stand a good chance of experiencing numerous other benefits, such as improving your cholesterol level, stabilizing your blood sugar, normalizing your weight, improving your energy, brightening your mood, becoming more fit, and feeling better overall. Keep these goals in mind every step of your way.

The "Why"

While obtaining a naturally normalized blood pressure with

its associated benefits might be your envisioned outcome, regular reminders of the deeper underlying purposes for your goal can help prevent you from being derailed by life's distractions.

Who cares if you have normal blood pressure? Why do you care? What's the point? For example, you may be motivated to see your six-year old daughter graduate from college one day, and not be watching from a wheelchair as your stroke-afflicted father was when you reached that milestone. Perhaps one of your underlying purposes is to get off the blood pressure medications that seem to be sapping your energy level. Whatever your reasons are, write them below.

My deeper underlying purpose for achieving normal blood pressure is:

_____

_____

_____

Don't be a distracted driver. Know where you are going, why you are going there, and how to get there. Let this book be your driving instructor.

Your Predecessors: They've Been There Before You

I've seen them over the years: Patients coming into medical practices and health care settings with long histories of high blood pressure. However, I've also seen some of those patients get motivated to make changes in their lifestyles, as well as utilize other natural therapies. Invariably they reduce their prescription medications or leave them off altogether. Among the programs I have worked with are the Weimar NEWSTART residential program, and the CHIP (Complete Health Improvement Program) community-based outpatient program. These programs are not only great ways to meet people who have gone there before you but also to work with people who are making lifestyle changes at the same time you are. Weimar is located outside of Sacramento, California (www.newstart.com). CHIP has numerous locations in many communities (www.chiphealth.com). Let me share a few real-life stories since many of you may never have the privilege of participating in either of these great programs.[32]

A Few CHIPPERS

Bill had elevated blood pressure, a fatty liver, chronic heartburn, excess weight, and high cholesterol. He had to stay on blood pressure medicine to try to "keep his numbers under control." He worked the program. His blood pressure normalized, liver tests improved, heartburn lessened, weight improved, and cholesterol normalized. He focused on his goal of better health and decided he didn't want to enter his retirement sick. It worked for him.

Joe couldn't get his blood pressure down. He was on blood pressure medicine, which had helped. He had a sedentary job, a lot of family stress, and a history of abandonment as a child. He worked the program. He focused on his goal and decided that his past was not going to determine his future. He took control. He wanted to be an example to his teenage children, didn't want to get sick and die the way that his father did, and he "wanted to make God proud." It worked for him.

A Weimar Alumnus Testifies

Ron's health had been declining for years. However, a decade ago, things had gotten so bad that, unless he made some major changes, he knew he wouldn't be around much longer. Survival was the underlying purpose that led Ron to enroll in Weimar's NEWSTART program. Looking back on what was essentially a *No Pressure* journey, Ron writes:

"I had extremely high blood pressure all my life. On a good day my blood pressure would be 160/95 and on a bad day it would run as high as 200/110. When I attended the NEWSTART program at Weimar, I learned a new lifestyle. In six days I discontinued all blood pressure medications and saw my blood pressure readings fall to around 130/80.

"Now, ten years later, my pressure runs 110/70 or less. In my 18-day stay at Weimar I lost 22 pounds. I have subsequently lost 100 pounds—and I'm still off all blood pressure medications."

When there is a deeper, heartfelt purpose, a clear vision of the desired outcome, and a good understanding of how to get there, a lot can happen. In addition to the stories above, thousands of people have gone through these programs and their clinical results have been recorded. Data from both these programs show what can happen to blood pressure in a month or less.

Realize too, the data tells only part of the story: Many of these individuals also decreased or eliminated their hypertensive medications. For an example of such results see Figure 4.1. What is remarkable about the results is the decrease in average blood pressure of 8 points systolic and 4 points diastolic occurred in a population whose blood pressure, on average, was normal at baseline.[33] Similar results have been seen in larger series involving over 5000 CHIP participants.[34]

NEWSTART and CHIP are examples of programs that have effectively used many of the *No Pressure* principles for decades. Other popular programs have employed these same principles and share similar success stories. These include residential programs like those offered at Wildwood Lifestyle Center and Hospital in Georgia, and Alabama's Uchee Pines Institute. (A newer community-based program that espouses similar strategies is Florida Hospital's CREATION Health initiative.)

I mention these examples to communicate an important point.

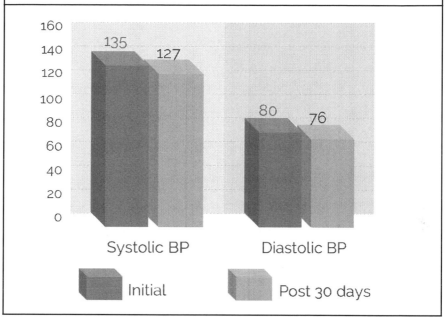

Figure 4.1 Decreases in Blood Pressure After 30 Days of CHIP
(Data represent average changes experienced by 836 participants from 18 different locations)

As we walk through the *No Pressure* construct, I'm not talking mere theory from the medical literature but describing solid approaches that have been employed successfully by thousands of people.

So How Do I Do It On My Own?

It's going to take more than a leisurely 30-day reading of this book to log serious blood pressure improvements. You'll need a plan and a series of commitments. I'll help you map out a strategy for optimal success. However, this is a *personal* program. If something doesn't seem to fit your situation, leave it off; or, better yet, modify it. However, the more of the elements you incorporate, the more success you're likely to achieve.

Okay, you have your goal and you're continually keeping "the why" in front of you. In addition, the following six steps will help you with accountability, organization, and brainstorming as you harness the *No Pressure* components. I recommend you put the following into place as soon as reasonably possible. In fact, I won't start the clock on your 30-day journey until you've committed to at least four of the following. Please, steps 2, 3, 4, and 6 are non-negotiable:

1. Find an accountability partner or support group with whom you will share your commitments. (A great way to use this book is in conjunction with Dr. DeRose's *Reversing Hypertension Naturally* DVD and related materials. For more information go to www.compasshealth.net).

2. Commit to reading the chapters in this book each week that deal with at least three of the *No Pressure* components. The goal is to cover all ten components in the span of three weeks, which means at least four chapters on one of the weeks.

3. Every time you read a chapter, look for at least one thing you can change that will bring you into conformity with the principles articulated in that chapter. Once you've chosen what you want to change, brainstorm ideas as to how to actually make those changes.

4. Now it's time to develop *a specific plan* that includes a definite, orderly approach to make the changes you've identified. Some of you may choose to start several new lifestyle practices at once; others may prefer to focus on one thing at a time. Be realistic. The more specific and well-thought-out your plan, the more likely you are to achieve it. This is something you can do on your own or in conjunction with your accountability partner or group. Whatever the case, make sure you *write down* your plan and the specific behavioral goals that you intend to practice throughout the 30 days. At this point, don't get too worried about this. Throughout

each subsequent chapter, I'll be seeking to encourage and inspire you when it comes to areas of behavioral change. Furthermore, at the end of each of the next ten chapters (where I cover the specific components in detail), I'll provide a *goal sheet*. There you'll be prompted to write out your chapter-specific behavioral goal or goals.

5. Track your progress daily towards your behavioral goals. The best way to do this is to transfer those goals to Appendix B each time you complete a chapter. That appendix thus becomes the one-stop location for tracking daily progress toward each of your behavioral goals.

6. Measure your blood pressure frequently during the 30 days. I recommend at least three times daily, and make sure you share those BP readings with your doctor or other health care provider. (In fact, I recommend you check in with that same health professional before embarking on your 30-day journey). It's always a good idea to keep careful tabs on your blood pressure (i.e., multiple daily BP checks) when using lifestyle modification or other natural therapies. Appendix A, at the back of this book, provides a place for you to log your blood pressures, three to four times daily, for one week before, and then all during your 30-day blood pressure journey.

    Don't be surprised by my desire for you to check your blood pressure three times per day the week before you start your 30-day program. I've been surprised by how few patients regularly check their blood pressure at various times throughout the day. Carefully charting your blood pressure for a full week before beginning the 30-day program will accomplish at least three things. First, you'll be in the habit of implementing this vital part of the program. Second, you'll have actual data to monitor yourself and share with your health care providers. Third, you won't be blindsided by surprising readings. Some of you likely have blood pressures that tend to run significantly higher or lower at different times of the day. It's best to know this before starting your 30-day journey. After all, if you've never checked your blood pressures in the evening, how would you (or even your doctor) know how to interpret a blood pressure that runs 20 points higher at night than in the morning when you're on the *No Pressure* program?

A summary of these six elements appears in Figure 4.2.

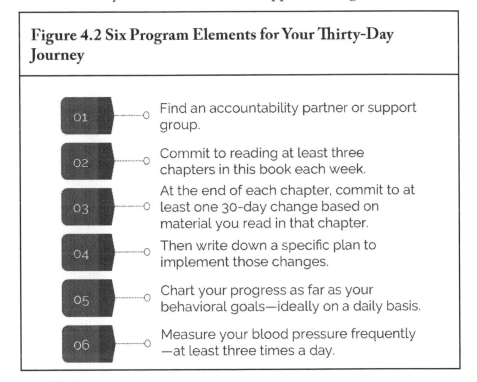

Figure 4.2 Six Program Elements for Your Thirty-Day Journey

01 — Find an accountability partner or support group.

02 — Commit to reading at least three chapters in this book each week.

03 — At the end of each chapter, commit to at least one 30-day change based on material you read in that chapter.

04 — Then write down a specific plan to implement those changes.

05 — Chart your progress as far as your behavioral goals—ideally on a daily basis.

06 — Measure your blood pressure frequently —at least three times a day.

SMART Goals

Now, let's assess. Let's say that during the first week you read the chapters on nutrition, optimal beverages and physical activity. You come up with behavioral goals for each one. However, give me a few minutes to provide some insights that will help you get the most out of your goal-setting activities. To make this practical, let's consider the example of exercise.

After finishing Chapter 8, you decide you're going to exercise more. This is a great commitment, but it doesn't constitute a specific plan. Qualities of a plan that is both specific and is likely to help you succeed are communicated by another acronym, SMART, as illustrated in Figure 4.3.

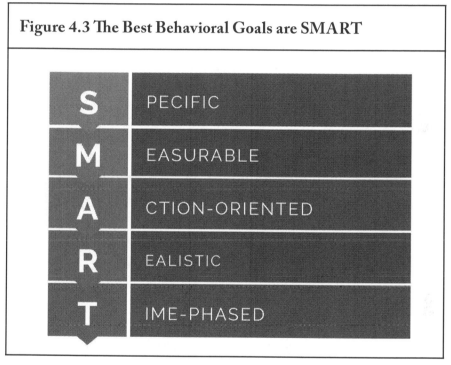

Figure 4.3 The Best Behavioral Goals are SMART

S PECIFIC

M EASURABLE

A CTION-ORIENTED

R EALISTIC

T IME-PHASED

Let's see what a SMART goal looks like using our example of exercise. You might decide that you're going to alternate days walking in your neighborhood with working out at the health club. (Good, you're being specific about your types of exercise). Furthermore, you commit to exercising at least 30 minutes every day. (Great. These are measurable commitments. So long as you're logging your progress, there'll be no guesswork as to whether or not you're on target. For example, if I called you in a month you could tell me whether or not you're reaching your goals.)

The third aspect of SMART goals, being action-oriented, is going to fit with most any exercise commitment. In fact, being action-oriented is really a check to make sure you have truly embraced a behavioral goal. Let me explain. When many people set health goals, they are really focusing on an end result rather than specific behaviors. For example, among denizens of the Western World, one of the most common health goals is to lose weight. However, losing weight is not a behavior. It is the result of behaviors.

This is an important point. If you're embracing a behavioral goal, then you're talking about doing something action-oriented. You can do it in the living room, or in your kitchen, or in the gym. SMART goals are behavioral goals, because those are the goals we have the highest likelihood of reaching.

The "R" in SMART stands for realistic. No one can tell you if a goal is realistic or not. However, past experience can be helpful. If, over a span of three years, you consistently exercised at the gym for 45-60 minutes a day, five days a week, I wouldn't be worried about a 30-minute daily commitment. On the other hand, if you've never been able to stick with an exercise program at a gym for more than a week and had never been able to consistently exercise in your neighborhood, other than a five-minute walk with your dog, then I'm getting worried.

Don't make the mistake of trying to please anyone else with your goals. First embrace something you are confident that you can do. For example, why not commit to walking a minimum of five minutes per day. *"Five minutes? What will that accomplish?"* A whole lot more than your zero minutes-a-day program has been accomplishing. I'm not saying five minutes of exercise daily is ideal, but it is a starting point if you've not been exercising at all.

Finally, we come to "time-phased." Although, ultimately, the best behavioral goals are ones that you stick with for the rest of your life, don't get bogged down with such thoughts. Right now,

I'm already setting the time phase for you: 30 days. Most of us can put up with some inconveniences for a month. That's especially true if it can help us achieve a better sense of health and well-being with less medication.

Now, here's the catch: Although I've already made an argument for you not setting yourself up for failure (by setting goals so lofty they're unattainable), there is an opposite danger. If your goals are all easily attainable, it's likely you're not making changes of sufficient magnitude to powerfully impact your blood pressure. Don't be afraid to stretch yourself. Don't shy away from bold commitments.

The ball is in your court. However, by all means, even if you won't have an accountability partner for the full 30-days (and, yes, that's the ideal), bounce your goals off someone you trust.

Another Behavioral Insight

In Dr. DeRose's popular DVD, *Changing Bad Habits for Good*, he addresses the dynamics of behavior change in greater detail. One of his most important principles can help protect you from the danger of aiming too low.

Specifically, DeRose points out that we all have the capacity to develop new enjoyments. If you realize this, then you have the key to stepping out more boldly during the upcoming month. When you tackle the subject of diet, don't ask, "How can I eat all the foods I like and still make progress?" Instead look in the mirror and say, "If I can develop an enjoyment for any menu, why don't I just try the best one for my blood pressure, at least for the next 30 days!"

Using the Natural Planning Model

At this point, you may feel you're ready to start the *No Pressure* program in earnest. If you're not a trained pilot, our dialogue in this chapter might feel similar to sitting in the cockpit alongside a captain prior to a cross-country flight. You're anxious to get going. However, he's meticulously checking a host of controls to ensure a satisfactory journey. If you don't really reflect on what's going on, it may feel like a lot of unnecessary preliminaries. However, we all know better.

Just as an airplane has backup mechanisms to try to ensure a safe flight even if certain components fail, it really behooves me to give you a few more mental tools just in case you run into unexpected turbulence on your 30-day flight. These tools are summarized in something called the natural planning model.[35] This model complements nicely what we've already learned about SMART goal setting. It presents some similar concepts with an aim of helping you achieve your goals. Experts assert that the natural planning model is actually the way your brain already automatically plans tasks. In your process of goal setting and implementation, I also encourage you to experiment with this 5-step approach as outlined in Figure 4.4.

Figure 4.4 Use the Natural Planning Model to Increase Your Likelihood of Success (Apply the following five steps to help define and achieve your behavioral goals)

1 Establish and keep before you your purpose and principles for the change you're making ("the Why").

2 Envision how you want your change to look when your goal is met (your SMART goal in action).

3 Brainstorm your options and the best way to get to your goal.

4 Organize the steps and ideas you wish to perform to implement the change.

5 Identify and set the next actions involved to proceed.

Consider Jennifer

Recently retired, Jennifer had just said goodbye to a successful career as a high school teacher. She was looking forward to enjoying her retirement. Unfortunately, she was 50 pounds overweight and was struggling with high blood pressure. Her readings typically averaged 150/90.

(#1) Jennifer's "Why": She didn't want health problems to interfere with her retirement plans, including time with her grandchildren. Her doctor told her if she didn't improve her blood pressure, then she would be at increased risk of stroke and heart attack, especially since strokes were common among her female relatives.

(#2) Jennifer envisioned herself as an active person with normal blood pressure who had achieved a normal weight through good eating and exercise habits. She found a picture of herself when she was 50 pounds lighter. She affixed it to her refrigerator. Before Jennifer stumbled across that old personal photo, she had put a picture of her friend Betty on the fridge. Betty was a good example of health. She maintained a normal weight and blood pressure and followed good eating and exercise habits. Jennifer decided she would emulate Betty's good qualities.

(#3) Jennifer recognized her bad habits. She regularly ate at fast-food restaurants. Her daily ritual of walking her dog had fallen by the wayside. However, Jennifer felt she could address these two bad habits and, thus, make progress toward her goal.

(#4) Jennifer decided she could take a healthy cooking class to help her break that fast-food-restaurant habit. She made a plan to eat 90% of her meals at home. Jennifer also felt that she could begin walking her dog every day with her friend Betty, who loved walking.

(#5) Jennifer called the organization running the healthy cooking program and learned the class wasn't starting for another two weeks. Still, she signed up. However, Jennifer then remembered that she had purchased a healthy cookbook a few years ago. She found that book, dusted it off, and decided to get a head start on her goal by preparing some of those recipes. (Jennifer was thus revisiting step #3). She would cut back her restaurant eating to twice a week for two weeks and then down to once or twice monthly once the class started (#3 again). She opened her cookbook and chose the meals she was going to cook for the next seven days. She also wrote down which days she was going to go to a restaurant (#4 again). Jennifer then went to the supermarket to buy the ingredients she would need for those home-cooked meals. Finally, she called Betty, who was excited to start walking with her. The two took their first walk the next day.

Before You Jump In

As her only son heads off to college, you can imagine the anxious mother giving her last pieces of "crucial advice" to the ambitious traveler. In the same way, here are some of my lingering concerns before you jump in.

The Most Important Rule

Let me say this once and for all, *never* stop your blood pressure medications abruptly! "*Why? Isn't this the goal of the book?*"

Yes, but the way to do that is not by dumping them down the toilet upon completing this chapter.

First, cessation of some blood pressure medications can cause "rebound hypertension," a situation where BP suddenly goes sky high (far higher than pretreatment levels) upon medication cessation. This grim fate awaited Wanda some years ago. She was emergently admitted to the hospital for a surgical problem. However, in the excitement surrounding her acute condition, no one thought to ensure that she received her morning dose of the antihypertensive drug, clonidine. The result some hours later was extremely high blood pressure in the 240/150 range, higher than Wanda had ever seen even before starting medications.

This scenario is not uncommon with clonidine, as well as

drugs in another antihypertensive class known as beta-blockers. Metoprolol, nadolol, atenolol, propranolol are common examples. Drugs like these lower blood pressure by interfering with the sympathetic nervous system, responsible for the stress, or "fight or flight," response. Among other things, your body has been trying to resist the effects of these drugs by increasing the sensitivity of its stress hormone receptors. (Although medications may have desirable effects, your body typically regards them as foreign substances that it tries to compensate for or neutralize.) Consequently, when these drugs are stopped abruptly, the now drug-free but overly sensitized receptors may over respond to even normal levels of stress hormones in your body. The result? The possibility of extremely high blood pressure, sometimes with disastrous complications like a stroke.

Even if you avoid the dangers of rebound hypertension, abrupt withdrawal of high blood pressure medications has, on occasion, triggered heart attacks. The bottom line is simple: you'll want to keep taking your medications, and keep in touch with the physician who prescribes your BP meds. However, don't wait until you're on the program before informing your doctor. Prior to embarking on your 30-day journey make sure your prescribing physician knows you are planning to make some major lifestyle changes that may well necessitate medication changes.

Clearly, the principles in this book are powerful. Your need for blood pressure medication is likely to decrease significantly over the next month. In most cases the best way to stop blood pressure medications is to wean the dosages and/or frequency of those meds as the diet and lifestyle principles in this book take effect. Again, working with your physician is important when adjusting medications.

As You Jump In: Measure Your Blood Pressure!

Careful, frequent blood pressure checks are a non-negotiable component of this program. (Remember Figure 4.2?) This is essential for your own safety. I recommend that you check your blood pressure at least three times every day, sometime during each "day part"; i.e., morning, afternoon, and evening. Although other expert groups sometimes recommend four daily readings, that's not typically necessary unless your BP is erratic. Remember, Appendix A is designed to keep you focused on this important task. If you'd rather use a computer program or spread sheet, that's OK. But faithfully record those three daily blood pressure readings *somewhere*.

However, it's not enough to merely check your blood pressure; you have to do it correctly. Yes, there is a right and a wrong way to check blood pressure. If you want accurate readings, I recommend the following:

1. *Minimize the white-coat effect.* When your blood pressure is checked at the doctor's office with a standard manual blood pressure monitor (a bulb squeezed by hand to inflate the cuff while listening with a stethoscope) it will tend to register 9/6 mmHg points higher than in research settings,[36] and as much as 15 points higher than in home settings.[37] The term *white-coat hypertension* is used when your blood pressure is high only at the doctor's office (with average home blood pressures <130/80) and normal almost everywhere else.

   One study showed that a hospitalized patient's blood pressure increases an average of about 27/15 mmHg when a doctor walks into the room.[38] If the doctor measures the blood pressure in the clinic setting, the pressure is 5-7/2-4 mmHg points higher than when the nurse does it.[39] In fact, the white-coat effect appears to occur in the vast majority of people with or without hypertension.[40] As a result, studies confirm that repeated home blood pressure measurement is usually more accurate than one or two blood pressure measurements done at the doctor's office.[41]

However, the condition is not innocuous. Studies show that white-coat hypertension is probably a precursor to full-blown hypertension. Furthermore, it appears to increase the risk of problems like artery narrowing and heart damage compared to people with normal blood pressures and no white coat effect.[42,43]

2. *Use an automatic blood pressure monitor.* Most people find it easiest, and most accurate, to monitor their BP at home using an automatic blood pressure monitor.[44] These units are convenient and require little skill and no assistant. However, even automatic blood pressure monitors can have problems with accuracy. One study showed that when an automatic monitor and a manual monitor were connected to the same blood pressure cuff on the same arm, the automatic monitor measured 2/1 mmHg points lower on average.[45] Although, those differences sound small, they were considerable in some groups. Consider the elderly. Their blood pressures varied up to 26/25 mmHg points. (The reason for differences in these blood pressure measurements is likely due, at least in part, to different things being measured. Conventional manual blood pressure testing relies on the examiner listening to sound changes in the artery. On the other hand, automatic blood pressure monitors measure wave changes that occur at lower pressures than the sound changes.)

To ensure you are using an automatic blood pressure device that is as accurate as possible, purchase a validated blood pressure monitor. This means the manufacturer has checked their device to ensure the measurements it gives are accurate. You can find a list of validated blood pressure monitors at http://www.dableducational.org.

It's true, manual blood pressure monitors, in some settings,

65

may be more accurate than automated ones. Actually, this is the case only if strict measurement protocols are followed.[46] Even in most doctor-patient situations, however, several factors impair the accuracy of manual blood pressure measurement. Some of these same factors can interfere with accurate manual blood pressure readings at home. Among the most important are: holding a conversation while performing a blood pressure check, checking only a single BP reading, allowing no period of rest before blood pressure measurement, performing an overly rapid deflation of the cuff, and engaging in "digit preference," where the recorder unconsciously rounds off the readings to end in a 0 or 5. Each of these factors tends to adversely affect the accuracy of manual blood pressure measurement.

3. *Make sure your blood pressure cuff fits properly.* The blood pressure cuff that you're using may be too large or too small. Too large a cuff will give you artificially low blood pressure readings; if the cuff is too small, you'll be looking at falsely elevated readings. However, most, but not all, home devices have indicators to help you know if the cuff is of proper size. If you have questions, you can visit your doctor's office (or a local fire department, county health department, etc.) and have your home blood pressure device checked to ensure it fits properly. If you still have concerns about your device's accuracy, this would be a great time to see how your device compares with other blood pressure measurement devices. Talk to your doctor about whether your blood pressure monitor appears to be accurate. Erratic readings are more problematic than readings that are predictably a few points too high or a few points too low, since you can correct for the latter.

4. *Obtain an automatic blood pressure monitor that digitally records the readings and stores those readings in its computer memory.* Studies show human bias is active when writing down blood pressure measurements to ultimately show a doctor. Some apparently want to show how high their blood pressure is and, thus, tend to write more of their higher measurements. Others tend to preferentially record lower measurements, apparently trying to make their blood pressure look good.

5. *Be mindful of the setting when checking your blood pressure.* Try to ensure your surroundings are not artificially elevating your numbers. For example, sitting in a cold or noisy environment are classic settings where BP will run higher. Similarly, you're likely to see artificially high readings if you're in the middle of rushing between activities, and then hastily sit down for a "quick BP check." Expressed positively, if you want the most accurate blood pressure readings you'll want to do the following:

   • Get yourself in a relaxed state of mind while sitting in a quiet, warm environment for five minutes before checking your blood pressure.

   • Ensure your back and arm are supported. This means sitting in a comfortable chair with a back and having the arm where you are measuring your blood pressure supported (e.g., resting on a desk or table).

   • Make sure your blood pressure cuff is at heart level. If your cuff is below the level of your heart, you'll get a falsely high reading. A cuff above heart level gives a falsely lower reading.

6. *To get an accurate reading, avoid substances that can elevate your blood pressure.* This includes:

- No smoking for at least 30 minutes.

- No caffeine for at least an hour (however, avoidance for at least four hours is optimal).[47]

- No adrenergic medications for 24 hours (this includes decongestant and pupil-dilating medications, such as phenylephrine). In other words, you'll either want to avoid these drugs completely during the 30 days, or if you have a medical need for any, check with your doctor to see if you can use them consistently at the same time every day during your one-month program.

- No illegal drugs. Drugs like methamphetamine and cocaine can also raise blood pressure.

Figure 4.5 summarizes the key points involved in your daily blood pressure checks.

Figure 4.5 Essentials of Proper Blood Pressure Measurement During Your 30-Day Journey

01	Obtain an automatic blood pressure monitor.
02	Relax for five minutes in a warm, comfortable environment—with your back and arm supported—before checking your BP.
03	Ensure you have not had any recent exposure to nicotine, caffeine or other blood-pressure-raising agents.
04	Always keep the blood pressure cuff at heart level.
05	Measure your blood pressure three times daily.

And, By All Means, Don't Forget...

All of the strategies I'll share in this book are powerful. A single one, consistently implemented, may lower your blood pressure so much that one or more of your medications might need to be adjusted by your physician. However, when it comes to other *No Pressure* components, your BP might be more resistant.

But don't get discouraged if your blood pressure readings don't seem to budge after implementing the first two or three components.

If you are like the average person, each of the ten *No Pressure* strategies may move your BP only a few points—small enough changes that you're not likely to notice them when superimposed on the other normal day-to-day causes of blood pressure fluctuation. However, remember this: Both addition and multiplication are powerful.

I say *addition is powerful* because, although any given aspect of lifestyle change may appear to have a relatively small effect on your blood pressure, the combination of multiple lifestyle changes—adhered to for the four weeks of this program—can have a large additive impact.

I say *multiplication is powerful* because even one or two positive changes can help set in motion a "virtuous cycle." A virtuous cycle is the opposite of that notorious "vicious cycle," where one or more deleterious factors start a process that sends you into a downward spiral (or, in the case of your blood pressure, an upward one). In a virtuous cycle, one good change promotes others that further aid you (in this case) of meeting your blood pressure goals. Consequently, through such virtuous mechanisms you can reap multiplicative benefits when it comes to blood pressure lowering.

If you like math, you'll appreciate Figure 4.6, where you see an illustration contrasting additive and multiplicative effects. (If you have an aversion to algebra, just skip that figure and move on.)

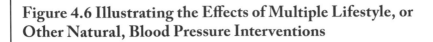

Figure 4.6 Illustrating the Effects of Multiple Lifestyle, or Other Natural, Blood Pressure Interventions

The Givens:

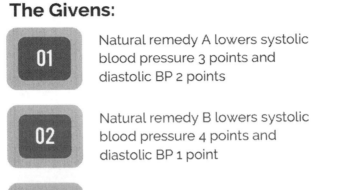

01 Natural remedy A lowers systolic blood pressure 3 points and diastolic BP 2 points

02 Natural remedy B lowers systolic blood pressure 4 points and diastolic BP 1 point

03 Natural remedy C lowers both systolic and diastolic BPs 2 points

The Examples:

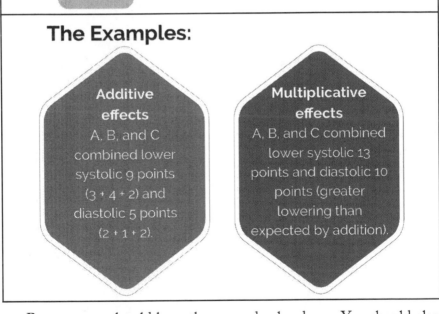

Additive effects
A, B, and C combined lower systolic 9 points (3 + 4 + 2) and diastolic 5 points (2 + 1 + 2).

Multiplicative effects
A, B, and C combined lower systolic 13 points and diastolic 10 points (greater lowering than expected by addition).

By now, you should have the ground rules down. You should also realize that we're about to discover some powerful material. In the next chapter, we begin our life-changing 30-day journey.

5

NUTRITION: EATING YOUR WAY TO LOWER BLOOD PRESSURE

DURING CHILDHOOD, I WAS being set up for a life of poor eating choices. After lecturing to thousands of people worldwide, I'm convinced my background is far from unique. Regardless of your cultural roots, I'd wager most of you unconsciously received the same indoctrination.

When I look back on my youth, at least two fundamental dietary principles were ingrained in my psyche, even though no one ever expressed them in words. The first was this: "If something tastes good, it must be bad for you." I was reminded of this on numerous occasions: being caught red-handed in the cookie jar or wanting ice cream before the main course provide examples. The second unexpressed principle was this: "If something tastes bad, it must be good for you." This message seems to have been powerfully inculcated in dinner table settings where I had trouble bringing things like green leafy vegetables to my youthful lips. "Eat those, they're good for you," was the messaging I received.

The problem with those two nearly-universal messages is this: they are false. The medical research studies don't lie. People who choose healthier foods (even if they are unpalatable at first!) actually have more enjoyment in food and in life than do people who don't. So even though certain "healthy" foods initially may seem distasteful, with careful preparation and continued exposure, you will tend to develop new tastes. In addition, when you leave off unhealthy foods, those items begin to lose their appeal. Just ask anyone who has decreased their salt intake for several months. There's a very good chance that heavily salted "favorite dish" began to taste excessively salty. Taste buds can change. (If you'd like more than this brief explanation on the power of making healthy choices, pick up a copy of Dr. DeRose's *Changing Bad Habits for Good* DVD.[48])

So, what can we do in the nutritional realm to help us get off those side-effect prone blood pressure drugs? Figure 5.1 provides an overview.

Figure 5.1 Three Key Nutrition Principles for Lowering Blood Pressure

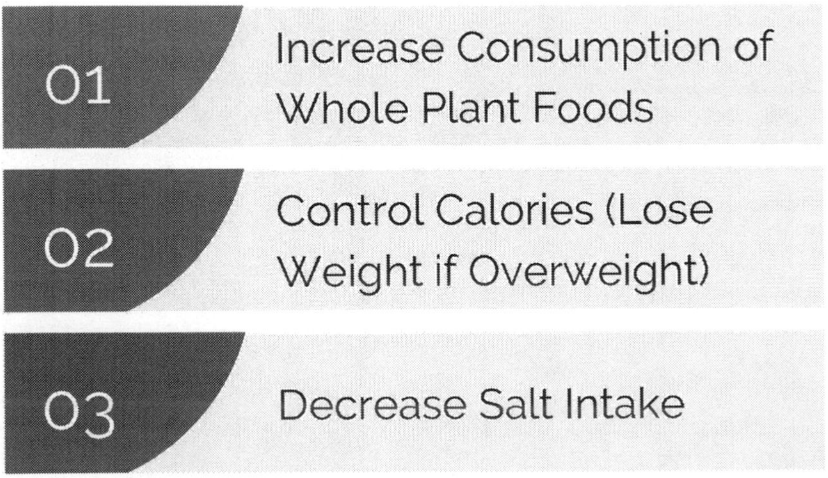

01	Increase Consumption of Whole Plant Foods
02	Control Calories (Lose Weight if Overweight)
03	Decrease Salt Intake

Boosting Your Consumption of Whole Plant Foods

Do typical dietary choices really make a difference? Definitely. Medical studies have clearly demonstrated that what we habitually eat strongly influences our blood pressure.

Some of the most fascinating research along these lines comes from a religious group known as Seventh-day Adventists (SDAs). Adventists are known for their healthful living and longevity. In November 2005, when *National Geographic* ran a cover story highlighting the healthiest people in the world, SDAs in Southern California took their position along with other societies boasting the oldest old people, in places like Sardinia, Italy and Okinawa, Japan.

What is relevant to our blood pressure discussion is this: Adventists have for over a century and a half emphasized the value of eating more whole plant foods. SDAs are not required by their religion to be vegetarians, but this historical health emphasis has resulted in many Adventists adopting a vegetarian lifestyle.

From a research standpoint, data from SDAs offers other advantages. First, Adventist populations feature not only many vegetarians but also an abundance of individuals who eat similarly to their non-Adventist peers. This allows researchers to draw statistically valid comparisons between different dietary practices. Second, Adventists are often integrated with the rest of society (i.e., they are not a reclusive or isolationist group). Consequently, their living circumstances are often similar to their peers, with the exception of their lifestyle choices such as diet. This makes it more likely that differences between SDAs and their neighbors will be due to lifestyle choices and not uncontrollable environmental factors.

The first Adventist study we'll examine involved a relatively small number of participants, 378.[49] These men and women were from two racial backgrounds, Caucasian and African American. Figure 5.2 shows the remarkable connection between diet and blood pressure in both races.

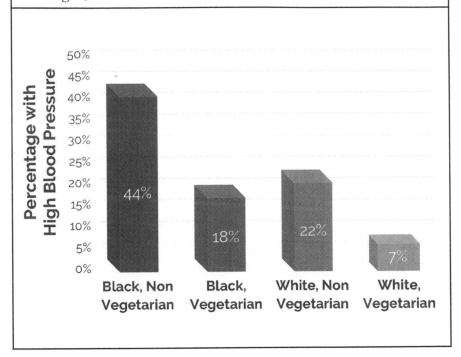

Figure 5.2 Do Typical Diet Practices Make a Difference?
(Data from a biracial sample of 378 Seventh-day Adventists in Michigan)

The data raise a number of questions. One obvious one is how comparable were the two racial groups? The white and black subjects were of roughly the same gender composition (roughly 80% of each group were female). Although similar in age, the black non-vegetarian subjects' average age was 3.5 years older than the white non-vegetarians (56.1 vs. 52.6). Perhaps the most striking difference occurred between these two meat-eating subgroups. Specifically, the white non-vegetarians ate, on average, only 3.6 servings of meat, poultry, and fish per week. Their fellow non-vegetarian church members from African American blood lines averaged 10.1 servings of flesh food weekly.

Some data, like these, raise concerns that certain races may be at greater risk for high blood pressure than others. However, it is likely that at least some of the differences in risk attributed to race are really due to lifestyle practices.

A more recent study of Seventh-day Adventists involved nearly 90,000 church members across the spectrum of age, gender, race, and ethnicity. No attempt was made to stratify the population based on demographics. However, a compelling relationship emerged when it came to diet and high blood pressure. Of interest, a similar pattern was noted between dietary practices and prevalence of diabetes. See Figure 5.3.[50]

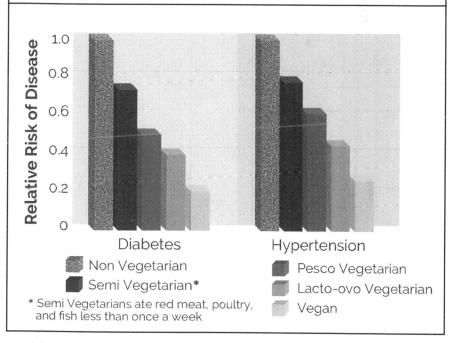

Figure 5.3 Diet Practices and the Likelihood of Hypertension and Diabetes (Data from 89,224 subjects enrolled in the Adventist Health Study-2)

If you're not familiar with the classification system used to delineate dietary practices in the Adventist Health Study-2, the researchers used a fairly straightforward nomenclature. Dietary categories were defined so as to denote progressively decreasing consumption of animal products:

- Nonvegetarians ate more than once a week from all the following categories: red meat, poultry, fish, milk, and eggs

- Semivegetarians ate milk and eggs, but fish, red meat and poultry less than once per week

- Pescovegetarians ate fish in addition to milk and eggs, but essentially no red meat or poultry (by definition, less than once per month)

- Lactoovovegetarians ate milk and/or eggs, but no red meat, fish, or poultry

- Vegans (also known as total vegetarians) ate no red meat, fish, poultry, dairy or eggs

The message of Figure 5.3 could not be clearer. The less animal products consumed—and the more plant products eaten—the less likely a person was to have high blood pressure. Yet, blood pressure is not the only parameter to benefit. Notice what one of this study's authors, Gary Fraser, MD, PhD, has to say about the benefit of vegetarian diets in general:

> "There is convincing evidence that vegetarians have lower rates of coronary heart disease, largely explained by low LDL cholesterol, probable lower rates of hypertension and diabetes mellitus, and lower prevalence of obesity. Overall, their cancer rates appear to be moderately lower than others living in the same communities, and life expectancy appears to be greater."

However, you may already have some questions about the data. If you're a scientist, you probably realize the data we've so far reviewed is "cross-sectional." That means we've looked at people at a single point in time to look for statistical connections, for our purposes, a correlation between dietary practices and high blood pressure. The problem with cross-sectional studies is that there may be other, unmeasured, differences between groups which affect the relationships. Consequently, a much more powerful research approach is the randomized clinical trial. For our purposes, we would want to search for studies of nonvegetarians who became vegetarians (or at least started eating more vegetables) and see what happened to their blood pressure.

Fortunately, this work has already been done for us. After reviewing 80 scientific studies, Drs. Susan Berkow and Neal Barnard concluded: "Randomized clinical trials have shown that BP [blood pressure] is lowered when animal products are replaced with vegetable products in both normotensives and hypertensives."[51] In plain English, these researchers found that it is never too late to get the benefits of a vegetarian diet. Make a priority to eat more fruits, whole grains, beans, and vegetables, and less meat, milk, eggs and cheese. Even cutting down on your poultry and fish consumption seems to have blood-pressure-lowering benefits.

I use the adjective "whole" before "plant foods" to make an important point. I'm not talking about eating more "refined" plant foods like potato chips or french fries. Think instead of baked potatoes, chopped potatoes used in a vegetarian stew, etc. If you understand what I mean by increasing your consumption of whole plant foods, you'll begin eating:

- more fruits, vegetables, nuts, legumes (beans), and whole grains
- less processed and refined grains, sugars, snacks, and sweets
- less red and processed meat

Application Time

Now this program involves not only information, but practice. Begin making a commitment to what we've just learned. It's actually the first of three fundamental nutritional principles I cover in this chapter. (That's right, you need only apply three nutritional principles to begin to substantially transform your blood pressure.)

So, in regard to the first principle: What could you do to boost your consumption of whole plant products and decrease your use of animal products? If you've already got a goal in mind, turn to the end of this chapter and begin to fill in the draft worksheet.

Each chapter from now on has such a sheet at its conclusion. I call each of those end-of-chapter worksheets a *draft*, because I want you to fill them out as *you're going through the chapter*. It thus becomes a work in progress. In fact, you can refine your goals as you learn more. However, once you've finished a given chapter, I want you to take your behavioral goals and transfer them to Appendix B at the end of the book. Once you put them down in Appendix B, you are saying you are really committed to following those practices for the duration of the 30-day program.

I should point out something that's obvious if you compare the end-of-chapter worksheets with Appendix B. Namely, you have space for up to five goals at the end of each chapter; however, I want you to transfer a *minimum of one* and *a maximum of three* goals from each chapter to Appendix B. You've also got more room at the end of the chapters to wax eloquent in writing your SMART goals. For example, you could write at the end of this chapter: "Eat vegetarian at least five days per week." You could then simply transfer this goal to Appendix B as "EV5."

If you feel that using abbreviations would make the process unnecessarily difficult, I can relate. For this reason, I've made available an enlarged version of Appendix B. Get it at the *CompassHealth Consulting* website (www.compasshealth.net) by clicking on the tab for "Free Materials," and then selecting the document, "Appendix-B-enlarged." It contains plenty of room to transfer, in their entirety, up to three of your behavioral goals for each chapter.

If you haven't already done so, turn to Appendix B and I'll point out a few other details. First, you'll see columns to the right of your behavioral goals. Those columns correspond to the four-plus weeks or thirty days of this program. Feel free to write the actual dates for the weeks of the program in the corresponding boxes. For example, in the box labeled "Week 1," go ahead and write "September 3 – 9" (or something similar) if that will be your first week on the program. Do this for all five of the weeks. This will help you keep focused. (Of course, you could make things really easy and simply start your program on the first day of a month. Then all your *program days* will correspond exactly to the dates of that month.)

Second, use the columns to check off your adherence to each behavioral goal on the day in question. Let's return to our example of eating vegetarian at least five days per week. At the end of Week 1, the relevant portion of Appendix B should look something like this:

Appendix B							
	Sept. Week 1 3-9						
	1	2	3	4	5	6	7
Ch 5							
EV5	✓	✓		✓		✓	✓

One last thing is worth mentioning. You've probably already realized that I included some of the columns representing the first two weeks on each of the end-of-chapter worksheets. Don't actually check off your behaviors on those sample worksheets. I recommend you only check off things in Appendix B. The reason for including those columns on the worksheets is to remind you why you're articulating your goals, and that you have a task to do at the end of each day (logging your progress).

So, it's time for the application. Flip to the end of the chapter and at least jot down (preferably in pencil) one idea of how you can improve your diet. If you're not yet convinced how important it is to move in the direction of a plant-strong diet, consider what follows.

Why Are Plant Foods So Powerful?

Manuel looked like the picture of health. He was a long distance runner who appeared younger than his thirty years. Yet, every time he came into the office his blood pressure was in the 150-160's / 100's. He checked it at home. It was the same. We reviewed his diet: it looked pretty good. True, he was eating red and processed meats once or twice a week, but that didn't seem all that egregious. I eventually felt compelled to put him on a blood pressure medicine, especially in light of the heart problems that ran in his family. A few months later he came into the clinic and told me that he was off his blood pressure medicine. I checked his blood pressure and it was normal. "What gives"? I asked him. "I completely stopped eating meat, not even once a week," he said. I was amazed. Of course, it made sense since meat tends to be high in calories and salt, lower in potassium, and high in saturated fat and other pro-inflammatory chemicals. Before my eyes, Manuel was improving the health of his blood vessels.

Indeed, for years medical evidence has pointed to a connection between dietary atherosclerotic risk factors and high blood pressure. In other words, the same dietary components that tend to foster higher cholesterol levels—and fatty buildup in our arteries—also predispose us to high blood pressure. Such a connection makes sense. Earlier in this book I already explained how stiffer arteries necessitate higher blood pressures in order to keep our blood circulating optimally.

What dietary factors worsen arterial health? For several decades the evidence has convincingly pointed to things like saturated fat and cholesterol.[52] Yes, the major source of saturated fat in the American diet is animal products. Looking for a zero-cholesterol diet? The only natural diet that has no cholesterol is the vegan, or total vegetarian diet. (That's right, even fat-rich plant products like nuts, avocados, and olives have not a single mg of cholesterol.)

Another area where plant products trump animal-derived

dietary constituents is in the "nutrient density" department. When you look at equal sized servings calorically, vegetable products typically give you more nutritional "bang for your buck." Consequently, your best sources for blood-pressure-lowering compounds come from the plant kingdom. Among those beneficial compounds are magnesium, potassium, and calcium. However, as we'll see shortly, the whole food benefits of plants have more going for them than simply a few isolated minerals.

Nonetheless, minerals (also known as micronutrients) like magnesium, potassium, and calcium are important, so some observations are in order. Before we look at the data on plant foods, let me address something that's likely already reverberating in your mind from the minute I mentioned the word "calcium."

In the United States, even most grade school children believe that dairy products are among the healthiest dietary choices. When it comes to blood pressure, it is true that diets containing dairy can be part of a blood-pressure-lowering program. The famous DASH Diet provides a good illustration. However, over the years I've found that patients with chronic diseases like high blood pressure generally do better the less dairy they consume.

I'm not trying to wrest that skim milk away from you. Yet dairy products lack many of the other blood-pressure-lowering compounds found in plants. Additionally, liberal consumption of dairy products may not help in the weight department (research suggests butter is especially bad for your waist line), and there are growing concerns about the toxin load contributed by milk and its derivatives.

But if I decrease or eliminate my dairy consumption aren't I destined for osteoporosis? Not necessarily. An excellent diet without dairy actually may be better for your bones than are typical diets liberally laced with milk products. In 2014 alone, a number of medical studies explored these relationships. Consider the following examples:

- Analysis of two huge data sets from Sweden (involving over 100,000 men and women who were followed for an average of 10-20 years) connected higher milk intake with greater mortality in both genders and with greater bone fracture risk among women.[53]

- Another two large data sets, this time from the United States, also found no evidence for the "drink milk-healthy bones" mantra.[54] An analysis of diet during the teen years of over 90,000 men and women in the Harvard University's Nurses' Health Study and male Health Professionals Follow-up Study showed that teenage milk consumption afforded no decreased risk of hip fractures in women and a significant increased risk of hip fractures in men. For each additional glass of milk per day consumed in the teen years, men increased their risk of hip fracture 9% later in life, with the highest milk consumers experiencing over a 20% increased risk of fractures.

If milk intake is not a guarantee of good bone health, then what about fruits and vegetables? If we eat more of those foods, are we likely to have stronger or weaker bones? Some of the same Swedish researchers who raised concerns with milk and bone health found a protective effect for fruits and vegetables. In a study of some 75,000 men and women they found that those consuming fewer servings of fruits and vegetables per day had a greater risk of hip fracture over the approximately 14 years covered by their study. The poorest fruit and vegetable eaters had an 88% increased risk of fracture compared to the men and women who had five or more servings daily.[55]

All of this is an aside, but an important one. I'm not going to recommend anything in this book for blood pressure lowering that would likely compromise your health in any other respect. When pointing you in the direction of eating more whole vegetarian foods—and less animal products—I'm not only offering you help for your blood pressure, but also for other health problems as well.

Plant Products: Mineral Powerhouses

There's a number of ways to look at nutrient content. One of the best sources for information is an amazing database maintained by the United States Department of Agriculture. Their "National Nutrient Database for Standard Reference Release 27" can be accessed at: http://ndb.nal.usda.gov/ndb/nutrients/index. The database allows you to search virtually any nutrient and rank foods according to the nutrient in question. I've done that with three blood-pressure-lowering minerals: magnesium, potassium and calcium. Diets with plant foods, such as beans, fruits and vegetables, that have high amounts of these minerals, can lead to significant improvements in blood pressure. In order to help you see why I rank plant products first when it comes to such compounds, I'll present the data from three different perspectives.

Figure 5.4 shows the top sources of magnesium among over 7500 foods listed in the USDA database. All these "champions" are from plant sources. Seeds, beans, nuts and grains steal the show. However, if we were to look at the same database in terms of nutrient density, we would again find that plant products dominate the field, even if this time a different set of plants tops the list. Among the leaders are Swiss chard (4.3 mg of magnesium per calorie), spinach (3.8 mg), dock (4.7 mg), beet greens (3.4 mg), seaweed (3.0 mg), purslane (3.7 mg) and lambsquarters (3.5 mg). In fact, of the top 100 whole foods on the chart, only two animal products made the cut. Raw snails ranked about 30th on the list, with 2.8 mg of magnesium per calorie, while baked conch (another shellfish) ranked around 70th, with 1.8 mg of magnesium per calorie.[56]

Figure 5.5 looks at potassium, another blood-pressure-lowering mineral, in terms of nutrient density. As with magnesium, when we rank foods by caloric density, the leafy vegetables tend to be at the top of the list. These plant foods are very low in calories but rich in a host of nutrients.

Figure 5.4 Magnesium Champions

Top food sources of magnesium in the 2015 USDA database based on amount of magnesium found in a one cup serving. (The data below is essentially unedited, deletions only being made for multiple forms of the same food item.*)

	Food Item	Weight (grams)	Magnesium content
1	Rice bran, crude	118	922
2	Molasses	337	816
3	Seeds, pumpkin and squash seed kernels, dried	129	764
4	Mothbeans, mature seeds, raw	196	747
5	Seeds, cottonseed flour, partially defatted (glandless)	94	678
6	Hyacinth beans, mature seeds, raw	210	594
7	Yardlong beans, mature seeds, raw	167	564
8	Seeds, watermelon seed kernels, dried	108	556
9	Cowpeas, catjang, mature seeds, raw	167	556
10	Mungo beans, mature seeds, raw	207	553
11	Soybeans, mature seeds, raw	186	521
12	Seeds, sesame seed kernels, dried (decorticated)	150	518
13	Soybean, curd cheese	225	513
14	Nuts, brazilnuts, dried, unblanched	133	500
15	Amaranth grain, uncooked	193	479

* For example, pumpkin and squash seeds occur once only in the "top 15 list," whereas in the actual database they appear several times, owing to different "forms" of these foods; e.g., salted vs. unsalted, roasted vs. dried.

Figure 5.5 Potassium Champions

Top food sources of potassium in the 2015 USDA database (in terms of nutrient density; mg of potassium per calorie). The graphic below is an unedited list featuring all whole foods (i.e., processed and combined foods were excluded, such as juices, mixed salads, etc.) Note: multiple forms of a given food were also excluded.

	Food Item	Serving Size	Wt (in g)	kcal	K in mg	K/kcal
1	Bamboo shoots, cooked, boiled, drained, with salt	1.0 cup (.5" slices)	120	13	640	49.23
2	Butterbur, (fuki), raw	1.0 cup	94	13	616	47.38
3	Beet greens, raw	1.0 cup	38	8	290	36.25
4	Cabbage, Chinese (pak-choi), cooked, boiled, drained, without salt	1.0 cup, shredded	170	20	631	31.55
5	Amaranth leaves, cooked, boiled, drained, without salt	1.0 cup	132	28	846	30.21
6	Taro shoots, raw	0.5 cup slices	43	5	143	28.60
7	Chrysanthemum, garland, cooked, boiled, drained, without salt	1.0 cup (1" pieces)	100	20	569	28.45
8	Cabbage, Japanese style, fresh, pickled	1.0 cup	150	45	1280	28.44
9	Watercress, raw	1.0 cup, chopped	34	4	112	28.00
10	Spices, chervil, dried	1.0 tsp	.6	1	28	28.00
11	Chard, Swiss, cooked, boiled, drained, with salt	1.0 cup, chopped	175	35	961	27.46
12	Purslane, cooked, boiled, drained, without salt	1.0 cup	115	21	561	26.71
13	Celtuce (a celery-lettuce cross), raw	1.0 leaf	8	1	26	26.00
14	Parsley, freeze-dried	1.0 tbsp	0.4	1	28	25.00
15	Squash, zucchini, baby, raw	1.0 large	16	3	73	24.33

Key: Wt (in g) = weight in grams; kcal = calories in the specified serving size; K in mg = mg of potassium per serving (note: "K" is the chemical abbreviation for potassium); K/kcal = mg potassium per calorie

When it comes to calcium per volume, the top food in the USDA database is fortified orange juice, with 1514 mg of calcium per cup. However, I generally avoid recommending fortified foods as ideal sources of any nutrient. If you "fortified" water with calcium it wouldn't change the fact that most water is intrinsically a poor calcium source. Fortified foods are often no different than sprinkling some vitamins or minerals on your meal.

If we limit our search to items naturally containing calcium, the top natural source per volume is a surprising one. Sesame seeds, with 1404 mg of calcium per cup, lead the list. After that, if you were wading through the USDA database, you would notice a host of dairy products, mostly cheeses. Yet these dairy sources are rich in animal protein, which is not optimal for calcium balance. Furthermore, as we'll see shortly, carrying extra pounds tends to raise blood pressure. Consequently, our goal should be to get as much high quality nutrition as possible, but with as few calories as possible. With this in mind, we'll again look at calcium in terms of nutrient density. That graphic appears in Figure 5.6.

Several foods that don't show up in Figure 5.6 are worth noting. Whole Grain Total® was excluded from my list because it is a fortified food, even though it would rank in the top ten with 10.4 mg of calcium per serving. Spices and other condiments are generally used in such small amounts as to make little difference in our total calcium intake. However, all of the following pack 6-8 mg of calcium per calorie: basil, chervil, savory, spearmint, and thyme.

Wondering what happened to the sesame seeds? Yes, they have over 1400 mg of calcium per cup. However, that one cup is loaded with 825 calories. Consequently, they don't even contain 2 mg of calcium per calorie.

When it comes to the blood-pressure-lowering trio of magnesium, potassium, and calcium, your best choices come from the plant kingdom. If that isn't' sufficient to motivate you to move more in the direction of a vegetarian diet (and begin filling out the worksheet at the end of this

Figure 5.6 Calcium Champions

Top food sources of calcium in the 2015 USDA database (in terms of nutrient density; mg of calcium per calorie). The graphic below is an essentially unedited list featuring all whole foods (i.e., processed and combined foods were excluded such as fortified cereals, etc.) Note: also excluded were condiments (due to their use in limited quantities) and multiple forms of a given food (e.g., the USDA database lists multiple preparations of mustard spinach, amaranth leaves, and pak-choi).

	Food Item	Serving Size	Wt (in g)	kcal	Ca in mg	Ca/kcal
1	Stinging Nettles, blanched (Northern Plains Indians)	1.0 cup	89	37	428	11.57
2	Nopales (cactus pads), cooked, without salt	1.0 cup	149	22	244	11.09
3	Butterbur, canned	1.0 cup, chopped	124	4	42	10.50
4	Tofu, various preparations, prepared with calcium sulfate	1.0 cup, block	11	13	135	10.38
5	Watercress, raw	1.0 cup, chopped	34	4	41	10.25
6	Amaranth leaves, raw	1 cup	28	6	60	10.00
7	Mustard spinach, (tender-green), cooked, boiled, drained, without salt	1.0 cup, chopped	180	29	284	9.79
8	Rhubarb, frozen, uncooked	1.0 cup, diced	137	29	266	9.17
9	Turnip greens, canned, solids and liquids	0.5 cup	117	16	138	8.63
10	Cabbage, chinese (pak-choi), raw	1.0 cup, shredded	70	9	74	8.22
11	Lambsquarters, cooked, boiled, drained, without salt	1.0 cup, chopped	180	58	464	8.00
12	Cheese, Swiss, nonfat or fat free	1.0 serving	28	36	269	7.47
13	Collards, raw	1.0 cup, chopped	36	12	84	7.00
14	Cheese, mozzarella, nonfat	1.0 cup, shredded	113	159	1086	6.83
15	Cheese, American, nonfat or fat free	1.0 serving	19	24	150	6.25

Key: Wt (in g) = weight in grams; kcal = calories in the specified serving size; Ca in mg = mg of calcium per serving ; Ca/kcal = mg calcium per calorie chapter), the most amazing subplot in the vegetable nutrition story is yet to come.

Fighting High Blood Pressure with Phytochemicals

Earlier in this book I spoke briefly about the kidney's role in high blood pressure. You may recall how, if the kidney senses lower than optimal blood pressure, or is in some way malfunctioning, it can pump out more of a blood-pressure-raising compound known as renin. Renin interacts with other compounds that can influence blood pressure, such as angiotensin and aldosterone. So important are these relationships that the so called "renin-angiotensin-aldosterone" system is the target for a number of classes of antihypertensive drugs. At the time of writing, some 40 different high blood pressure medications target this system, in whole or in part.

Now here is something remarkable about plant products: these foods are loaded with "phytochemicals." This designation should refer to any plant chemical, but it is used in medical circles to refer especially to biologically active compounds that are not vitamins or minerals. Among these plant chemicals are compounds that have "ACE inhibitory effects." Now, "ACE" stands for angiotensin converting enzyme. ACE inhibitors work to lower blood pressure by interfering with the blood-pressure-raising effects of the renin-angiotensin-aldosterone system.

Perhaps you are taking a medication for your blood pressure like enalapril (found in Vasotec® and Vaseretic®), lisinopril (found in Prinivil®, Prinzide®, Zestril®, and Zestoretic®), moexipril (found in Uniretic® and Univasc®), trandolapril (found in Tarka®), or some other antihypertensive drug whose generic name ends in "pril." If so, then you are taking an ACE inhibitor. But there are other ways to get ACE inhibitors besides taking drugs. Guess? Yes, these "drugs" are found in small quantities in fruits and vegetables. Figure 5.7 provides a list of foods identified as containing ACE inhibitory compounds.[57]

Figure 5.7 Angiotensin Converting Enzyme (ACE) Inhibitory Compounds in Foods

The following foods have been found to contain blood-pressure-lowering ACE inhibitors

Broccoli	Mung Beans	Soybeans
Buckwheat	Mushrooms	Spinach
Chickpeas	Peanuts	Sunflowers
Corn	Potatoes	Wheat
Garlic	Rice	

Don't let Figure 5.7 worry you. In my decades of medical practice, I've never seen anyone admitted to the hospital in shock (i.e., with profoundly low blood pressure) from eating too many plant products. Granted, if you are highly allergic to any food, you can develop anaphylactic shock, one cause of profoundly low blood pressure and even death. So, by all means, if you're allergic to peanuts, don't start eating them to try to lower your blood pressure!

Such extenuating circumstances aside, I've never seen someone who was not taking medications develop hypotension (too low a blood pressure) because of a healthy diet. But remember this: because of the powerful effects of nutrition on blood pressure, you may develop blood pressure that is too low if you change your diet dramatically and don't work with your doctor to change your medications in the face of improving blood pressure numbers.

Don't Be Misled

While we are on the topic of health-enhancing food constituents, don't let anyone hoodwink you into boosting your intake of animal products by trying to convince you of their healthy constituents. Yes, many beneficial compounds exist in animal products. And there are situations where some of these foods should be included in the diet. I would never think of a telling a person in poverty, just barely getting by calorically, to give up the milk, eggs or poultry that was helping sustain his life.

However, the population data is clear when it comes to blood pressure. Eat more plant foods, lower your pressure. Eat more animal foods, raise your pressure.

So how could anyone obscure such a clear message? Here's how the argument goes: "There's a blood-pressure-lowering compound X in generally unhealthful food Y. Therefore, you should eat food Y to get this compound." It's true; scientists have been able to find some good things even in the most health-destroying of foods and habits. For example, is it any surprise that in tobacco smoke with over 7000 identified chemicals, that at least one of them might have some beneficial property? For example, smokers actually decrease their risk of a serious bowel problem called ulcerative colitis. However, before you rush out and grab a pack of cigarettes, realize that smoking increases your risk of a more extensive bowel disorder called Crohn's disease. (We'll find later in this book, tobacco also has powerful blood-pressure-elevating effects.) Solid research data indicates, in the U.S. alone, some 300,000 to 500,000 people die annually from cigarette smoking. Don't let anyone fool you into thinking you should be smoking for your health.

Ironically, we haven't learned our lessons from tobacco. Despite the literature showing the blood-pressure-lowering effects of eliminating animal products in favor of plant sources of nutrition, powerful corporate interests, in concert with the scientists they fund, are trying to tell us we should eat more of these BP-raising foods because of "healthful constituents" found therein.

Dangers of Extremes

As powerful as the vegan diet is in lowering blood pressure, you can take a good thing too far. I don't recommend further narrowing your diet and going to excessive extremes. For example, a water-melon-only diet may help lower your blood pressure, but it is not a prudent strategy for long-term health. (Nor, might I add, is it usually a good short-term strategy for individuals with diabetes. Melons often raise blood sugar significantly.)

Other potential problems with the vegan diet relate to two nutrients: vitamin B_{12} and vitamin D. Vitamin B_{12} is made by bac-teria and is found reliably only in animal products and fortified foods. Nonetheless, many vegans never run into obvious trouble with B_{12} deficiency. However, some do. Because of this, I recom-mend that if you embrace a total vegetarian diet, you take a vita-min B_{12} supplement daily. If you are young and healthy, you prob-ably can get by with 50 micrograms or less daily. If you are older, you may require more. Unless prescribed by a health practitioner, I don't recommend anyone take more than 1000 micrograms daily.

If that data seems sufficient to convince you to embrace a "semi-vegetarian" diet as opposed to a vegan program, think about this: The majority of Americans who develop B_{12} deficiency are eat-ing plenty of animal products. Here's the message: don't eat ani-mal products to ensure you're getting B_{12}, take a supplement. If you have questions, ask your doctor to check your B_{12} level.

When it comes to vitamin D, vegans lose a degree of protec-tion offered by the public health community, at least in the United States. Milk sold in the U.S. is required to be fortified with vitamin D. However, to urge milk consumption on these grounds is disin-genuous. Dairy products are a notoriously poor source of vitamin D in and of themselves. You can just as well take a vitamin D sup-plement, for much less expense in terms of both dollars and poten-tial side-effects. Furthermore, soy milk as well as some other vegan products is often supplemented with vitamin D. We'll talk more about vitamin D later in this book.

Summarizing Things Thus Far

The amazing synthesis of the data is this: we need to be optimizing our intake of fruits, whole grains, vegetables, beans, nuts and seeds. In scientific research these foods help to lower blood pressure. Medical data suggests those benefits are likely due, at least in part, to their helping us optimize our status with respect to minerals like magnesium, potassium, and calcium. Plant foods often have modest drug-like effects mediated through ACE-inhibitory compounds that can help normalize blood pressure. Finally, plant foods can help you lose weight if you're carrying extra pounds. So far, we have only touched on this latter relationship. We now take a closer look at how even a modest amount of excess body fat can be undermining your blood pressure control efforts.

Lose Weight if Overweight

For years physicians and researchers have been aware of the strong connection that exists between body weight and blood pressure. The heavier a person is, the higher his or her BP tends to be. And these relationships between blood pressure and weight don't wait until adulthood to manifest themselves. Even children who are heavier than their peers tend to have higher BPs.[58]

In the early 1990s, researchers compared just how much difference selected lifestyle changes could make in blood pressure.[59] Merely supplementing with blood-pressure-lowering minerals like magnesium, potassium and calcium (without the comprehensive dietary changes I have emphasized) had relatively little effect. Most impressive, however, were changes effected by weight loss and sodium (salt) restriction. These are depicted in Figure 5.8.

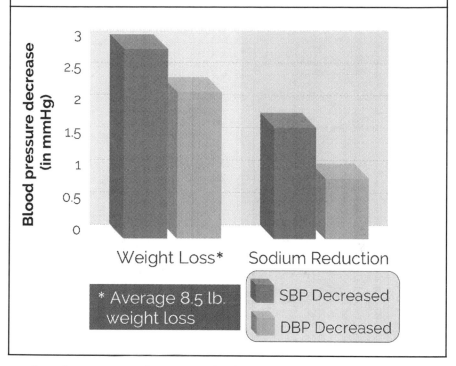

Figure 5.8 The Blood Pressure Lowering Effects of Sodium Reduction and Weight Loss

I realize some of you might be underwhelmed after looking at Figure 5.8. After all, how much will you accomplish by dropping your blood pressure a few points? First, evidence indicates you lower your risk of stroke by 2.8% for every one mmHg you lower your blood pressure.[60] Second, and perhaps most important: We're looking at multiple natural interventions to improve your blood pressure control. Even if you only lower your blood pressure a few points through nutritional means, the same magnitude of change for all the *No Pressure* components would result in your blood pressure falling 20 or 30 points. Furthermore, the higher your blood pressure, the more it tends to fall when you make lifestyle changes—it's possible for blood pressure values to drop 40 points or more. I have seen this happen many times in the lifestyle intervention programs I've conducted.

Okay, so you're overweight and now you feel like you've got some book author (in addition to those "well-meaning" friends and family members) nagging you to lose weight. If you're like most individuals who are carrying more pounds than optimal, you would be happy to shed that excess weight. But how?

I'm not going to tell you that losing weight and keeping it off is easy. However, there's an often-overlooked truth which most overweight individuals fail to fully harness: Over the long haul, temporary changes are difficult to maintain, while new lifestyle commitments are much easier to internalize. In other words, if you want to lose weight and keep it off, then I challenge you to make decisions that you plan to embrace for the rest of your life. Don't get too hung up on this "rest of your life" bit. Right now I want you to focus on just 30 days. But to get the most long-term benefit from this book—especially on a matter like weight loss—you won't be planning a party 31 days from now when you can throw off all lifestyle restraint.

If you haven't already visited the closing pages of this chapter, each chapter is designed to challenge you to do things differently. What might you choose to do for the next month (and, I hope, longer) that might help you finally get the upper hand in "the battle of the bulge"? Figure 5.9 presents seven lifestyle principles that can be powerful aids in the weight loss arena.

Points 1 and 3 in Figure 5.9 put in a practical context what I've already been trying to communicate. Expressed in other words, don't fall into the trap of embracing a "diet" for a few weeks or months, only to return to your old lifestyle. The real power in this battle comes when you are willing to make long-lasting changes. If you get serious about eating more whole plant foods—for the rest of your life—you're already well on your way to a healthier life. This truth was recently documented in the *New England Journal of Medicine* as illustrated in Figure 5.10.[61]

Figure 5.9 Seven Weight Loss Keys

1. Focus on habits not short-term diets.

2. Never make weight loss your sole focus.

3. Don't be afraid to make lifestyle changes.

4. Exercise daily.

5. Make clean breaks with "problem foods."

6. Eat a good breakfast—and don't snack.

7. "Eat to satisfy simple hunger, not appetite."

Figure 5.10 shows which foods have the biggest impact on weight. If the bars are going to the right, *avoid* that food! If the bars are going to the left, you can generally assume that food is a reasonable choice when it comes to body weight.

Point 2 of the Seven Weight Loss Keys is also critical to keep in mind from the beginning. When you focus on the scale, you put your energies in the best place to sabotage your program. Let me explain: weight fluctuates for many reasons. Some are uncontrollable (e.g., a woman's monthly cycle causes greater fluid retention just prior to menses). Others are the side-effects of good behaviors (e.g., if a new exercise program causes muscle soreness, the affected muscles are somewhat inflamed and thus retaining more fluid). So, yes, you have to pay some attention to the scale (just to make sure you are moving in the right direction). But I don't recommend you check your weight more than once weekly. Instead, focus on healthy behaviors.

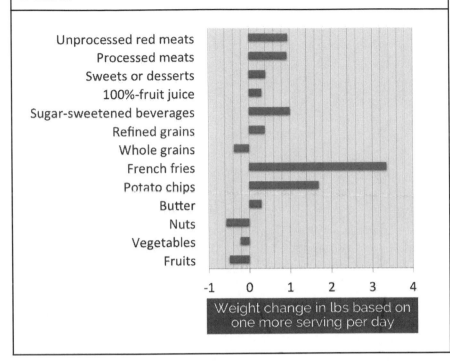

Figure 5.10 The Relationship between Changes in Dietary Habits and Weight Change Over Successive Four-Year Periods

Points 4 through 7 may sound simple, but they can pay huge dividends. Regular physical exercise and proper meal timing are two of the most important principles when it comes to optimizing one's weight. I'll devote a whole chapter to exercise shortly, but for now, start thinking about what you can do daily in the physical activity department. Studies demonstrate the weight losing benefits that accrue from making breakfast your main meal of the day and decreasing caloric intake as the day progresses.[62] (Eating little or no supper has been one of the most powerful weight loss strategies for many of my patients.) And if you haven't heard: today fewer and fewer dietitians and nutrition experts are recommending the "grazing" pattern for weight reduction. For many overweight individuals, eating seven times per day merely provides more opportunities to overeat. I side with the evidence recommending two or at most three meals daily.

The Power of Clean Breaks

Point 5 may seem counterintuitive. However, most individuals find that the path to freedom in the weight reduction realm requires making clean breaks with those foods that have been undermining your success. Think about it. If someone can't control their alcohol consumption, what do we tell them? No more alcohol. If someone is addicted to cigarettes, what's the medical message? Make a clean break: Quit smoking.

But why do we have such a hard time telling someone who can't control their consumption of chocolate or ice cream or potato chips to make a clean break with one or more of those foods? (I'm not picking on any specific foods; I've chosen some common examples from my patients over the years.) Now, please understand: I'm not telling every reader to swear off of chocolate, ice cream, and chips. However, if you can't control your consumption of a certain food category, treat that category as an addiction, and make a clean break with it.

What is "uncontrolled consumption"? You're feeling lonely one night, and decide to try that chocolate sampler you had saved for a special occasion. You determine to eat "three or four" only. Thirty minutes later you're looking at an empty box. When you can't exercise normal restraint in the face of a given food, you're likely dealing with "a problem food" and the result is "uncontrolled consumption." A clean break is in order.

Marie came to our clinic some years ago. She was frustrated in her attempts to really take charge of her lifestyle. Then one day, during a group lecture, something finally clicked. For years, Marie had been struggling with her ice cream consumption. She would cut down for a while, only to see her consumption gradually rise to previous levels. During that lecture she determined she would make a clean break with ice cream. Sometime later Marie confided that this represented a critical juncture in her lifestyle change journey. With ice cream now on her "forbidden" list, she was free to develop new enjoyments. She was reaching her health goals, and no longer missed the ice cream!

Yes, you *can* develop new enjoyments.

Learning to Differentiate Hunger from Appetite

Over the years I've learned that Point 7, "Eat to satisfy simple hunger, not appetite," immediately resonates with some patients, while others are left clueless. If you find yourself in the latter category, a few words of explanation are in order.

When I refer to "hunger" I'm talking about a true physiologic need for food that is perceived by your brain. I use the term "appetite" to indicate a desire for food that may or may not be in harmony with your body's actual needs.

Imagine you haven't eaten for 24 hours. There's a very good chance that you will be both hungry and have a good appetite. Fast forward now to the end of a one-hour meal. Odds are, your hunger has long been sated, but if someone brings out a delectable dessert, there's a good chance appetite will clamor for some.

The premise behind Point 7 is this: as infants we all knew when our hunger was satisfied, and we stopped eating. (Have you ever tried to get an infant to overeat? Your futile attempts were likely met with turned heads, or spit out foods.) However, most of us were educated from an early age to eat even when not hungry. You showed up at Grandma's house 45 minutes after a meal and she offered you cookies and milk. Whenever you skinned your knee, your mom gave you something to eat (regardless of the proximity to mealtime). Celebrations, a tough day at school, a neighborhood friend visiting, all were settings for eating, whether or not you were hungry.

The key here is to again get in touch with when you are eating to satisfy hunger, and when it is merely appetite clamoring for more. I'm told the Okinawans from Okinawa, Japan, have incorporated this concept into a traditional teaching, referred to as "Hara hachi bu." The common translation is "eat until you are 80% full."

Surprisingly, a number of simple things can help you get back in touch with your brain's signals that your hunger is satisfied. They basically center either on slowing your tempo of eating or becoming more mindful of your eating habits. Figure 5.11 provides a list of several concrete strategies.

Some of the advice in Figure 5.11 may seem intuitive. However, the rationale for other aspects of those recommendations may seem at least a bit elusive. Thus, an explanation is in order.

The reason for avoiding the old practice of serving foods in courses is relatively simple. If you feel satisfied and then the host brings out another palatable food item, you are more likely to be driven by appetite to eat more. Seeing all the food options up front puts you in the driver's seat.

Serving fewer options at a given meal will generally help you be more sensitive to hunger's soft voice. To illustrate the other extreme, think of dining at an all-you-can-eat buffet. The abundance and variety of palatable foods sets you up for appetite-driven eating.

The slower your pace of eating, the more likely hunger will be able to get your attention; that is, if you are not too engrossed in something else. (This is why it's typically a bad idea to eat while watching TV, a movie, or engaging in some other captivating activity.) Putting your fork down between bites and chewing your food thoroughly are time-honored principles of slowing one's eating pace.

Figure 5.11 Strategies for Learning to Differentiate Hunger from Appetite

- Never serve food in courses. Always put out all the meal options before eating.

- Limit the number of options served at any meal.

- Drink plenty of water between meals. (Thirst is often misperceived as hunger.)

- Eat slowly.

    o Put your utensil down between bites.

    o Chew your food thoroughly.

        ▪ Emphasize foods that must be chewed.

        ▪ Be careful of caloric beverages, soups, etc.

        ▪ Don't drink with your meals (a common substitute for adequate chewing is using beverages to help "wash down your food").

    o When eating, don't be overly engaged in another activity (e.g., watching a TV program, reading a captivating book, etc.).

- Don't serve food from your table.

    o Serve the food from a counter or even the range if necessary.

    o Initially take a smaller amount than you would normally choose.

- If you have a question as to whether you are still eating because of hunger or appetite, leave the table until the next meal.

- Use *the substitution principle* (see text).

This brings me to one corollary. Medical research reveals that—compared to eating whole foods—you get much less satisfaction from eating your calories in a liquid or pureed state. Your brain's hunger signaling mechanisms work best when you eat an apple rather than eating apple sauce or drinking apple juice.

Although putting your serving dishes on the table seems so convenient, it makes it very easy to ignore hunger's cues. When the serving dish is just an arm's length away, it is easier to eat just a little more, then a bit more, then still just a tad more. If the food is on a counter where you have to physically rise to obtain more, you give yourself the opportunity to ask, "Is this really hunger (i.e., physiologic need) calling for more food, or is it just appetite?"

This all brings us to perhaps the single most important principle if you want to learn to differentiate hunger from appetite: If you think your hunger *might* be satisfied, simply stop eating. What's the danger? You say, "If I really am hungry I won't get enough calories." Now, in some settings this could be a problem. (For example, if you are taking insulin or other medications that lower blood sugar, you may need to eat a given number of calories to avoid hypoglycemia.) However, for the vast majority of us, there is no risk from leaving the table hungry.

Give it a try. If you think your hunger is satisfied, simply stop eating. If you are worried about what your blood sugar might do before eating the next meal, make sure you have a glucometer. If your blood sugar gets too low then, of course I advise my patients eat before their next formal meal time.

Sound too austere? Then try the substitution principle. This strategy is based on a simple fact: if you are truly hungry you will eat anything that is acceptable. In contrast, appetite generally calls for specific foods.

Here's how you apply the substitution principle. Let's say you excuse yourself from the dinner table to get a fourth serving of the vegan lasagna from the counter. As you look at the food options available, you notice there's still some cooked broccoli, tossed salad, and whole wheat bread remaining as well. Then, rather than immediately taking more lasagna, ask yourself: Would I be willing to eat some more broccoli or whole wheat bread if that were all that was left? If you say "No" (and assuming broccoli or bread is something you find palatable enough to eat) then you have just told yourself appetite, not hunger, is calling for the lasagna. On the other hand, if you say, "Sure, I'd eat the whole wheat bread if that were all that was available," then feel free to have the fourth serving of the lasagna.

Weight Loss in Perspective

By offering a few pages for your consideration, I haven't meant to trivialize the challenges of weight loss. There are whole books written on the subject; many, no doubt, well worth your time and attention. However, my aim was to give you some solid, simple pointers to help you make serious progress. Consider one or more things you would be willing to commit to in order to shed some of those unwanted pounds, then hasten to the end of this chapter and add them to your list of behavioral goals.

The Great Sodium Debate: Or Is It?

I've been a physician since the mid-1980s. For as long as I can remember, the medical community has continued to debate the pros and cons of sodium restriction. A quick internet search will reveal individuals with similar medical credentials arguing for, or against, the value of sodium restriction when it comes to high blood pressure.

So, let's make it simple. When the average person with high blood pressure cuts his or her sodium intake, blood pressure decreases. (Figure 5.8 provided some such data.) Major expert groups concur with such observations and, consequently, recommend that individuals with high blood pressure curb their sodium intake. For example, the United States' Centers for Disease Control and Prevention, lists a "low in salt (sodium)" diet among their lifestyle strategies for controlling hypertension.[63] The World Health Organization has gone on record as strongly recommending "a reduction to <2 g/day sodium (5 g/day salt) in adults" as a prevention strategy aimed at hypertension-related conditions like heart attack and stroke.[64] These conclusions are supported by comprehensive analysis of the research literature, including a 2013 meta-analysis of 34 different studies.[65]

Sure, some people don't seem to be "salt sensitive." Others, due to medications or metabolic needs, could run into trouble with excessive salt restriction. However, these realities don't militate against the *general value* of cutting back on sodium.

Ironically, the fact that some individuals' blood pressures don't seem to be helped much by salt restriction is one of the greatest reasons to give the low sodium diet a 30-day trial. Why? Although, across the board, sodium restriction may appear to make only a small blood pressure difference, realize *salt-insensitive* individuals are included in that data. Therefore, if you were to exclude those who don't benefit from salt reduction, you would be left with a population whose BP responds more markedly to limiting salt intake, and you may be among that population! So I recommend that most of you seriously consider a sodium-restricted diet. I say "most" because some of you need to exercise caution, as I'll explain shortly.

Societal Benefits from Sodium Restriction

Not long ago, one of the world's most prestigious medical journals, the *New England Journal of Medicine*, provided more evidence clarifying the sodium consumption-high blood pressure connection. Researchers from Stanford, Columbia, and the University of California at San Francisco, examined some of the best data available and came to a striking conclusion. In the United States alone, small changes in sodium consumption could save tens of thousands of lives and billions of dollars annually.[66] The life-saving implications are shown graphically in Figure 5.12.

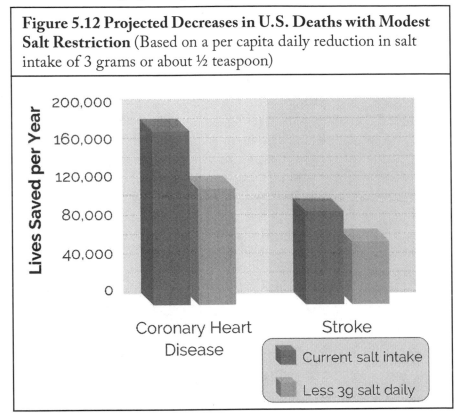

Figure 5.12 Projected Decreases in U.S. Deaths with Modest Salt Restriction (Based on a per capita daily reduction in salt intake of 3 grams or about ½ teaspoon)

As I've already mentioned, the authors did not only provide concrete evidence of lives saved, they also looked at cost savings to the U.S. health care system. Their statistical modeling indicated that nationally we could reap savings of $10 billion to $24 billion in health care costs annually.

The graphic indicates that these calculations were based on the average American decreasing his or her salt intake by 3 grams (about ½ teaspoon) daily. Such a goal seems very reasonable when you consider that the average American today consumes some 8.6 grams of salt each day. We're talking then about a roughly 30% decrease population wide.

If you're already having trouble following along with the numbers, even health professionals sometimes get confused when it comes to the different ways we measure sodium. Figure 5.13 provides some needed perspective on these nuances.[67]

Figure 5.13 Decoding Sodium Lingo

- 1 mmol (millimole) sodium = 23 mg (milligrams) of sodium

- 1 g (gram) sodium = 1000 mg sodium = 43.5 mmol sodium

- 1 g salt (sodium chloride) = 390 mg sodium

- 1 teaspoon of salt is equal to 6 grams of salt and approximately equivalent to:

  - 2400 mg of sodium

  - 104 mm sodium

  - 104 mEq (milliequivalents) sodium

As indicated in Figure 5.13, some of the sodium terminology is simplified by recalling that 1000 milligrams (mg) is the same as 1 gram (g). Other key points are related to a basic chemistry fact; namely, salt is made up of both sodium and chloride. Some health professionals talk about salt intake, while others just look at the sodium. If you want to convert between the two, multiply the sodium content by 2.5 and you'll have a very good approximation of the total salt content. The graphic in Figure 5.14 puts some of these figures in the context of current intake and recommendations.[68,69,70]

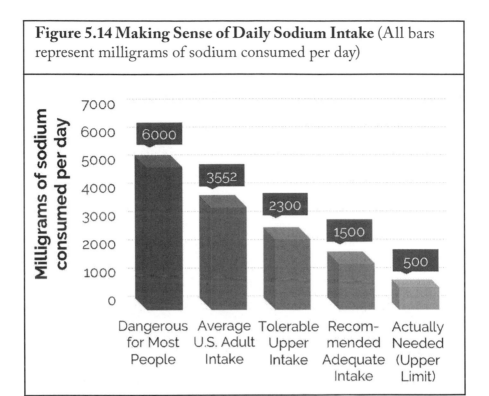

Figure 5.14 Making Sense of Daily Sodium Intake (All bars represent milligrams of sodium consumed per day)

If you're still wondering about whether it's worth the effort to decrease sodium intake, consider what the *New England Journal* researchers concluded from their work:

- "The cardiovascular benefits of reduced salt intake are on par with the benefits of population-wide reductions in tobacco use, obesity, and cholesterol levels."

- "A regulatory intervention designed to achieve a reduction in salt intake of 3 g per day... would be more cost-effective than using medications to lower blood pressure in all persons with hypertension."

If you think it is important to control your cholesterol, lose weight or stop smoking for your circulatory health (and all these things *are* very important), then you've got to be serious about your salt intake. Also, if as a society we're thinking costs alone, we'd be better off ditching all our high blood pressure medication and just focusing on curbing our salt intake.

By now you should realize that I'm not telling you to eliminate your blood pressure medications from day one. However, by now too, I hope you realize the data suggests many of you can be aided on the path toward drug-free hypertension control by maintaining safe levels of sodium consumption.

Who Should Be Concerned About Sodium Reduction—and Who Shouldn't?

I've already intimated that some people are "salt-sensitive" and others not. Simply put, salt-sensitive adults tend to experience a rise in blood pressure with higher salt intake. Individuals who are salt sensitive also tend to be at greater risk of cardiovascular events, strokes, and deaths. In other words, the data suggest that the benefits detailed in the previously cited *New England Journal of Medicine* study might accrue primarily—or exclusively—to individuals in this salt-sensitive group.

Unfortunately, no current test can diagnose salt sensitivity, although promising tests are under development.[71] Nevertheless, the research suggests you may well be salt-sensitive if you have any of the following characteristics: older age, black race, obesity, metabolic syndrome, lower renin levels or higher urinary microalbumin levels (technical kidney-related tests), family history of sodium sensitivity, cholesterol problems, or chronic kidney disease.[72] Many American adults have at least one of the above characteristics, making them more likely to be salt sensitive. Nonetheless, only about 25% actually are.

So, if you're already eating less than 6000 mg of sodium per day[73] and are not salt sensitive, you're not likely to reap any benefit from cutting back on your salt intake. Furthermore, some could actually face significant danger from further sodium reductions. This dialogue has become heated in medical circles especially when it relates to those with congestive heart failure (CHF). Some research indicates those with CHF might benefit from eating less sodium,[74] while other data suggests they might experience higher death rates![75,76]

These conflicting studies, however, make an eloquent point: if you have been diagnosed with congestive heart failure, don't decrease your salt intake without first checking with your doctor. Figure 5.15 includes congestive heart failure among the characteristics of individuals who should exercise caution before cutting back on sodium.[77]

Figure 5.15 Caution Warranted for Some When it Comes to Sodium Restriction

The following classes of people may be at special risk of overzealous sodium restriction:

- Individuals being treated for heart failure
- Those taking medications that already predispose to sodium loss; these include
  - Pure diuretics (e.g., furosemide, hydrochlorothiazide)
  - Other blood pressure medications (note: many contain diuretics in addition to another drug from which the pill derives its name; e.g., Diovan HCT® contains Diovan® plus a diuretic)
- Those prone to significant sodium losses
  - Working in heat with large amounts of sodium-free fluid replacement
- Individuals with excellent blood pressure already (<115 systolic and <70 diastolic)

If the preceding discussion or, perhaps, your previous experience, suggests you might be salt sensitive—and you don't see any red flags in Figure 5.15—then planning to decrease your sodium intake may well be a reasonable conclusion. If you have questions about whether or not a trial of salt restriction is a good idea, please consult with a health care provider.

How to Decrease Salt Intake

If you're going to make a break from high sodium living, you first need to know where the enemy is hiding. Consequently, it is vital to recognize where sodium typically creeps into our menus. Dietary sources of sodium include table salt, salt added to food during its preparation, monosodium glutamate, baking soda, and baking powder. However, as illustrated in Figure 5.16, over three quarters of our salt intake comes from two sources: processed foods and restaurant fare.[78]

Figure 5.16 Most Sodium Comes from Processed and Restaurant Foods

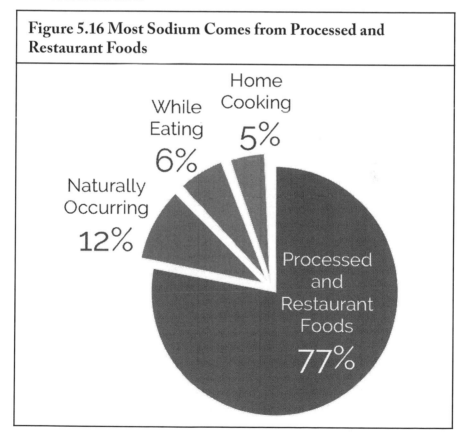

Home Cooking 5%

While Eating 6%

Naturally Occurring 12%

Processed and Restaurant Foods 77%

So how do we apply this information? It begins by reading labels. A good rule of thumb is to eliminate any food items that have more sodium than calories per serving. Think about it this way: if you consume 2000 calories per day, such advice would ensure you are eating less than 2000 mg of sodium daily.

This recommendation also provides a bit of a window of safety for the salt you may consume from other sources, such as that used in cooking. However, even on this front there's probably room for improvement. Try gradually cutting down on the salt in your favorite recipes. And here's a trick that may also help you in the weight control department: cut back on sweeteners in recipes and you'll find you need less salt. That's right, sweetness tends to mask saltiness. So if you decrease the honey, or white sugar, or even juice concentrate that you're using as a sweetener, you can cut back on the sodium without missing the salt.

Don't think you need to read labels? Think again. Most of us underestimate the amount of salt in our foods. One good example is intimated by a question that usually stumps my audiences: "Which typically has more sodium, a serving of corn chips or an equal caloric serving of corn flakes?" Yes, I know: the way I asked the question gave away the answer (corn flakes typically have at least double the sodium of the chips). But my point is simple. We can't trust our taste buds to tell us how much sodium we're eating.

What about eating out? There are two main options here. First, see if you can decrease your dependence on restaurant dining. Second, when preparing to patronize a public eatery, do some homework first. Many larger restaurants and chains already have analyzed their recipes for sodium. Before you sit down and look at a menu—before you even make the reservation—have a plan that will help you stick with your lower-sodium-eating resolve.

Dealing with Perhaps the Biggest Objection
The biggest obstacle for many in the way of sodium reduction

lies with preferences. A dramatic decrease in salt intake is likely to be met, at least initially, with a menu that is no longer palatable.

If you're sitting at the table after a few bites of your first low sodium meal, you may be tempted to throw in the towel. It's normal to raise questions like, "How much is this really going to help lower my blood pressure?" or "Who cares if I avoid a stroke at 75 years of age, if I have to be miserable, with no enjoyment of my food for the next 30 years?"

Here's the key message: Don't attempt to judge the quality of the rest of your life based on your first few days of low sodium eating. When it comes to salt intake, we have had concrete evidence for years regarding the truth of a central tenet of this book: You can develop new enjoyments.

In the 1980s a fascinating study was conducted that looked at what happened to sodium preferences after individuals dramatically decreased their salt intake.[79] As illustrated in Figure 5.17, you'll notice that within a matter of days, salt preferences changed. But maximal changes did not occur for some three months. However, pay careful attention to the graphic. The average participant in that study began the intervention with a taste for sodium that would find the typical commercial soup of that day palatable. Three months later, the subjects preferred soups with half as much salt.

This is an incredibly encouraging study. Many of us likely could decrease our salt consumption by 50% with no loss of palatability in the long term.

Yes, the sodium restriction message is compelling. Make changes in your salt intake and your food will gradually return to its former palatability. Although I'm calling on you to make changes for only 30 days (initially), you'll need to stick with your sodium reduction commitment for longer before realizing just how good lower sodium foods can taste.

113

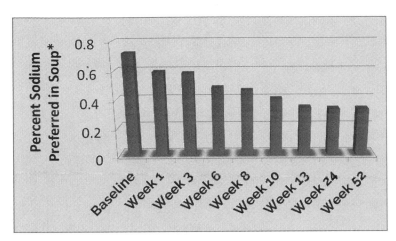

Figure 5.17 Changes in Sodium Preference Over Time After Adopting a Low-Salt Diet (Percentage of sodium preferred in soups, graphed according to study week)

*At the time of this study,
commercial soups had .8 to 1.1% sodium

Putting it All Together

We've covered a lot of ground in Chapter 5. However, for this book to actually make a difference in your blood pressure, you have to determine to make some changes. I ask you to commit to at least one SMART goal based on the material in this chapter. Of course, the more changes you make, the greater the benefits you're likely to obtain. In fact, because this is among the most extensive chapters in the book, you're most likely to get the full benefits from my 30-day approach by committing to at least three behaviors based on the material in this chapter.

Don't forget. Check with your doctor first before making any of the changes advocated in this book. You definitely want someone looking over your shoulder as you put these blood-pressure-lowering principles into practice. And keep up with your daily BP checks, recording them in Appendix A or in a similar spread sheet or table.

Now, make sure you finish filling out the draft worksheet that follows. Since I hadn't mentioned it yet, you're more than welcome to use the examples I provided—or modify them as you see fit. But remember, the most powerful goals are the ones you commit to yourself—and that are SMART for you. Once you've finalized your behavioral goals, transfer up to three of them to Appendix B. That's where you'll be headed at the end of each day to track your progress.

Chapter 5 Diet - Draft Worksheet

(Work on this as you read through the chapter. When you've completed the chapter and finalized your goals, transfer no more than three of them to Appendix B.)

	Week 1							Week 2						
Day #	1	2	3	4	5	6	7	8	9	10	11	12	13	14
Behavioral Goals														
Example 1: Every week have at least 3 meat-free days (days where I eat no meat at all)														
Example 2: Eat less than 2000 mg of sodium each day														
My Goal 5:1														
My Goal 5:2														
My Goal 5:3														
My Goal 5:4														
My Goal 5:5														

6

OPTIMAL CHOICE OF BEVERAGES: ANOTHER KEY TO NATURAL BLOOD PRESSURE CONTROL

WITHIN THE SPAN OF a year, two unrelated patients came through my office with similar stories. Both had dropped some thirty pounds in a matter of months. Both attributed some or all of their success to a simple change in beverage choices: they had eliminated—or dramatically curtailed—soft drink consumption. Those results might not be all that surprising. After all, most of us realize our beverage choices, like our food preferences, affect our weight. However, what we drink also powerfully impacts our blood pressure.

Indeed, those two patients who were opting for water rather than soda were moving their bodies toward more optimal blood pressures. Conversely, some of your blood pressure problems may lie no further away than your favorite drinks.

If you want to have the best blood pressure, what should you be drinking? Let's begin by looking at some of the beverages that aren't our allies when it comes to optimal BP. I'll conclude with some very good news about blood pressure's "best friend" on the beverage aisle.

Bad News About The Beverage Alcohol

Although it was once fashionable to talk about potential health benefits accruing from alcoholic beverages, a growing body of research evidence lends serious doubts to the health claims made for these drinks. (For example, many studies now document an increased risk of cancer even with moderate drinking.[80])

Some, even in the medical community, still try to advocate the "benefits" of moderate alcohol consumption. However, they're having an increasingly difficult time maintaining such a stance, because more data testifies to alcohol's toxicity. This fact was highlighted in 2015 when the physician website, *Medscape*, announced its most widely read article by Internal Medicine specialists was an evidence-based review entitled "No Amount of Alcohol Is Safe."[81]

Although attempted rebuttals seem to follow each new disclosure of alcohol's risks, when we confine our focus to the topic at hand, there is no question alcohol raises blood pressure. As expressed nearly a decade ago by Australian researchers Beilin and Puddey, "A relation between average weekly alcohol consumption, blood pressure level, and hypertension prevalence has been consistent worldwide."[82] In plain English: the more you drink, the higher your blood pressure, and thus the greater your risk of hypertension.

In addressing research that alleged red wine was free of blood-pressure-raising effects, the same researchers asserted: "moderate alcohol consumption raises blood pressure regardless of source." Finally, the duo reminded the medical community of a 2003 World Health Organization study that attributed 16% of global hypertensive disease to alcohol. Figure 6.1 lists some of the connections between alcohol and high blood pressure.

Figure 6.1 Avoid Alcohol if You Want the Best Blood Pressure
<ul><li>More than three drinks at a time raises blood pressure significantly.</li><li>Regular binge drinking can lead to long-term BP increases.</li><li>"Moderate" drinking is also a problem:<ul><li>It can interfere with BP medication effectiveness.</li><li>It can increase side effects of some BP drugs.</li><li>It can undermine weight control efforts: Alcohol packs a big caloric load.</li></ul></li><li>Alcohol decreases willpower.</li></ul>

Sure, these connections might be impressive, but what is it about alcohol that actually elevates blood pressure? Researchers have found evidence for a number of biochemical explanations. Beverage alcohol has been linked to all of the following blood-pressure-raising abnormalities:[83,84]

- stimulation of the fight-or-flight sympathetic nervous system
- activation of the renin-angiotensin-aldosterone system
- impaired baroreceptor function (biological sensors that help to normalize blood pressure)
- elevated levels of blood vessel constricting substances like endothelin 1 and 2
- interference with blood vessel relaxing substances like nitric oxide
- magnesium and/or calcium depletion
- increased oxidative stress (due in part to acetaldehyde, a product of alcohol metabolism)

Granted, some of the items are quite technical. My goal is not to explain them now but merely to paint a picture: For many reasons, alcohol is bad news for blood pressure.

The last few points in Figure 6.1 also deserve special notice, for they are sometimes the most underestimated. I find it surprising that so few individuals comprehend just what caloric bombshells alcoholic beverages are. By weight, alcohol packs nearly twice as many calories as pure sugar (approximately 7 calories per gram compared to 4 calories per gram). Clearly if you are trying to trim down, you don't need the calories served up by beer, wine, or any other alcoholic beverage.

But, perhaps, most importantly, even small amounts of alcohol adversely affect judgment and will power. There is a reason why society doesn't tolerate any alcohol in the bloodstream of commercial airline pilots. With many lives riding on their performance, we demand optimal cognitive functioning.

Should it be any different with us individually? At a minimum your own life is riding on your ability to make sound decisions—and execute them. For example, failing to take full advantage of this 30-day journey may contribute to a stroke, heart attack or kidney failure somewhere down the road. I've already begun to encourage you to take bold steps to get *once and for all* your blood pressure under control. I'll continue that approach throughout this book. What chances do you think you have of following a dramatically healthier lifestyle if you compromise your willpower with alcohol?

I can unequivocally state you'll want to exclude all non-prescription mind-altering drugs during this 30-day program. In fact, when it comes to prescription drugs that affect motivation or willpower, check with your doctor to see if even these can be decreased or eliminated. I have special concerns about the motivation-impairing effects of marijuana (I'll share more about this in Chapter 11).

When it comes to anti-anxiety drugs, don't make changes on

your own but check with your doctor to ensure you're in the best possible position to get the full benefit of this month-long blood pressure focus.

Soft Drinks: More Problems in Blood Pressure Land

Another popular beverage category that can contribute to blood pressure problems is soft drinks. You've probably assumed as much given the illustrations at the opening of this chapter. Let's look at the incriminating evidence, first as it relates to the so-called "sugar-sweetened beverages." (Granted, many of these sodas are now sweetened with high fructose corn syrup.) When it comes to this class of soft drinks, as well as their non-carbonated cousins, the evidence points strongly in the direction of their promoting weight gain, which in turn raises blood pressure.

Harvard researchers examined these relationships in 30 medical publications. They reported their conclusions in the *American Journal of Clinical Nutrition*: "The weight of epidemiologic and experimental evidence indicates that a greater consumption of SSBs [sugar-sweetened beverages] is associated with weight gain and obesity."[85]

Medical researchers are not concerned merely with associations; we look for causal linkages. In other words, we want to find solid evidence that a factor was more than an "innocent bystander." We want evidence that the risk factor actually contributed to a given condition. In order to establish such a chain of causation we look for something called "biological plausibility." Do we have this kind of evidence incriminating soft drinks?

We do. Here's how the Harvard team put it: "Experimental studies have suggested that the likely mechanism by which sugar-sweetened beverages may lead to weight gain is the low satiety of liquid carbohydrates and the resulting incomplete compensation of energy at subsequent meals." In other words, when you consume your calories in liquid form, you get relatively little satisfaction, at least from a nutritional standpoint. For example, down 200 calories in soft drinks, then sit down to a meal an hour later. You're not likely to eat 200 calories less as a result of those soft drink calories. The bottom line is this: You eat more calories and those calories make it more likely you'll add to the current international epidemic of overweight and obesity. This comprehensive publication shared additional details relating to the incriminating evidence linking sugar-sweetened sodas and overweight. These are summarized in Figure 6.2.

Figure 6.2 Sugar-Sweetened Sodas: Their Burden in America

- The World Health Organization recommends added sugars provide no more than 10% of a person's calories.
- However, United States residents exceed that recommendation by over 50%, consuming some 15.8% of their calories from such sugars.
- Non-diet soft drinks are the single largest source of those added sugars, accounting for 47% of the total.
- It's easy for the calories to add up. Consider these facts about the average 12-oz can of soda:
  - It contains 40–50 grams of sugar in the form of high-fructose corn syrup (which is the equivalent of 10 teaspoons of table sugar).
  - This equates to 150 calories.
- Furthermore, we're not making progress in curbing our use. Non-diet soft drink consumption swelled 135% between 1977 and 2001.

Susie came up to me after one of my lectures. She shared how she had made a single lifestyle change. You probably guessed it. Susie, like my two patients at the beginning of the chapter, made a clean break with all her sugar-sweetened soft drinks, and that's the only change she was conscious of making. The result? She too had lost over 25 pounds.

Can such a small change really make such a big difference? Just do the math. Figure 6.2 indicates the standard can of soda contains 150 calories. Just two cans per day would, therefore, give a person 300 extra calories. When you realize it takes 3500 calories to make a pound of fat, 300 calories may not sound like a lot. But over the course of a year, just 300 calories extra per day would add up to 30 pounds of weight.

Should We Then Choose Diet Soft Drinks?

Dr. Hannah Gardener and colleagues from the University of Miami Miller School of Medicine and Columbia University Medical Center looked at the connection between diet soft drinks and one of high blood pressure's leading complications, stroke.[86] The team evaluated 2,564 participants from the National Institutes of Health-funded Northern Manhattan Study, an investigation designed to look specifically at stroke in a multi-ethnic (20% white, 23% black, 53% Hispanic) city-dwelling population. Daily soft-drink users were significantly more likely to report a history of hypertension. However, the most sobering results are summarized in Figure 6.3.

As depicted in the graphic, in addition to the connection with high blood pressure, regular diet soft drink use was linked to a 44% increased risk of serious vascular complications like stroke. Not illustrated in Figure 6.3 were other connections with diet soft drink use that may have helped to explain the association: increased caloric intake and greater body weight. Although the medical literature is mixed, some studies suggest that consumption of sugar-free sodas may actually result in greater intake of foods at subsequent meals.

Figure 6.3 Soft Drink Consumption and Vascular Disease
(e.g., stroke, heart attack, or vascular death)

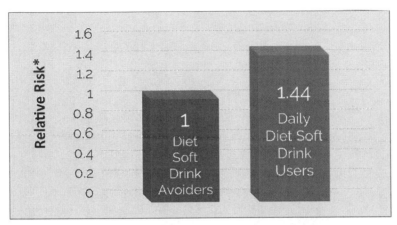

* controlled for pre-existing vascular conditions such as metabolic syndrome, diabetes and high blood pressure

---

Many of these diet soft drinks are, also, caffeinated. Might caffeine play a role in their connection with high blood pressure and stroke? We turn our attention to the caffeine story next.

Caffeine: Another Blood Pressure Foe

There is no question caffeine raises blood pressure. As Drs. Mort and Kruse summarized in a 2008 issue of *The Annals of Pharmacotherapy*: "Reviews of caffeine's acute effect on blood pressure indicate changes of 3-15 mm Hg systolic and 4-13 mm Hg diastolic. Typically, blood pressure changes occur within 30 minutes, peak in 1-2 hours, and may persist for more than 4 hours."[87] These are not insignificant changes. Think about it. In a worst-case scenario caffeine alone could raise someone's blood pressure from 136/79 to 151/91.

So, if caffeine is a known *pressor* (the medical term for an agent that raises blood pressure) then why do even professionals spar over the BP effects of this popular beverage constituent? Where the argument lies is here: Does a habitual user become "immune" to caffeine's blood pressure-boosting effects? Although coffee and soft drink devotees may try to present such a case, the evidence indicates otherwise.

Over a decade ago, psychologist Jack James, PhD, published a telling review aimed at his professional colleagues. The title of the paper was, in itself, a rebuke to the health care community: "Critical review of dietary caffeine and blood pressure: a relationship that should be taken more seriously."[88] What Dr. James was telling his peers was simply this: You've become too cavalier when it comes to caffeine and blood pressure; as a profession, let's get serious about this important issue.

The rationale behind James' conclusions included the following:

- "There is extensive evidence that caffeine at dietary doses increases BP." In other words, it doesn't take mammoth doses of caffeine to boost blood pressure. Common amounts ("dietary doses") can make a significant difference.

- "When considered comprehensively, findings from experimental and epidemiologic studies converge to show that BP remains reactive to the pressor effects of caffeine in the diet." Translation: formal experiments as well as population studies are in agreement, demonstrating that humans do not become immune to caffeine's blood-pressure-elevating effects.

Dr. James strengthened his case with a final salvo, showing the life-or-death impact of caffeine on blood pressure. He wrote: "population studies of BP indicate that caffeine use could account for premature deaths in the region of 14% for coronary heart disease and 20% for stroke."

What Then Should We Drink?

By now, we've crossed most of the world's favorite beverages off the good-for-your-BP list. So what do I propose you drink? It probably comes as no surprise that I advocate making or keeping water as your primary (if not sole) beverage.

Sound boring? Well to some extent it is, at least from a medical standpoint. Drinking more water is of demonstrated benefit when it comes to keeping you out of the hospital, and the morgue.

Consider the work of Dr. Jacqueline Chan and colleagues at Loma Linda University. Some years ago, Chan had a hunch that those who drank more water might be able to stave off heart disease. Before she actually conducted research on the topic, many health professionals, no doubt, thought such a connection was fanciful at best. However, no one was laughing when Dr. Chan published her research in the *American Journal of Epidemiology*.[89] Some of the data she uncovered is depicted in Figure 6.4.

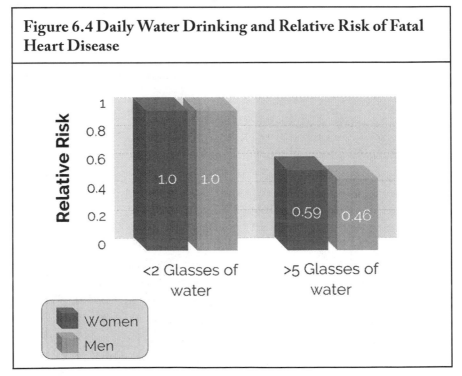

Figure 6.4 Daily Water Drinking and Relative Risk of Fatal Heart Disease

What Chan had uncovered was this: independent of gender, the likelihood of dying from a heart attack fell about 50% in those drinking just a bit more water. That's right. We're not talking huge amounts of fluid consumption. The difference between the high risk and low risk groups was just over three glasses of water per day. Why, you ask? Among the possibilities are improved blood pressure and better blood fluidity. Both of these factors have been connected to less risk of clogged blood vessels.

If you're like many in my public audiences or clinic rooms, I know what you're likely thinking at this point. "What happens if I prefer to get my fluids from other sources like soft drinks, alcoholic beverages—or even milk and juice?" Well, Dr. Chan's team helped answer this very question. Figure 6.5 reveals their findings.

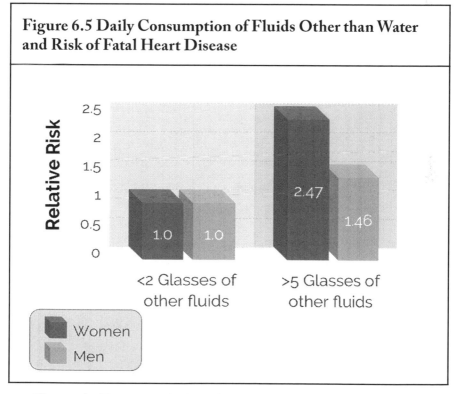

Figure 6.5 Daily Consumption of Fluids Other than Water and Risk of Fatal Heart Disease

Granted, Figure 6.5 doesn't give as much detail as any of us would like. Clearly, this paper doesn't permit our drawing conclusions about specific beverages other than water. (In order to draw valid comparisons with statistics you have to have an adequate number of data points. The Loma Linda team could accomplish this only by aggregating all other beverages.)

The bottom line? If milk is your favorite beverage, and you drink an average of six glasses per day, this data *does not* prove you're hastening your early demise. However, it should at least have you asking some questions. In general, beverages other than water are less desirable when it comes to optimal blood pressure—and, by extension, heart health.

Does Water *Really* Lower Blood Pressure?

So does water really lower blood pressure, or are the entirety of its benefits found in keeping us away from things that worsen our BP? Actually the evidence suggests water intrinsically improves blood pressure. Among the likely explanations are the following:

1. Water keeps us hydrated, and thus prevents excess sodium retention. If we're skimping on water, our bodies move into conservation mode. In this scenario we hold onto sodium (wherever sodium goes, water tends to follow). We've already seen that excess sodium may predispose to hypertension in some individuals.

2. Abundant water flushes out excess sodium. When we drink more water than our body needs, we excrete the excess in the form of urine. However, urine always contains some sodium. Therefore, drinking water liberally actually flushes excess sodium from our bodies. However, beware: copious amounts of water (probably somewhere in the range of three to five gallons for healthy, non-medicated adults) can flush out so much sodium that a life-threatening condition known as dilutional hyponatremia can occur.

3. Liberal hydration keeps our blood vessels relaxed. If we are

dehydrated, another part of conservation mode involves our bodies shutting down some of our tiny capillaries. Clamping down some of those small vessels ensures enough circulating blood volume to satisfy critical organs like the brain and heart. However, these same microvasculature changes increase resistance to blood flow, which, in turn, leads to higher blood pressure.

4. Optimal hydration improves blood fluidity. When a person drinks sufficient amounts of water, the blood becomes less viscous. Expressed another way, the blood can flow more smoothly. Medical research suggests that less viscous blood is easier for the heart to pump, thus contributing to lower blood pressure.[90,91,92]

5. Individuals who are deficient in healthy minerals like magnesium and calcium may get a blood-pressure-lowering effect by drinking spring water or other mineral-containing waters. In one study, blood pressure decreases of 6 points systolic and 4 points diastolic were registered over a one month time frame.[93] Practical corollary: although charcoal-prefiltered, distilled water may be free of contaminants, it provides no insurance against mineral deficits, unlike pure spring water.

However, water has a paradoxically beneficial effect on those with *abnormally low blood pressure*. Individuals who have impaired blood pressure regulation and are thus prone to fainting, actually have *less* risk of lightheadedness and passing out following the ingestion of pure water. The physiology is complex, but has been well studied.[94,95] The practical message is this: Every member of your family can enjoy water, regardless of whether they have normal blood pressure or are prone to higher or lower readings.

More Amazing Evidence of the Power of Water

One of the most amazing applications of water has been that

used in fasting regimens to rapidly improve blood pressure. I personally have supervised patients on water-only fasts and have seen impressive blood-pressure-lowering results. However, I do not recommend such an approach without medical supervision.

Dr. A.C. Goldhamer and colleagues published data on 174 consecutive hypertension patients who they treated in a medically-supervised inpatient setting.[96] The participants were given a fruit and vegetable diet for two to three days before being placed on a water-only fast (lasting 10 to 11 days on average). After the water fast the subjects were placed on an approximately week long "refeeding" program that featured a low-fat, low-sodium, vegan diet. Almost 90% of the subjects achieved a blood pressure of less than 140/90 mm Hg by the end of the program. The average participant dropped his or her blood pressure a whopping 37/13 mm Hg!

Give Your Blood (Pressure) Away

Further testimony to water's prowess in the hypertension arena is provided by a look at an underutilized blood pressure remedy. Recent data is adding to evidence that there are other ways to improve blood fluidity—and thus lower blood pressure—besides water drinking.

A team of researchers from Germany studied 292 blood donors.[97] Exactly half of these unselected donors (146 of them) had elevated blood pressure at the beginning of the study. Following four blood donations over the course of one year, the participants logged incredible benefits. These are illustrated in Figure 6.6. The investigators concluded: "Regular blood donation is associated with pronounced decreases of BP in hypertensives. This beneficial effect of blood donation may open a new door regarding community health care and cost reduction in the treatment of hypertension."

If the connection with water drinking is not apparent, both liberal hydration and blood donation help to improve blood fluidity. It is likely that this is at least one of the common denominators in these two inexpensive approaches to blood pressure regulation.

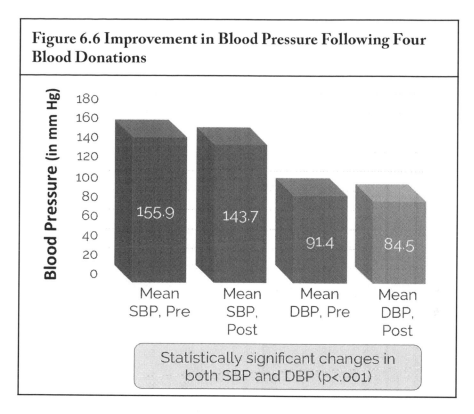

Figure 6.6 Improvement in Blood Pressure Following Four Blood Donations

Blood Pressure (in mm Hg)

155.9   143.7   91.4   84.5

Mean SBP, Pre   Mean SBP, Post   Mean DBP, Pre   Mean DBP, Post

Statistically significant changes in both SBP and DBP (p<.001)

Other Benefits of Water Drinking

Water rises to the top of the list of beverages, but not only for its cardiovascular benefits. The evidence indicates that drinking more liberally of nature's most abundant fluid can help you avoid a number of other health problems. Figure 6.7 offers a partial list.

Consider one final example of water's far-reaching benefits: that of helping shed unwanted pounds. Earlier in this book, I pointed to the well-recognized connection between being well hydrated and a decreased tendency to overeat. (Remember, your body can have a hard time telling the difference between thirst and hunger.) And, yes, your mother probably told you that if you drank a lot of water before sitting down at the table, you wouldn't eat as much. (I actually don't recommend that one. For many people it just lays the foundation for eating more between meals since they're less likely to satisfy their hunger at mealtime.)

Figure 6.7 Other Conditions Potentially Helped By Drinking More Water

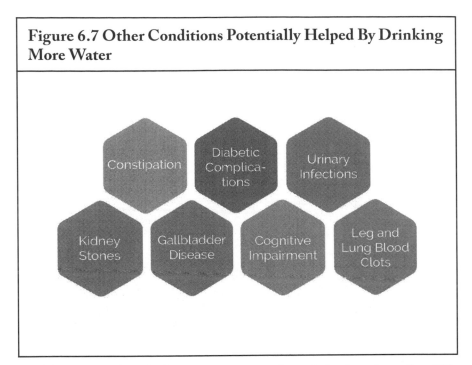

However, there's far more to water's weight loss benefits. We owe this insight to German researchers under the direction of Michael Boschmann, MD. Boschmann and colleagues demonstrated that drinking modest amounts of water actually revs up your metabolism.[98] Specifically, they found that drinking as little as 500 ccs (about a pint) of pure water raised metabolism 24% for one hour. Vitamin-fortified waters and other flavored waters probably do not offer this benefit. Why? When the researchers added just a small amount of salt to the water (to make it equal in concentration to the blood) there was no such metabolic augmentation. The evidence suggested that anything added to the water undermined its fat-burning benefits.

Resolving to Shop Better (or Less) in the Beverage Aisle

The data is compelling. What we drink has a profound influence on our blood pressure. Indeed, by ignoring our beverage choices, we are neglecting a key to optimal blood pressure.

Now it's your turn. What changes will you make in the beverage department to help you be more successful on your month-long journey to better blood pressure? A beverage worksheet awaits you on the next page.

Chapter 6 - Beverage – Draft Worksheet

(Work on this as you read through the chapter. When you've completed the chapter and finalized your goals, transfer no more than three of them to Appendix B.)

	Week 1							Week 2						
Day #	1	2	3	4	5	6	7	8	9	10	11	12	13	14
Behavioral Goals														
Example 1: Leave off all caffeinated beverages														
Example 2: Limit my soda consumption to no more than twice per week (with 2 cans or less on those occasions)														
Example 3: Go to my local blood bank and begin a process of regular blood donation														
My Goal 6:1														
My Goal 6:2														
My Goal 6:3														
My Goal 6:4														

7

SOCIAL SUPPORT: THE BLOOD PRESSURE BENEFITS OF SOCIAL CONNECTEDNESS

CARLOS, TO ME, WAS a hero. He first showed up in my medical office with Harold, an emaciated man three decades his senior who had come to get established as a new patient.

As Harold's medical history unfolded, I learned that nearly a year before he had been evicted. As a dejected Harold sat on the lawn in front of his apartment on that fateful day, his old friend Carlos showed up with his pickup. Carlos brought him—and all his meager earthly belongings—to his own, already crowded, home.

Carlos' home had, before this, become a refuge for other struggling family members. Every bedroom was filled. Nonetheless, Carlos put a divider in his basement and quickly fitted up a "room" for Harold.

As I looked through Harold's medical records, I was struck by something of particular interest to our blood pressure journey. Harold's records described a man with a history of hypertension who had been on daily blood pressure medications. However, his blood pressure was now perfectly normal, and he reported not having had any medications whatsoever for five months.

Was Harold's normal blood pressure—in the face of serious social stressors—due to the support he was receiving from Carlos? There's no way to know definitively, but research suggests that such social support was likely playing an important blood-pressure-lowering role. To this important connection we'll soon turn our attention.

Regaining Our Bearings

If I were slavishly following the *No Pressure* mnemonic like a certified error-free map or GPS system, I would have launched into a discussion of *physical activity* at this point. However, as the story of Carlos and Harold indicates, the topic of social connectedness is so crucial that it begs to be addressed right now. This ensures that those following my prescribed roadmap for the journey (reading at least three chapters per week) will be exposed to this material during the first week.

Why is social support so vital? Researchers in Switzerland studied 22 individuals with high blood pressure and compared them to 26 subjects who were normotensive (had normal blood pressure). They found those with hypertension had significantly lower levels of perceived social support than did those with good BP readings.[99]

Furthermore, researchers uncovered *why* social connectedness helped lower blood pressure. By actual measurement, they discovered that low social support was associated with higher levels of the stress hormone epinephrine (adrenaline), a compound known to raise blood pressure.

Several years later, researchers at Johns Hopkins University took these insights one step further. Caryn Bell and her colleagues examined whether social support helped explain racial differences in high blood pressure.[100] They used data from a representative sample of the U.S. population found in NHANES (the U.S. National Health and Nutrition Examination Survey).

Bell and colleagues noted something we observed earlier: a higher likelihood of hypertension among those with African blood lines. In looking deeper into racial and ethnic disparities, they found something that may be surprising to the uninitiated: Mexican Americans had significantly *lower* rates of high blood pressure than did whites.

The authors found that social support helped explain these differences. The striking conclusion is that social connectedness impacts blood pressure, and that those benefits cut across racial and ethnic lines.

Are Healthy and Unhealthy Lifestyles Contagious?

This may sound like a ridiculous question, but don't dismiss this possibility out of hand. Researchers published a fascinating article in the June 14, 2012 issue of *Science Reports* (from the prestigious *Nature* publishing group).[101] There, Lazaros Gallos of the City University of New York and his collaborators made a stunning observation: if you look at the temporal distribution of obesity in the United States, it looks similar to the spread of an infectious disease. The team went so far as to map this "spread," using a scientific technique called "spatial spreading analysis." If obesity were an infectious disease, the team's data suggested "the outbreak" would have begun in Greene County, Alabama.

Of course, most of the factors that predispose to obesity are not *literally* contagious. Indeed, the researchers were not arguing for a viral or bacterial determinant of weight problems. How then do we explain the data in this provocative article? One of the most compelling explanations is that we are subtly being molded by those around us. Put another way, social and societal factors may ultimately be greater determinants of obesity than are our personal habits. Viewed from a societal level, the authors expressed it this way: "individual habits may have negligible influence in shaping the patterns of spreading [of obesity]." In other words, if you want to gain weight, spend time with those who are overweight. Conversely, if you want to lose weight, hang out with thin people.

This message applies to more than girth; it applies to the entire lifestyle framework upon which this book is built. Look at it this way: If we surround ourselves with people who do not apply the *No Pressure* principles, we are unlikely to apply them ourselves. I want you to succeed, and know that your success will be greatest if you take this 30-day journey with others who have the same destination in mind.

Personally Connect

Earlier in this book, I talked about six program elements, four of which I said were non-negotiable (see Figure 4.2). However, at the time, I let you off the hook when it came to the first program element: finding an accountability partner or support group. I'm not going to change the ground rules on you midstream, and now require such social support. But I urge you to become part of a movement larger than yourself over the next thirty days. Just reading this book and joining me and literally a worldwide movement of many others on this journey accomplishes this in some respects, but personally helping someone accomplish these goals, and also receiving their support, may make more of a difference for you than you realize.

How Are You Doing When it Comes to Social Support?

Denizens of the United States are sometimes stereotyped as fiercely independent at the expense of close, nourishing relationships. Yet the U.S. is clearly a "melting pot" when it comes to cultures and individuals. We've already observed that one segment of the U.S. population—those of Latin-American ancestry—often have cultural roots that more highly prioritize social relationships.

However, stereotypes and generalizations are not particularly helpful when it comes to any individual—and particularly when it comes to you. So how do you fare when it comes to social connectedness?

We can each get a pretty good idea of how we stand in this domain. A variety of social capital or social connectedness assessments have been designed, typically with specific target groups in mind. For example, specific assessments have been used to evaluate adolescents in Brazil,[102] adults in China,[103] and individuals with significant online social contacts.[104] Figure 7.1 draws questions from these and other assessment instruments to provide an estimate of your social connectedness.[105] If you want a more precise personal evaluation, use a quiz designed specifically for your age group and region of residence.

Finding Social Support

One of my motivations for writing this book relates to people like you—my patients, seminar attendees and others—who have asked for more information. I have also been encouraged by favorable evaluations of an earlier DVD series that covered many of the elements found in this book. (If you want to check it out, you can pick up a copy of my "Reversing Hypertension Naturally" at www.compasshealth.net.)

The advantage of having a DVD resource that is already widely available is that I can help you cover the main principles of this book in an engaging format suitable for viewing as a group or with your accountability partner. And you don't need a special license to show "Reversing Hypertension Naturally" to a group of any size. In other words, you can convene your own support group. And it will take less than a $100 investment in DVDs, a place to meet, and a one-hour session once a week for six weeks. You choose the place: It could be your home, your workplace, a house of worship, or a community center.

Figure 7.1 Assessing Your Level of Social Connectedness

Instructions:

- Answer each of the twelve questions below with the best response to the right.
- Scoring: Give yourself between 1 and 5 points for each question based on your response (e.g., answering "Strongly Disagree" gives you 1 point for a given question).
- Higher scores indicate higher levels of social connectedness. (Minimum Score: 12; Maximum Score: 60.)

Statement	Strongly Disagree	Disagree	Neither Agree nor Disagree	Agree	Strongly Agree
	1	2	3	4	5
Offline, I come into contact with new people frequently.					
I regularly interact with people who make me feel like part of a larger community.					
During my leisure time I frequently connect with other people through personal visitation, or telephone or internet communication.					
I regularly attend a place of worship (church, synagogue, mosque, etc.), club, or voluntary business or social organization in my community.					
I regularly volunteer my time in my community.					
When I learn of people in need in my community, I often give them some type of assistance or encouragement.					
People living in my community or neighborhood support me and get along with me well.					
When I feel lonely, there are several people offline I can talk to.					
I know specific people who, if I asked, would help me solve problems or make important decisions.					
There are people I interact with who would put their reputation on the line for me.					
There are people I know who would help me fight an injustice.					
If I needed an emergency loan of $500, I know people I could turn to.					

Yet this book is designed to stand alone. You don't need any additional resources to harness this program. Find a friend and read through this book together, calling each other to be accountable. If you are interested in the ancillary DVD-based resources, you can get all the information you need at www.compasshealth.net.

More Opportunities for Social Support

A number of great community-based programs can help you feel supported as you make lifestyle changes to improve your blood pressure. I've provided three examples below.

- The *Complete Health Improvement Program (CHIP)*. Like this book, CHIP is a scientifically-based program. Additionally, CHIP boasts a wealth of scientific data actually documenting its efficacy. Although it is one of the most intensive community programs available, CHIP is a high-quality program boasting over 60,000 graduates. It has been generally well received by community groups and patients alike. You can get more information at www.CHIPHealth.com.

- *CREATION Health*. Developed by the multi-campus Florida Hospital Health System, this quality program is also based on a solid medical platform with highly qualified presenters. *CREATION Health* covers eight health-enhancing elements similar to those in the *No Pressure* mnemonic, meeting once per week for eight weeks. You'll find more information and CREATION Health resources at www.creationhealth.com

- *The Nedley Depression and Anxiety Recovery Program*. This is perhaps the most surprising of the three programs I'm highlighting. After all, how could a program targeting mental health provide a fitting social environment for those interested in optimizing their blood pressure? Actually, Dr. Neil Nedley's once-per-week, 8-week community program dovetails very nicely with the elements I emphasize in this program. And as we've already seen in this chapter, elevated stress hormone levels can raise your blood pressure. Get more details about Dr. Nedley's programs at www.drnedley.com.

Tap Into the Benefits of Social Connectedness

Social support can come in myriad forms. Some find it in a close nuclear family unit. Others gain considerable strength from associations in the workplace. Still others gain their main support from friendships with individuals who have no kinship or occupational ties. Along these latter lines, I have already highlighted the tremendous benefits of having an accountability partner. Additionally, personal experience with the three programs reviewed above has convinced me of the great value of making changes in concert with a group of people who have embraced similar goals.

Indeed, social support is vital. It can enhance motivation, provide new and deeper insights into information we're studying, and inspire us to accomplish things we've never before attempted. As seen in the studies cited in this chapter, better social connections also promote lower blood pressure.

It's one thing to talk about the benefits of social connectedness; it's another thing to put it into practice. I challenge you to deliberately cultivate more supportive relationships. It may make sense to do that specifically in the context of hypertension. I've already given you some ideas on how to do this. However, you can ramp up your social connections in other ways that don't directly involve high blood pressure interventions, and still benefit your blood pressure. When Kamiya and colleagues looked at a representative sample of the British population over 50 years old, they found evidence of blood pressure benefits from participating in activities as diverse as environmental groups, neighborhood watch programs, religious organizations, arts or music groups, evening classes, and social clubs (e.g. Rotary Club, women's groups).[106]

In short, share your social influence with others. You'll benefit your community, you'll help yourself, and you're likely to see better blood pressure readings.

Chapter 7 Social Connectedness – Draft Worksheet

(Remember, after you've completed the chapter and finalized your goals, transfer no more than three of those goals to Appendix B.)

	Week 1							Week 2						
Day #	1	2	3	4	5	6	7	8	9	10	11	12	13	14
Behavioral Goals														
Example 1: Call my accountability partner at least once per week to review my progress and challenges														
Example 2: Reconnect with the faith community of my childhood by attending weekly services														
My Goal 7:1														
My Goal 7:2														
My Goal 7:3														
My Goal 7:4														
My Goal 7:5														

8

PHYSICAL ACTIVITY: LOWERING PRESSURE THROUGH MOVEMENT

THE CLAIM OF THE American College of Sports Medicine is far-reaching: "Any amount of physical activity, even low-intensity exercise such as walking, can lower your blood pressure."[107] Docs this sound too good to be true? Can you really walk (or run) your way to normal blood pressure? Medical research answers with a resounding "yes."

Pooled studies (called meta-analyses) show that regular exercise typically lowers systolic blood pressure by 4 to 6 points and diastolic BP by 3 points. Although this, like any other single lifestyle component, may seem underwhelming, there's more to the story. Selected individuals may lower their blood pressure by as much as 15 mmHg. That's right, regular exercise alone can directly lower your blood pressure by 4 to 15 points. However, regular exercise improves multiple other factors that can *indirectly* improve your blood pressure. These factors include better brain function, improved stress control, higher quality sleep, and a tendency toward smarter dietary choices.

What else makes the difference? Why do some individuals reap large benefits, while others only register modest improvements? One thing is clear: the younger you are, the more you can expect exercise to lower your blood pressure.

Is this good news or bad? If you consider yourself young, great. However, some of you may think your best years, thus your best chances to lower your BP with exercise, are behind you. If you've placed yourself in such a category, I'd prescribe a change in perspective.

Think about it this way: you'll never again be as young as you are today. So, if you aren't yet on a regular exercise program, the time to start is *now*. Metaphorically speaking, you'll reap more benefit than if you waited until you were older *tomorrow*.

Even if you have an aversion to the very word *exercise*, I have some good news: you don't have to be on a formal exercise program to improve your blood pressure. Any form of physical activity counts. This means you can move toward a better blood pressure by standing (rather than sitting) while talking on the phone, opting for the stairs rather than an elevator or escalator, or walking a bit more by choosing a parking spot further from the mall entrance.

Don't miss my point. Although any activity is good, planning structured bouts throughout your week is still better. In addition to looking for ways to incorporate more activity into your daily routine, I want to challenge you to plan some exercise sessions as well. The latter may include an exercise class, a pick-up basketball game, or a 30-minute walking session, for example. And, if you've never been on one, such an exercise program may be a lot less painful than you've imagined.

How Much Do I Need to Exercise?

Many non-exercising individuals may think the very term "exercise program" seems onerous. But you may be surprised by just how big a difference a relatively small amount of exercise—engaged in consistently—can make. Over a decade ago, Dr. Ishikawa-Takata looked at the impact of exercise on blood pressure. His team's conclusions are illustrated in Figure 8.1.[108]

Note that Figure 8.1 lists exercise in minutes per *week*, not *day*. Merely thirty to forty minutes per week can lower one's systolic blood pressure seven points. Double the duration and you double the effect. Sixty to eighty minutes per week can drop your systolic BP in the range of 14 points.

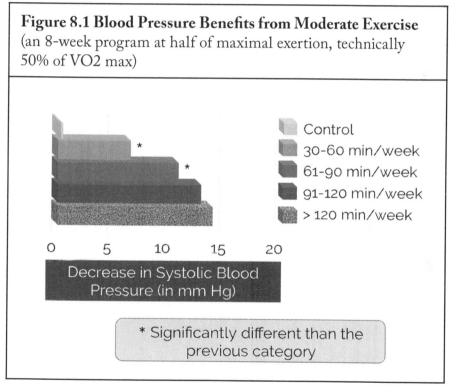

Figure 8.1 Blood Pressure Benefits from Moderate Exercise (an 8-week program at half of maximal exertion, technically 50% of VO2 max)

Control
30-60 min/week
61-90 min/week
91-120 min/week
> 120 min/week

0   5   10   15   20

Decrease in Systolic Blood Pressure (in mm Hg)

* Significantly different than the previous category

There is no question about exercise's blood-pressure-lowering powers. However, what is problematic is harnessing exercise's capabilities. Along these lines, we've learned some secrets from indigenous peoples.

Consider Native Americans. Before European contact they didn't need parks, swimming pools, or fancy health clubs in order to keep fit. Exercise was simply part and parcel of their daily life. Whether they were farming, hunting, fishing, walking, canoeing, playing sports, or a hundred other things, they were an active people.

Their example speaks to us today. Often I'm asked *"How much should I exercise?"* However, the better question is, *"How often should I exercise?"* And the answer to that latter query is simply "daily." The single most important thing you can do is establish the habit of exercising on a daily basis. Although, in most cases, more exercise increases the blood pressure benefits, making exercise a regular habit is paramount. Once the practice of daily exercise is ingrained, you can always ramp up *how much* exercise you do.

Here's another reason why I first encourage my patients to make a *daily* exercise commitment rather than committing to a specific *amount*. For sedentary people with heart disease risk factors (remember, high blood pressure is one of them), recommending an arbitrary amount of exercise is a potential prescription for trouble. Although as a physician, I've made many specific exercise prescriptions in the context of personalized cardiovascular evaluations, I will never have the opportunity to do that for most of you. So, for now, focus on making exercise a part of your daily routine.

Along these lines, consider another set of questions...

- Are you wondering if you are going to eat today? Are you right now wrestling with a decision as to whether you should fast for the next 24 hours? Possibly, but more than likely you at least have tentative plans for your meals today. Although you might opt to fast for a day, if you're like most of us, on any normal day, it's a given that you are going to eat.

- How many of you are wondering if you're going to sleep this evening? I'm not talking about struggling with insomnia but rather about whether or not you plan to try to get some shuteye after nightfall. Sure, on rare occasions you might choose to stay up all night. Perhaps you're dealing with a looming deadline; a family emergency might occasion an all-night car ride. However, if you're like most of us, on any normal day, it's a given that you are going to sleep.

Where I'm going with this line of questioning is perhaps already transparent. I'm arguing that just as eating and sleeping are "givens," when it comes to daily living, so should exercise be.

More Exercise Questions

Once someone signs onto that daily exercise commitment, some very practical questions still remain. After all, we earlier observed that the best lifestyle decisions are "SMART" ones—and that includes being specific and measurable. So ask yourself these kinds of questions, "Who can I exercise with?" "What kind of exercise would I enjoy?" "How long a session is safe, practical, and appropriate?"

Let's consider exercise safety for a moment. How many people really need a doctor's prescription to go shopping at the mall? If it's a sizable complex of stores, you'll likely be getting a goodly amount of exercise. However, physical activity at such modest intensity is usually not problematic. If it is, a person has likely already become aware of his or her limitations. Nonetheless, even if you are unaware of serious heart issues, significantly ramping up your exercise commitment could be dangerous, even life threatening. Perhaps you have an unknown heart or other physical problem that would deleteriously affect you during a high-intensity workout. Expert groups have developed a seven-question, simple quiz, found in Figure 8.2, that I recommend you use before significantly increasing the intensity or duration of physical activity. The PAR-Q evaluation that follows was originally designed for individuals between the ages of 15 and 69. If you're 70 or older, I side with those experts who recommend that even if your PAR-Q is perfect, you should still check with a physician before significantly increasing your physical activity.

Figure 8.2 Physical Activity Readiness Questionnaire (PAR-Q)

A. Answer yes or no to the following questions:

Question	Yes	No
1. Has a doctor ever said that you have a heart condition and that you should only perform physical activity recommended by a doctor?		
2. Do you feel pain in your chest when you perform physical activity?		
3. In the past month, have you had chest pain when you were not performing physical activity?		
4. Do you lose your balance because of dizziness or do you ever lose consciousness?		
5. Do you have a bone or joint problem that could be made worse by a change in your physical activity?		
6. Is your doctor currently prescribing drugs for your blood pressure or heart condition?		
7. Do you know of any other reason why you should not do physical activity?		

B. Interpretation:

A "Yes" answer to even one of the questions above necessitates a physician's evaluation before increasing your physical activity—or even taking a fitness test. Tell your physician about any questions above where you answered "Yes." After your medical evaluation, ask your doctor for medical clearance along with information about specific exercise limitations you might have.

Other Exercise Cautions

One of the world's foremost exercise advocacy groups is the American College of Sports Medicine. It reminds us of the caution needed when ramping up physical activity when individuals begin a typical "exercise program":

"Prior to beginning any exercise program… individuals should seek medical evaluation and clearance to engage in activity. Not all exercise programs are suitable for everyone, and some programs may result in injury. Activities should be carried out at a pace that is comfortable for the user. Users should discontinue participation in any exercise activity that causes pain or discomfort. In such event, medical consultation should be immediately obtained."[109]

Exercise? Yes—but exercise caution.

Is All Exercise Created Equal?

The type of exercise is important. Years ago, I was collaborating with researchers at the Lifestyle Center of America. In one study, our team looked at two basic approaches to exercise: continuous vs. intermittent. My curiosity regarding these differing approaches stemmed in part from my work with indigenous people groups. Remember how, earlier in this chapter, we reflected on the traditional lifestyle of Native Americans? Whether speaking in terms of the Americas, Europe, Africa, or Asia, those living in traditional cultures generally obtain their exercise from practical physical labor and other, often unstructured, activities.

To this day, the Chinese living in rural venues might find themselves tending fields, herding sheep, or working at various trades. Although living in a nation of phenomenal technological progress, those following more traditional lifestyles are often physically active even when recreating. Whether they are walking or bicycling to a social event, playing sports, or attending outdoor festivals, activity is part and parcel of their "time off" as well as their work.

Put yourself in the shoes of such an indigenous laborer. If you are doing useful, practical work, such as farming, gardening, or chopping wood, what do you do if you get tired? Unless you have a belief that you must maintain your activity at a certain intensity— or are confronted with a looming deadline (e.g., an approaching storm that would compromise your hay crop)—you probably will take a rest. Indeed, intermittent exercise (activity interspersed with periods of rest) seems to be the type of activity prioritized by indigenous people across the globe.

Other researchers have examined differences between intermittent and continuous exercise in their quest for optimal fitness strategies. Both of these streams of interest (indigenous values along with fitness benefits) converged in the 1990s at the Lifestyle Center of America. There, our team recruited 31 sedentary individuals from our community. All were between the ages of 45 and 75. These subjects were randomly assigned to one of three groups for a ten-week intervention: a continuous training/exercise group (CT); an intermittent (interval) training/exercise group (IT); and a control group.

Members of the control group were asked to maintain their sedentary lifestyle for the duration of the study. On the other hand, both the IT and CT groups exercised five days per week. Participants started at 20 minutes per day and increased their sessions by three minutes each week. By the end of the ten weeks, each subject had worked up to 47-minute exercise sessions.[110]

Because it was a carefully regulated study, we elected to have the subjects exercise in a gym where they could be directly monitored. Rather than engaging in indigenous activities like gardening or chopping wood, they used conventional exercise equipment like treadmills, rowing machines and stair machines.

Of note, both the IT and CT group members spent equal time in the gym. The only difference was this: those in the CT group exercised continuously at their individual target heart rates (THRs) while each person in the IT group alternated between exercise (until one's heart rate went five beats above his or her THR) and "active rest"—a sort of "cool down" activity (until heart rate fell five beats below THR).[111] Specifically "active rest" referred to slow movement using the same muscle groups employed in the preceding aerobic activity.

To help you better visualize the intervention, imagine what you would have seen if you had walked in on IT and CT participants exercising during the final week of the study. Those on the CT program would be exercising virtually non-stop for 47 minutes. They would be rotating between a variety of fitness devices: stair machines, bicycles, and treadmills. The IT group members would be utilizing the same pieces of equipment. However, every minute or two they would stop their moderate activity and go into what looked like "cool down" mode.

For example, an IT participant on a treadmill would be going along at a good clip, walking briskly up a steep grade. Suddenly, in response to a beeping pulse rate monitor (indicating she was five beats above her target rate), she would take the grade or slope off the treadmill and drop her speed from perhaps 3.5 miles per hour to 1 mile per hour. Perhaps 30 seconds later, you witness that same individual ramping her treadmill back up to 3.5 mph with a 10 % grade. Why? Her heart rate has just fallen five beats below her target heart rate, indicating it was time to return to moderate activity.

Realize that eight or nine weeks earlier that formerly sedentary IT participant might have spent as much—or more—time in "active rest" as in actual exercise. However, as she became more fit, her heart rate increased more slowly with exercise and "recovered" more rapidly during active rest.

So what happened after ten weeks on those various exercise programs? Both exercise groups, IT and CT, improved their fitness levels equally. Not surprisingly, members of the control group who remained sedentary made no such improvements. However, Figure 8.3 shows that significant differences emerged when it came to body weight and fat.

The control group actually gained 3.5 pounds during the ten-week program. No surprise there. Those in the CT group were over five pounds better off, losing 1.9 pounds on average, rather than gaining. However the CT exercisers did not lose any body fat. On the other hand, those in the IT group lost, on average, 5.3 pounds, and actually lost body fat.

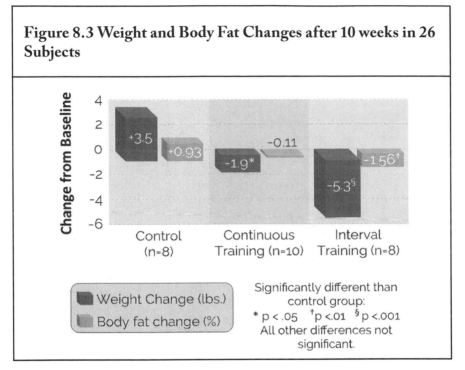

Figure 8.3 Weight and Body Fat Changes after 10 weeks in 26 Subjects

Why the differences? Taking breaks as part of one's exercise program appears to offer metabolic advantages. For example, it is likely your tissues will be better oxygenated if you don't overdo things. The lesson? You don't have to follow a rigid, austere exercise program. Simply make a point *not* to push yourself unduly. Listening to your body and taking breaks is not only a safer approach to exercise but it can ramp up your benefits!

The "How Much" Question

So far I've conveyed my perspective that two aspects of optimal exercise for high blood pressure control involve engaging in physical activity daily, and ensuring you don't overdo it. Yet some other questions remain. In fact, exercise goals are generally best expressed using at least four variables. These are illustrated in Figure 8.4.

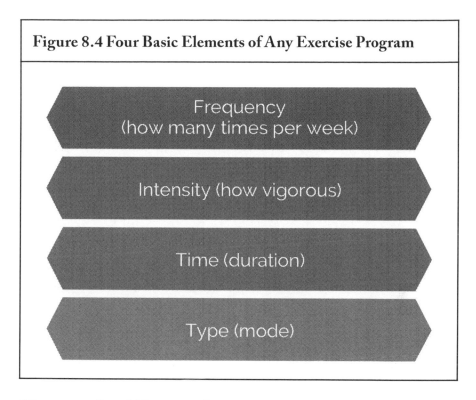

Figure 8.4 Four Basic Elements of Any Exercise Program

Frequency
(how many times per week)

Intensity (how vigorous)

Time (duration)

Type (mode)

"Frequency" and "Intensity"

We've already nailed down the "Frequency" element. We're focused on *daily* exercise. Habits are best made if consistent. And having a regular time for exercise is a tried and true way to help you develop a consistent program.

What about "Intensity"? If no red flags turned up on the PAR-Q test (see Figure 8.2), a good rule of thumb is to start with an amount of exercise that doesn't feel taxing. Many fitness experts recommend doing "the talk test." If it is difficult to carry on a normal conversation, then you're pushing too hard.

Not sure what constitutes "a normal conversation"? Then try another approach. Researchers at the University of Wisconsin asked exercise participants to recite the Pledge of Allegiance during their workouts. If they had difficulty reciting those words, then they were working too hard.

Recent research sheds some further fascinating light on the questions of frequency and intensity. Srinivasan Beddhu, MD, and colleagues at the University of Utah analyzed data from the 2003-2004 U.S. National Health & Nutrition Examination Survey (NHANES) in an attempt to find connections between exercise frequency, exercise intensity, and mortality. They discovered that individuals could cut their risk of death by approximately 33% simply by adding a mere two minutes of light activity, like walking, into each hour devoted exclusively to sedentary activities.[112]

This research speaks eloquently to the intensity debate. Just do *something* physical, don't worry if it's not enough. It also speaks to the topic of frequency, underscoring the need for physical activity during every day that finds us mired in sedentary activities. The only days you don't need to add a couple of minutes per hour of activity are days where you are already being physically active.

Exercise "Duration"

Dr. Beddhu's research takes us one step further. It actually moves us to the third element of an exercise program; namely, "Duration." The implications of his work include this: Small amounts of exercise can pay big dividends.

I'm not suggesting that you max out on the blood-pressure-lowering benefits of exercise by adding 16 minutes of activity to a day that has you sitting for eight hours. We've already seen that more exercise can give you more benefits. However, I share the NHANES data to emphasize the importance of not getting paralyzed by the "Duration" question. Start by doing *something*.

You can increase your exercise time and intensity in small increments. Remember how the Lifestyle Center of America study participants increased their exercise sessions by three minutes per week? This is often quite reasonable.

One other caveat is in order. Another way of planning for exercise is based on a measurable duration. If you are a very schedule-conscious individual—or if you have a job that is not conducive to small breaks—sneaking two minutes of exercise into every hour isn't likely to happen. In such scenarios, the most certain way for exercise to occur is by adding it to your daily schedule. Many middle-aged people can plan on twenty minutes a day when starting out. But if that seems like too much physically—or too much in terms of time commitment—set a smaller goal. Then do it.

"Type" of Exercise

For years the opinion dominant in the cardiovascular community was that exercise had to be aerobic to reap the most circulatory benefit. "Aerobic" may conjure up ideas of moving to music in a gym, but it is far more. Any activity that both uses large muscle groups like your arms and/or legs and stimulates your heart and lungs is considered aerobic. Walking, running, cycling, ice skating, cross country skiing, dancing, swimming, and rowing are all aerobic activities. Research indicates that aerobic exercise does, indeed, lower blood pressure.

Consider a now classic meta-analysis (compilation of studies) performed by Belgian researchers Robert Fagard and Véronique Cornelissen. These two investigators examined over 70 exercise studies and found a compelling blood-pressure-lowering effect that occurred with aerobic exercise. Blood pressure benefits occurred regardless of whether or not a person had high blood pressure. However those with hypertension benefitted the most, lowering their numbers an average of 6.9 points.[113]

Of interest to our dialogue about intensity, subsequent research by the same Belgian team found that among those 55 and older, light exercise and moderate exercise were equally efficacious in lowering blood pressure. So long as the participants exercised for equal duration (in their study, three hours per week), they experienced equal blood pressure benefits.

Another category of exercise, resistance activity, also has been documented to offer blood-pressure-lowering benefits. When it comes to resistance exercise we're talking about things like weight lifting, exercising with elastic bands, or machine-based activities where your muscles are working against a resistive force.

One special type of resistance exercise is called "isometric" activity. In such activities your muscles do not shorten and lengthen like they do when you do repetitions of lifting a barbell. Instead, your muscles contract and hold their position against a constant resistive force. An example is seen with isometric grip exercise, where you hold a steady grip on a towel or other device for one to two minutes or until your hand becomes fatigued.

If that explanation is still lacking something, call to mind those old grip strength devices, like the one illustrated in Figure 8.5. When I was a kid I seem to recall trying to see how many times I could "pump" that device before I fatigued. Well, that was *dynamic* resistance exercise; my hand muscles were repetitively shortening then lengthening. On the other hand, *isometric* resistance exercise occurs when you squeeze the device and hold its two arms together for, perhaps, a couple minutes. Your hand muscles are holding a fixed, contracted posture for that entire time.

Figure 8.5 A Typical Grip Strength Device

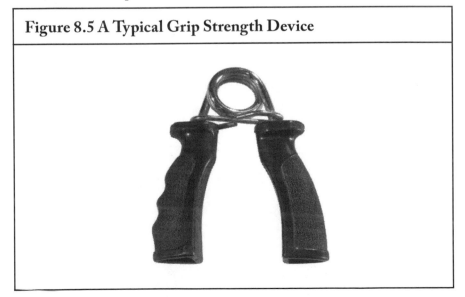

By now it's perhaps not surprising to learn that Véronique Cornelissen and her Belgian colleagues also assessed the literature relating to resistance exercise and its effects on blood pressure.[114] They identified 28 trials with over 1000 total participants. The evidence showed that resistance exercise had a significant blood-pressure-lowering effect. The studies analyzed revealed an approximately 4 point lowering of blood pressure in both individuals with high blood pressure as well as those with normal blood pressure. Of particular interest, the three studies that looked at isometric handgrip exercise yielded some of the most impressive results, with an approximately 13 point systolic and 6 point diastolic drop in blood pressure.

Exercise in Perspective

All this research points us in several important directions:

1. Get physical activity on a daily basis.

2. Start at a safe level, appropriate to your level of health (check with your health care provider if you have questions).

3. Include both aerobic and resistance exercise.

One more aspect of "Mode" or "Type" of exercise is worth noting. Although one tenet of this book is that you can develop new enjoyments, you'll get off to a better start if you commit to activities you already enjoy. If you can't think of an activity you find pleasant, why don't you make a less than palatable exercise more enjoyable by doing it with a friend?

Now it's your turn. What are you willing to tackle? Is the first step for you a trip to your doctor's office? Or can you commit now to a regular exercise program? List your behavioral goals in the worksheet that follows.

Chapter 8 Exercise – Draft Worksheet

	Week 1							Week 2						
Day #	1	2	3	4	5	6	7	8	9	10	11	12	13	14
Behavioral Goals														
Example 1: Walk for a minimum of 15 minutes per day (outside if possible, on treadmill if not)														
Example 2: Accumulate 5,000 steps per day using a pedometer.														
My Goal 8:1														
My Goal 8:2														
My Goal 8:3														
My Goal 8:4														
My Goal 8:5														

9

REST: SLEEPING YOUR WAY TO BETTER BLOOD PRESSURE?

OVER THE YEARS, it has ranked among my patients' most pressing concerns: insomnia. And it's an ironic concern, isn't it? Many of us try to squeeze as much as possible into our days, seemingly begrudging the hours we have to spend in sleep. But just take away one's ability to *choose* to sleep, and the average person will become extremely frustrated, if not agitated.

Indeed, sleep and rest may seem like passive, relatively unimportant activities. However, it usually takes only a night or two of missed sleep before most people become acutely aware of the profound physiologic importance of rest. In fact, it seems our bodies are programmed as much to rest as they are to function during waking hours.

Consider your digestive system. If you go to bed on an empty stomach, your intestinal tract will soon come under the control of something called the "migrating motor complex." This orchestrated system serves to cleanse—or provide a "housekeeping role" for—your bowels.[115] The intricate multi-staged process includes something called *retroperistalsis*, when contractions in the upper small intestine (the duodenum) move in the reverse direction.[116] The reason? To help care for your stomach lining. The duodenum contains a substance called bicarbonate that helps tone down (or more technically, "neutralize") acidity. Presumably, this gives the stomach lining a break from the high acidity with which it is typically bombarded.

This anecdote from the annals of digestive physiology may be of special importance if you have ulcers or gastritis. (I hope you have taken my hint about going to bed on an empty stomach. That's right, bedtime snacks are not gut-friendly.)

What does all this have to do with high blood pressure? A huge amount. There are literally thousands of things that happen during rest and sleep which, like your intestinal tract's "migrating motor complex," are vital to keeping your body in optimal health, which is important for optimal blood pressure.

I'll later discuss more about the emerging connections between intestinal health and blood pressure. For now, there is a far more compelling angle to the sleep deprivation-high blood pressure story. When we cut ourselves short on rest, not only do we miss out on sleep's restorative benefits, but we also push our body into overdrive. How can you keep going if your body is calling for sleep?

One common strategy is to reach for the caffeine. We've already observed what that does to blood pressure. No doubt you recall how America's favorite drug ramps up your stress hormone levels, giving a boost to your energy level, as well as your blood pressure.

Others stimulate stress hormone output more transiently, jarring themselves awake with a strident alarm clock or a cold shower. However, even if you forego the java and other sources of external stimulation, your body simply cannot keep going without adequate sleep unless something revs up your metabolic machinery. Whether you've thought about it or not, some of us are good at ramping up our stress hormones simply by mental drive.

If you don't feel you're a highly disciplined person, you might be wondering, "Mental drive? Me?" Well, let me assure you: if you went to bed at 2 AM and got to work on time at 8 AM, you exercised considerable discipline (in order to override your body's desire to sleep). And you boosted your blood pressure in the process.

Simply put, lack of sleep raises blood pressure. And part of that elevation is likely due to elevated levels of stress hormones like cortisol.[117]

Beware of Sleep Apnea

They come through my office regularly, complaining of fatigue, often dozing at inappropriate times. A careful medical history (complemented by the observations of a family member) will often nail the diagnosis. If you snore, struggle with daytime wakefulness, and have been observed by your partner to stop breathing, then you have the tell-tale signs of sleep apnea. And sleep apnea often contributes to high blood pressure.

Sleep apnea refers to the absence of breathing while asleep. Of course, no one with the condition actually stops breathing all night and lives to tell about it. Those afflicted with sleep apnea may stop breathing hundreds of times each night. Fortunately—or unfortunately—the individual with sleep apnea is usually oblivious to these awakenings.

How could someone awaken myriad times each night and not realize it? The affected individual wakes on a subconscious level only. If you're not breathing, chemical signals reach your brain, triggering a state of alarm and, in that alarmed state, the brain arouses just enough to take a breath. It then dozes off.

On a chemical or electrical level, as attested to by an EEG (electroencephalogram), the brain is indeed waking every time this occurs. Restorative sleep is eroded. When the affected individual arises the next morning, he may think he just got eight or more hours of sleep. Nonetheless, he probably still feels fatigued.

Thus, when sleep apnea short-changes your body of restorative sleep, your body will ramp up stress hormones to keep you going. Hence, you'll likely reach for the caffeine or find some other way to jolt your body into action. Our systems can, however, handle only so much. If you have sleep apnea, you're likely waging a perpetual war with fatigue.

The bottom line? If you have high blood pressure and seem unduly fatigued, think sleep apnea. The condition is more common in men, and is more likely if you are overweight. Many women, and thin individuals of both genders, also have the condition.

The best news about the most common form of sleep apnea (called obstructive sleep apnea, abbreviated OSA) is that it is generally easily treatable. If you're wondering about the terminology, *obstructive* indicates something is obstructing the flow of air through your respiratory tract when you sleep. The obstruction is typically caused by your upper airways "collapsing." Think of it this way: if the tissues are more lax in the region of your wind pipe—a situation that commonly occurs in individuals carrying extra weight—those tissues can "crimp" your wind pipe and obstruct or restrict the flow of air.

The standard treatment for OSA utilizes a CPAP machine. This device delivers "continuous positive airway pressure" (thus the abbreviation) which keeps your airways open—and prevents the apneic (breathless) episodes.

Tried CPAP but didn't like it? Don't give up. Most people at first find the devices awkward (most of us are not used to having something on our faces during sleep). However, if you persist (and work with your provider to experiment with different masks or other delivery devices), you'll likely find what most of my patients have found. Namely, a little bit of hassle is surely worth the incrementally better sleep. But the sleep benefits don't stop there. Well-treated sleep apnea can make it easier to shed unwanted pounds.

Furthermore, treating sleep apnea typically improves blood pressure control.

The data really is compelling when it comes to the difference between treated and untreated obstructive sleep apnea. Perhaps this was shown most elegantly by a research team in Spain who looked at the development of high blood pressure in nearly 2000 individuals who were followed for a minimum of ten years.[118] The data, collected as part of the Zaragoza Sleep Study, showed a remarkable difference in risk of developing hypertension depending on whether or not a person had OSA—and, if present, whether or not that OSA was treated. The results are depicted in Figure 9.1.

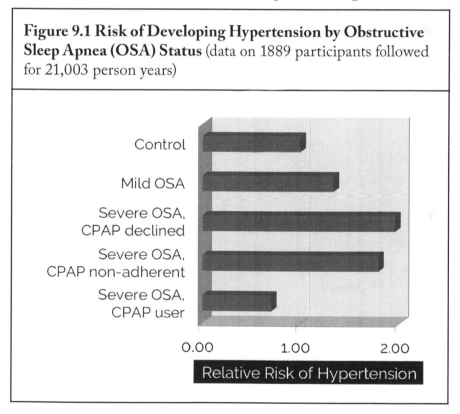

Figure 9.1 Risk of Developing Hypertension by Obstructive Sleep Apnea (OSA) Status (data on 1889 participants followed for 21,003 person years)

Figure 9.1 demonstrates something that at first is counterintuitive: the individuals who fared the best in the blood pressure arena were those with OSA who were faithfully using their CPAP machines. They were less likely to develop hypertension than were those who did not meet the criteria for sleep apnea (the control group), or those who had mild disease and, thus, were not considered candidates for CPAP. Not surprisingly, the groups who did the worst were those with severe sleep apnea who either refused to use CPAP or started treatment but did not stick with it.

Why did consistent CPAP users do the best? The data revealed an interesting finding: even those who had "no sleep apnea" and were thus designated the control group, still had occasional episodes of either breathing stoppage or decreased air flow (on average 2.6 events per hour). These episodes of decreased or absent air flow are captured in a measurement called the apnea-hypopnea index (AHI) which records the number of such episodes per hour. Theoretically, those getting optimal treatment with CPAP would have an AHI of zero—indicating no episodes of decreased or absent airflow. Figure 9.2 illustrates the AHI for each group prior to CPAP treatment. This data provides further insight into the findings already depicted in Figure 9.1.

Figure 9.2 pulls back the curtain on several relationships. First, as I've already pointed out, even the control group had some nightly episodes of sleep apnea. However, second, the mild OSA group had over five times more, logging an average of 14.2 such events per hour. Third, we have an explanation for why there was more hypertension among those who declined CPAP than those who started but didn't stick with it (see Figure 9.1). Do you see the answer? Figure 9.2 reveals those who declined CPAP just happened to have had worse sleep apnea (37.1 events per hour) than those who were non-adherent (31.3 hourly events). Finally the group that stuck with CPAP had the very worst apnea of all. It definitely leaves you wondering, doesn't it? Could their severe OSA have been a factor in motivating them to start treatment and stick with it?

The data leaves us with an inescapable conclusion: sleep apnea is bad for blood pressure. And the worse your sleep apnea is, the more likely you are to have trouble with hypertension. This all argues for discussing the possibility you might have sleep apnea with a health professional. A diagnosis of OSA may put you on the road to getting your BP under control without medication.

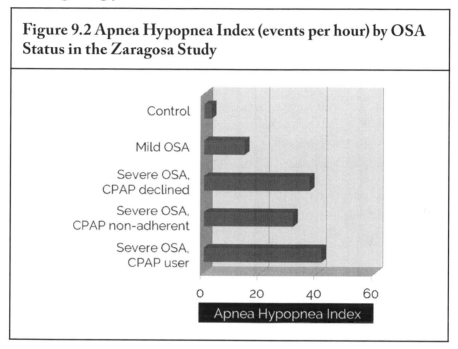

Figure 9.2 Apnea Hypopnea Index (events per hour) by OSA Status in the Zaragosa Study

The Sleep-BP Plot Takes Another Turn

I began the chapter with an illustration of the complex restorative processes that occur each night as we sleep, as illustrated by the "migrating motor complex" (sometimes simply referred to as the MMC), because it bears some fascinating connections with blood pressure.

For example, some data indicates that individuals with high blood pressure may be at higher risk of stomach and duodenal (upper intestinal) ulcers.[119] Some have speculated this is due to the damaging effects of high blood pressure itself; e.g., taking a toll on the blood vessels responsible for nourishing the intestinal lining. However, other data raises concern that some medications used to treat high blood pressure may put individuals at greater risk for intestinal disorders. Certain high blood pressure drugs, by interfering with the MMC may actually undermine the health of the digestive tract.[120] If you have problems with gastritis or ulcers, this material should further up the ante to do all you can *naturally* to control your BP.

Nonetheless, one of the most fascinating connections between sleep, your gut, and your blood pressure relates to a hormone called melatonin. The first link is this: if you forego that evening snack and retire with an empty stomach, your intestinal lining makes an abundance of melatonin.[121] In this context, melatonin helps to stimulate the MMC with its intestinal health-enhancing properties.[122] However, as we'll see in some detail shortly, the third link in the chain is perhaps most fascinating: melatonin helps to lower blood pressure. Some of this BP benefit may be mediated through healthier intestinal processes, but melatonin may also have direct anti-hypertensive effects.

More About Melatonin

In addition to its production in the gut, melatonin is made by your pineal gland, a small gland in the lower regions of your brain. (Don't confuse the pineal with the pituitary gland—another small structure which, in this case, hangs by a narrow stalk from the base of your brain.) Melatonin is involved with more than the MMC. It is an important hormone that helps restore our bodies from the tolls exacted by daily living. That's right, our bodies take quite a bit of abuse during our waking hours. Hormones like melatonin and growth hormone help rejuvenate our bodies while we snooze.

A somewhat crude illustration is seen daily in the airline industry. At the end of every flight, and then more comprehensively at the end of each day, a team of laborers seeks to return the plane to the fully functional, more hygienic state it was in when it began its daily duties. Whether flight crew members, mechanics or janitorial workers, their job is to get the plane back to a "renewed" state of functioning.

A similar thing happens with your body. Each evening, a whole team of players, from the migrating motor complex to melatonin, seek to renew every aspect of your physiology.

Melatonin and Blood Pressure

Some of what we know about melatonin's blood-pressure-lowering effects comes from research on the isolated compound. In 2011, after an exhaustive review of thirty years' worth of medical research, Ehud Grossman and colleagues found seven high quality melatonin studies suitable for collective analysis.[123] The seven studies were about equally divided into those that used fast-release melatonin and those that used a controlled-release preparation (theoretically delivering something more akin to your body's production of this hormone throughout the night). Specifically:

- Three studies used controlled-release melatonin at a dosage of 2-3 mg/day
- Four studies used fast-release melatonin in a dosage of 5 mg/day

What the researchers found was fascinating. Their data, summarized in Figure 9.3, reveals that only the physiologic (controlled-release) melatonin product had blood-pressure-reducing efficacy. Furthermore, the magnitude of that benefit was remarkable. Systolic blood pressure dropped an average of six points while diastolic levels fell nearly four points.

Grossman's review left at least one key question unanswered: Is controlled-release melatonin merely a substitute for what our bodies would normally produce were we on an optimal lifestyle?

This is more than an academic query. About fifteen years ago, Neil Nedley, MD, in his popular, *Proof Positive: How to Reliably*

Combat Disease and Achieve Optimal Health Through Nutrition and Lifestyle, analyzed the melatonin research literature. Nedley came to an amazing conclusion: a number of simple lifestyle strategies can boost a person's intrinsic production of melatonin, without taking a supplement. Not surprisingly, one of the connections Dr. Nedley found is the one I have already discussed—the importance of going to bed on an empty stomach. His list, however, included a host of strategies as summarized in Figure 9.4. [124]

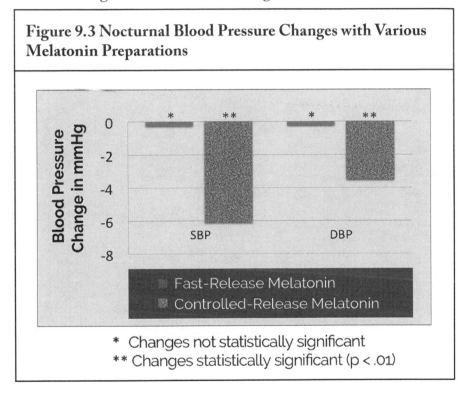

Figure 9.3 Nocturnal Blood Pressure Changes with Various Melatonin Preparations

* Changes not statistically significant
** Changes statistically significant (p < .01)

Sleep and Digestive Processes: The Discussion Comes Full Circle

Among the most common causes of interrupted sleep in America are those relating to the gastrointestinal tract. A person might be awakened by colon spasms connected with irritable bowel syndrome (IBS), intractable pain from the inflammatory bowel diseases (IBD) Crohn's and Ulcerative Colitis, heartburn triggered by gastroesophageal reflux disease (GERD), or gnawing pain from an ulcer or gastritis. Melatonin may help a number of these processes.[125] Furthermore, a number of these conditions may have linkages with high blood pressure. I gave the example of gastritis, ulcers, and impaired MMC function earlier in the chapter. However, data also links uncontrolled high blood pressure to heart burn and GERD (a condition where acid flows backwards from the stomach into the swallowing tube or esophagus).[126]

This data together makes an eloquent plea: take care of your body by getting adequate sleep. Better sleep will not only help lower your blood pressure but will also decrease your risk of a host of problems (like intestinal disorders), which can, in turn, further erode your sleep and raise your blood pressure. If your sleep is already compromised by a digestive disorder, get proper diagnosis and treatment. You may find that a healthy lifestyle— with adequate rest—will be an important part of the equation, allowing you to ultimately be free of medications for the intestinal disorder.

If you think I've belabored these connections more than necessary, hold your judgment until we come to Chapter 12. There we'll pick up these lines of research as we'll learn that improving the health of your digestive tract with probiotics seems calculated to lower your blood pressure. And you guessed it: Those same natural strategies can help conditions like IBS and IBD as well as ulcer disease.[127]

Waves of Healing

Interrupted sleep's blood-pressure-boosting qualities transcend elevated stress hormone levels and undermined melatonin production. Here alcohol again raises its ugly head. If you've ever partaken of a nightcap, you realize that alcohol's sedative effects may seem to be a boon to insomniacs. However, the opposite is true.

Alcohol interferes with restorative sleep by undermining what is called "normal sleep architecture." You see, sleep is not an all-or-none phenomenon. We go through stages during sleep—and that normal progression through sleep's various stages is impaired by beverage alcohol. Alcohol can also directly raise blood pressure.

Figure 9.4 Boosting Melatonin Naturally*

- Get outside daily during daylight hours

- Sleep in total darkness

- Avoid caffeine, alcohol and tobacco

- Get at least two hours of sleep before midnight

- If possible, avoid drugs that can impair melatonin production including:

  - Nonsteroidal anti-inflammatory drugs (see Chapter 13)

  - Sleep aids

  - Antianxiety agents

  - Antidepressants

  - High dose vitamin B_{12} (≥3 mg/day)

  - Selected blood pressure pills such as beta- and calcium-channel blockers

- Don't overeat (restrict food intake in general)

- Practice fasting, especially in the evening (i.e., eat your last meal early, and don't snack)

- Eat foods rich in tryptophan like tofu, pumpkin, sesame seeds, almonds, and walnuts

- Ensure adequate dietary intake of calcium and pyridoxine (vitamin B_6)

- Don't skimp on rich sources of dietary melatonin like whole oats, corn, and rice

*adapted from N. Nedley, *Proof Positive*

Consider our old friend the sympathetic nervous system. You'll recall that this facet of our unconscious nervous processes is responsible for the fight-or-flight response. Alcohol ramps up the sympathetic nervous system, at the same time raising blood pressure[128] and upsetting the necessary nervous system balance[129] required for optimal sleep.

Consequently, alcoholic beverages trigger mechanisms that intrinsically raise blood pressure in the short term as well as contributing to high blood pressure chronically through deprivation of quality sleep.

Don't be duped into thinking that alcoholic beverages compensate for their short-term blood-pressure-raising effects by helping you in the sleep department. To make it very practical: If you really want to maximize lifestyle approaches for high blood pressure, you'll opt for grape juice instead of wine.

Persistent Troubles with Evening Rest?

At this point, some of you might be getting frustrated. If you already struggle with insomnia, this chapter may be raising your blood pressure. After all, you were already distressed about your poor sleep. By now I've probably convinced you that your insomnia is bad for your blood pressure as well.

If so, I have good news. Although the research is not totally harmonious, a midday nap appears to be beneficial, particularly if you are not sleeping sufficiently at night. One of the more recent chapters in this emerging research was presented by Dr Manolis Kallistratos at the European Society of Cardiology's annual meeting in August 2015.[130]

Kallistratos and his colleagues looked at the effects of midday napping in individuals with high blood pressure. In their study of 386 middle-aged men and women (average age 61.4 years) they found a significant benefit for the nappers. When compared to those who got no midday sleep, those who napped had systolic blood pressures that were 5 points lower during the day and 7 points lower when they slept at night.

Such impressive results have not been shown in all cultures and in all environments, raising concerns that just napping to nap may not necessarily be health enhancing.[131] Where I come down on the research is simple: If your energy and concentration are waning at midday, don't hesitate to take a nap if you can fit it in. However, the consensus of most researchers is that a nap should ideally be kept to 30 minutes or less.[132] Indeed, even naps of such short duration have been shown to have far-reaching benefits as far as improving alertness, learning and concentration, if not blood pressure.[133]

Introducing Sleep Hygiene

No chapter on the importance of rest would be complete without a discussion of what health professionals call "sleep hygiene." In fact, if you've read much in the sleep field, you realize I've basically begged the question with the preceding discussion about napping. You see, some health professionals discourage naps for fear it will erode evening sleep. I side with the experts who tell those not getting adequate nightly sleep to nap if you can squeeze it into your schedule.

With that background, I've adapted some of the best insights on sleep hygiene—behaviors that help improve sleep quality—from a number of international sources.[134] If you have trouble sleeping, why not align your behavioral goals with some of the recommendations in Figure 9.5? Because melatonin is a key substance involved in healthy sleep, you'll notice some striking similarities with the list found in Figure 9.4. Rather than condensing the two figures into a single graphic, I've included the repetition to help reinforce areas you may want to prioritize when it comes to setting your goals.

Weekly Rest and Blood Pressure

Our examination of rest's blood-pressure-lowering efficacy has largely focused on getting sufficient sleep. However, might our blood pressure benefit from other forms of rest as well? For example, could a weekly day of rest further aid in blood pressure lowering?

When we consider that hypertension is a leading contributor to many cases of sudden death such as heart attack and stroke, a fascinating study from Israel raises interesting implications. In 2001 Jon and Ofra Anson of Ben Gurion University of the Negev analyzed all deaths in their nation over a ten-year period from 1983 to 1992.[135] Their goal was to see if there was any pattern to morality rates that might differ during certain holidays or days of the week.

The Ansons' remarkable finding was that death rates dropped significantly during the Bible Sabbath (from sundown Friday to sundown Saturday).[136] On the surface, this might not seem all that surprising as during the era in which their study was done, Saturday was an enforced national day of rest such that beginning early afternoon on Friday "businesses, services and public transportation close[d] down, with very few exceptions." However, the same was true of other national holy days, and no similar decrease in mortality was observed. Additionally, this decrease in mortality was not seen among those who only had a day off to which they attached no significant social or spiritual connection. Young Jewish children as well as non-Jews reaped no mortality benefits. Figure 9.6 presents some concluding insights from the Ansons.

The very language of the Ansons, invoking words like "sacred" and "holy," might lend one to conclude that the study is looking purely at the impact on blood pressure of devoting one day a week to spiritual pursuits. However, I think we need to be careful about making such a connection. In a traditional Jewish context, the Sabbath is not merely a day where one ceases from secular labor but where he or she spends time with family, worship, and other spiritual concerns. All "secular" activities such as shopping, balancing the check book, focusing on scholastic assignments, etc. are proscribed. In this sense we are really talking

181

Figure 9.5 Sleep Hygiene Principles

- **Exercise Regularly** for at least 30 minutes daily, preferably more than four hours prior to bedtime. Exercise closer to bedtime stimulates some individuals and will make it more difficult for them to sleep.

- **Get Bright Light Exposure During the Day.** Bright light exposure early in the day helps you fall asleep. Bright light exposure just prior to sunset helps individuals sleep through the night.

- **Keep Evening Meals Light – at Least Four Hours Before Bedtime.** Although late night eating can make you feel sleepy, a rising blood sugar will undermine the production of growth hormone, a compound that even adults need to get peak rejuvenation from sleep.

- **Avoid Caffeinated Beverages.** Caffeine after lunchtime may erode sleep quality. Even earlier in the day, caffeine may affect sleep by lowering melatonin levels.

- **Avoid Alcohol.** Late afternoon and early evening alcohol intake interfere with sleep architecture (the normal rhythmicity of sleep which is necessary for optimal restoration); alcohol at other times erodes resolve, making it easier to neglect to practice good lifestyle habits throughout the day.

- **Avoid Nicotine Intake.** Nicotine isn't your friend when it comes to blood pressure, or health in general. If you still haven't made a complete break, avoid this stimulant for at least four hours before bedtime to get the best sleep.

Figure 9.5 Sleep Hygiene Principles (continued)

- **Avoid High-Risk Naps.** Naps that are longer than 30 minutes or later in the day (after 3 PM) are more likely to interfere with sleep.

- **Maintain a Regular Sleep Schedule,** even on the weekends. Your body functions best when it can lock into a daily *circadian* rhythm. If you get up at the same time each day, your body will properly time the release of hormones like cortisol, so you'll be ready to hit the ground running.

- **Have a Sleep Routine.** Your body does best if you give it cues to wind down. Examples include listening to soothing music, praying, meditating and reading inspirational material. Also consider taking a warm or tepid (lukewarm) bath or a hot shower.

- **Mentally Prepare for Sleep.** Wind down mentally before bedtime; don't take anger, worries or concerns with you into the bedroom. (Incidentally, watching the news is generally not an effective way to do this.)

- **Refocus Your Brain.** If you can't mentally wind down, go to sleep listening to something that is engaging but not stimulating. This is best accomplished by listening to something familiar. Such an activity can focus your brain on something other than unpaid bills, tomorrow's meeting, your retirement account, or other waking activities.

- **Avoid Late-Night Light-Emitting Screens.** For an hour before retiring, avoid any significant use of light-emitting screens (laptops, tablets, smartphones, etc.).

Figure 9.5 Sleep Hygiene Principles (concluded)

- **Go to Bed Early.** Because restorative hormones, like growth hormone and melatonin, peak earlier in the night, sleep before midnight may be better sleep than after. Some experts recommend turning in by 10 pm.

- **Rethink the Alarm Clock.** Depending on an alarm is usually an indication that you're shorting yourself on sleep. After all, if you get to bed early enough, you should be able to get your required sleep and still be up in time for your morning routine. However, tossing your alarm clock may be premature. For example, anxiety-prone individuals may sleep more fitfully without the assurance of an alarm preventing their oversleeping. Bottom line: you may be better off, sooner or later, without an alarm clock.

- **Ensure Restful Surroundings.** Cool, dark, comfortable and free of excessive noise are all qualities of an optimal sleeping environment. Wearing earplugs or blinders may be necessary in certain circumstances.

- **Get Up and Try Again.** Don't try to "force sleep." If you've been lying in bed for more than 20 minutes, get up and do something non-stimulating. Then try to go back to sleep again. Such non-stimulating activities include low intensity exercises, like stretching or marching in place at your bedside. If you can do this safely with the lights out, so much the better. (Avoid doing things that are stimulating or interesting as this can increase wakefulness.)

about truly taking a break from the pressures of life. Might this have health benefits for more than just those of the Jewish faith?

The study is of further interest to those advocating a legislated "day of rest," using rationale from various perspectives including spiritual, physical, political, and economic. The work of the Ansons suggests that legislating such a day really does nothing as far as reaping its most profound health benefits. (After all, the Palestinians, like the Jews, were required to cease working on the Sabbath yet logged no mortality advantages.) Health benefits came only to those who internally regarded the day of rest as having special significance on a moral and/or social level.

Figure 9.6 Death Rests a While: Reflections of researchers Jon and Ofra Anson on decreased death rates in Israel during the hours of the weekly Sabbath (from sundown Friday to sundown Saturday)

"the sacred nature of the Sabbath, its being set apart from all the mundane work-days of the week, creates a special situation in which the probability of death is reduced. We have argued that this special nature derives not from what the Sabbath is not—a workday— but from what it is..."

"If the essence of a holy day is that it is differentiated from the mundane rest of the week, then Saturday in Israel is a holy day par excellence. Indeed, by Jewish tradition, the Sabbath is the most important festivity in the Jewish year."

Introducing Circaseptan Rhythms

We still have much to learn about the health benefits of "a Sabbath rest." What is clear is that human beings (as well as many other creatures) have hormonal rhythms that operate even when cut off from light-dark cues. For example, put a man or woman in a cave without any timekeeping devices and his or her metabolic and hormonal processes will still exhibit about a 24-hour rhythmicity. We call these circadian rhythms.

While circadian rhythms have been popularized in the lay press, the general public is largely unaware of circaseptan rhythms. However, these seven-day rhythms are equally part of our physiology.[137] Most important to our dialogue, some of these weekly rhythms affect blood pressure.[138] Chronobiologists have even demonstrated that certain natural blood pressure interventions may be more efficacious on the weekends than during the week. We will see a good example of this in the next chapter when we examine a deep breathing intervention.[139]

Could, then, we improve our blood pressure by honoring this hormonal rhythmicity and resting every seventh day? When we explore further the subject of stress and blood pressure, one might conclude that such a weekly rest would have stress-relieving benefits of great value to our culture today, regardless of whether or not it helps us harness circaseptan rhythms.

Indeed, the jury may be out as to whether a day of rest is a boon to blood pressure. However, there's no doubt most of us need more rest and sleep. Make a commitment to doing better in this department, and don't be surprised if you reap blood pressure improvements.

Setting Behavioral Goals

If you've not already been working on your behavioral goals for this chapter, it is time to think about doing so. However, our last topic has definitely injected a note of good news into our dialogue.

If you're feeling a bit overwhelmed by the *daily* commitments you're making, why not set a *weekly* goal for rest? Example 2 below illustrates just such a goal. Best of all, in a sense, you are keeping that goal all week long, just by honoring that one-day-in-seven for a "Sabbath." So, when you're charting your progress in Appendix B, if you've set such a goal, feel free to check off each daily box—so long as you kept a day of rest that week.

Not good enough news? Let me then give you one other simple thing you can likely set as a goal. If you're currently taking blood pressure medications, why not talk to your doctor about taking them all at bedtime? That's right. Recent data indicates you will get more blood-pressuring lowering benefit from your meds if you take them late in the day as opposed to early in the morning.[140]

Chapter 9 Rest & Sleep – Draft Worksheet

	Week 1							Week 2						
Day #	1	2	3	4	5	6	7	8	9	10	11	12	13	14
Behavioral Goals														
Example 1: Ensure I get at least 7 hours per sleep each night (even if I don't sleep that long, I will spend that long in bed)														
Example 2: Plan to set aside one day per week for a "Sabbath" where I truly take a break from all the pressing cares of my life.														
My Goal 9:1														
My Goal 9:2														
My Goal 9:3														
My Goal 9:4														
My Goal 9:5														

10

ENVIRONMENT: FRESH AIR, QUIET, SUNSHINE AND NATURE ITSELF AS HYPERTENSION REMEDIES

WHILE ATTENDING MEDICAL SCHOOL, Richard and I lived in the same suburban apartment building. He was in his early 20s, like me, yet had a different perspective on what I thought was our relatively quiet environment. Richard's conclusion: it was "noisy."

Richard underscored his verdict with an unusual train of logic. He asserted that his blood pressure was always higher when living in our apartment than when school was out and he returned home. To him, this provided implicit evidence of our "noisy" environment.

I remember being taken aback by his assessment. Our apartment was not in a noisy area of town. I had roots in big city living, and this didn't even come close. Furthermore, I was quite skeptical about Richard's purported link between noise and his elevated blood pressure readings.

I'm not sure if I wondered whether academic stress would be a better explanation for his high BP numbers. I don't recall whether my mind went through a list of other possible "confounders" (alternate factors that would explain Richard's school-related hypertension). What I do know is this: his comments made such an impression I didn't forget them.

Years—and, ultimately, multiple scientific studies—later, I was forced to agree with Richard's conclusions.

Road Traffic Noise Linked to High Blood Pressure

In 2011 German researchers published a synthesis of existing medical studies (called a "meta-analysis"), looking at the connection between road traffic noise and blood pressure.[141] They came up with some striking conclusions, as illustrated in Figure 10.1.

Figure 10.1 Connections Between Noise and High Blood Pressure

"Noise annoyance" due to road traffic was convincingly linked to high blood pressure. The greater the noise exposure, the greater one's risk of hypertension.

The closer a person lived to a major road, the greater the noise stress on his or her blood pressure.

Seemingly small changes in noise exposure could make a big difference. Sleeping in a bedroom facing a road (as opposed to one on the opposite side of the house) was associated with higher blood pressures.

I found the connections between noise and hypertension astounding. Other than Richard, I'd never had a lay person make this important connection between noise and blood pressure. Think about it. Simply moving your room to another side of the house might decrease your need for high blood pressure medications.

Why would noise have such a blood-pressure-elevating role? Evidence suggests noise exposure and/or noise annoyance stimulates the autonomic nervous system. As I've noted earlier, this arm of your unconscious nervous system activates the fight-or-flight response. Once you trigger this system, your body raises levels of stress-related hormones, bearing technical monikers like *catecholamines* and *cortisol*.

Noise and Childhood Health

Noise is not only of concern when it comes to blood pressure in adults. It is a pediatric issue as well.

This consideration takes on special import as public health professionals raise concerns about the current generation of children being outlived by their parents. Consider recent research published in the *Journal of Research in Medical Sciences*.[142] The article's title essentially tells the whole story: "Overweight, air and noise pollution: Universal risk factors for pediatric pre-hypertension." In the paper, the authors make a point that is sobering, yet probably already obvious; namely, under a barrage of noise pollution, our kids are running higher blood pressures.

Such a relationship is particularly worrisome. Biometric parameters like blood pressure tend to track throughout the lifespan. In other words, a child with prehypertension today is likely to have overt high blood pressure down the road.

The authors' sobering analysis goes deeper, as illustrated in Figure 10.2. Clearly, when we survey the data, we must be concerned about noise exposure. Even if we don't think it makes a big difference for ourselves, it is seriously impacting the youngest members of society.

Take-Home Lessons

Our first lesson from environmental health is relatively simple conceptually: *prioritize quiet*. Application is, of course, more difficult. What can you do to limit noise in your life? Have you been contemplating a major relocation? Could you move to an apartment on the other side of the complex? Is a move to a different bedroom in your house in order?

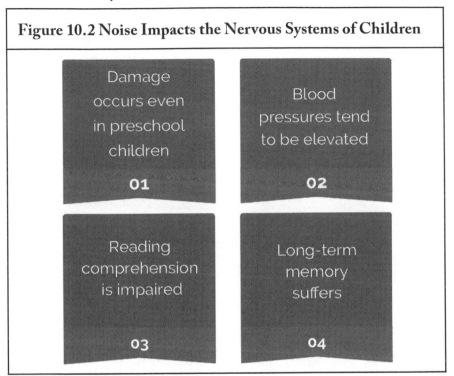

Figure 10.2 Noise Impacts the Nervous Systems of Children

Damage occurs even in preschool children 01

Blood pressures tend to be elevated 02

Reading comprehension is impaired 03

Long-term memory suffers 04

Perhaps you have come up with some other strategies to quiet your environment. I challenge you to commit to at least one such behavioral goal. Once you've formulated a plan, record it in the log at the end of this chapter.

Gut Feelings: One Last-Ditch Noise-Protection Strategy

I know some of you may be at a loss to know how to quiet down your environment. Even if your strategy includes a change of residence, that's not likely to happen overnight. A recent trip reminded me of the power of a simple, inexpensive noise reduction technique.

The first evening of our excursion, my wife had a terrible night of interrupted sleep. I was sharing the same hotel room but didn't wake up with the same level of frustration. Perhaps I was simply more sleep deprived, or maybe just less aware of my surroundings. However, even I had a dim recollection of what seemed like an all-night party in the parking lot below our third-floor hotel room.

The next night found my wife in somewhat different attire. Her sleeping clothes were the same, but her ears were now highlighted by some neon green accoutrements: foam earplugs. I don't know if the noise level outside the room was much different our second night in the hotel, but the conclusion the next morning was strikingly different. My well-rested wife credited the superior night's sleep to those ear plugs.

Such simple articles as earplugs and eye masks have been shown to improve sleep—and biological markers connected with high blood pressure—in even the most difficult environments. One recent study was conducted in a simulated intensive care unit, known as one of the least restful places on the planet. There Hu and colleagues from Fujian Medical University in China found the use of earplugs and eye masks resulted in significantly better sleep—as well as improved melatonin levels.[143] Five years later, another Chinese team conducted a similar study. However, they added supplemental melatonin to the equation.[144] Their results suggested that if you had to choose between earplugs with an eye mask and melatonin supplementation, you would be better to choose the latter. Additional research has shown that melatonin supplementation can actually reduce adverse hormonal effects caused by noise stress.[145]

My conclusion is simple: sleep in as quiet an environment as possible. If you can't escape a high noise or brighter light setting at night, then seriously consider using an eye mask, earplugs *and* supplemental melatonin.

Sunshine and Blood Pressure

Although bright light at night can undermine hormonal processes and health, sunshine during the day is health enhancing.

195

Specifically, ample exposure to sunshine can be a boon to our blood pressure. If dermatologic considerations stand in the way of greater sun exposure, we may be able to reap many of these same benefits by ensuring adequate vitamin D intake.

Figure 10.3 Indirect Epidemiologic Evidence Suggests a Link Between Low Vitamin D Levels and High Blood Pressure

 **01** When exposed to similar amounts of sunshine as lighter races, people with darker complexions (especially those of African origin) have a harder time making adequate amounts of vitamin D. Those same darker races tend to have higher BPs.

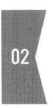 **02** Racial factors being equal, the further one lives from the equator, the greater his or her tendency for high BP.

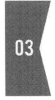 **03** BP tends to be higher in the winter than in the summer.

Figure 10.3 presents some of the indirect evidence from population studies which link deficient vitamin D levels to higher blood pressure readings as synthesized by noted integrative medicine researcher, Richard Nahas, MD.[146]

Although the epidemiologic data is provocative, basic science—perhaps more compellingly—suggests a link. Consider some of the following lines of evidence, also summarized by Dr. Richard Nahas and encapsulated in Figure 10.4.

Figure 10.4 Basic Science Linking Low Vitamin D Levels and High Blood Pressure

Activated vitamin D (1,25-OH vitamin D) blocks production of the blood pressure-raising hormone, renin.

Adequate vitamin D status is important for the health of tiny blood vessels known as the microvasculature.

"The sunshine vitamin" blocks proliferation of vascular smooth muscle cells; when smooth muscle cells proliferate, our small arteries are narrowed, leading to:
- increased resistance to blood flow.
- elevated blood pressures to move blood through these narrower vessels.

Messages from the Sun

The implications of this research seem clear: we need to prioritize judicious sun exposure. Experts indicate we can do well in the vitamin D arena by daily exposing our face, arms and hands to ¼ to ½ of a minimal erythemal dose.[147] What exactly is a "minimal erythemal dose"? It is the amount of sunshine necessary to turn your skin a light pink. Remember, however, you need only ½ to ¼ that exposure.

Let me illustrate. If it takes 15 minutes of noonday sun in mid-July to turn your skin a light pink, then all you need is a maximum of 8 minutes of exposure to your face, hands, and arms at that hour. The above guidelines apply to summer months, and other times of year, when sunshine exposure is adequate for vitamin D production.

Unfortunately, if you live far from the equator, sun exposure may be insufficient for many months. Figure 10.5 provides data from three illustrative cities.

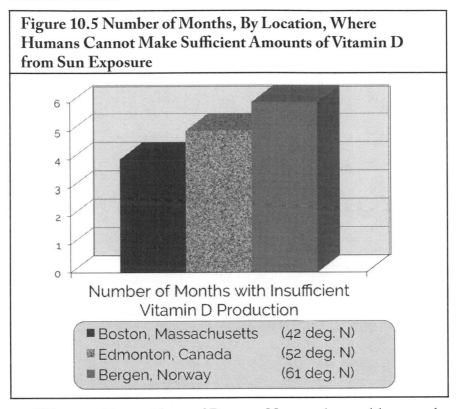

Figure 10.5 Number of Months, By Location, Where Humans Cannot Make Sufficient Amounts of Vitamin D from Sun Exposure

Number of Months with Insufficient Vitamin D Production

- Boston, Massachusetts   (42 deg. N)
- Edmonton, Canada   (52 deg. N)
- Bergen, Norway   (61 deg. N)

Why would a resident of Bergen, Norway be unable to make vitamin D for fully half the year? The answer lies with simple physics. The particular ultraviolet B waves needed to make vitamin D are blocked by the atmosphere unless the sun comes up sufficiently far above the horizon. As you get closer to the poles, the sun in winter never rises far enough. The bottom line is this: If you live at a latitude further than 35 degrees north or south of the equator you will need to take a vitamin D supplement at least during some portion of the winter.[148]

Can You Get Too Much of a Good Thing?

There is no question that too much vitamin D can be toxic.

198

Typical vitamin D toxicity sets in around the 100-150 ng/ml level. It is not hard to avoid this level of toxicity. The research indicates it takes at least 10,000 IU (international units) per day or more to run the risk of such dangerously high levels. For this reason, I've been educating audiences for years to never take more than 5000 IU per day without a doctor's orders.

On the other hand, sunshine exposure, in and of itself, will never produce toxic levels. Theoretically, however, ample sun exposure could render even moderate supplementation of vitamin D dangerous. The bottom line is this: if you have a question as to your status, simply ask your doctor to run a 25-OH vitamin D level (the most accurate test for vitamin D).

Despite these considerations, a growing body of research suggests that lesser levels of vitamin D (than the 100-150 ng/ml mentioned earlier) may also cause deleterious effects. The bottom line is ensure adequacy, but guard against overenthusiasm. Although I formerly suggested shooting for levels greater than 50 ng/ml, today, in view of concerns for over-exuberance, I recommend goals in the 40 – 50 ng/ml range. If your lab uses international units of nmol/liter, the target range would be 100 – 125 nmol/l. And remember to ensure adequate levels of vitamin D year round.

Fresh Air and Blood Pressure

When it comes to public enemy Number 1 on the air pollution front, we have to go no further than tobacco.

Although my Native American friends might want to take issue with this, even sporadic ceremonial use may be problematic for those with high blood pressure. Pay special attention to Figure 10.6 before concluding that small amounts of tobacco are innocuous when it comes to blood pressure.[149] Granted, this is looking at cigarette smoking, so it doesn't fully answer the ceremonial tobacco question (where the smoke is typically not inhaled).[150] However, it does give cause for concern.

Figure 10.6 First Cigarette of the Day Raises Blood Pressure

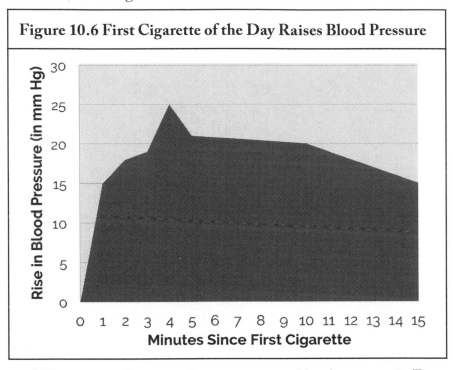

Why is smoking so devastating to blood pressure? First, smoking impacts one of the common pathways to blood pressure elevation; namely, the sympathetic nervous system. Nicotine ramps up the fight-or-flight hormonal mechanisms that not only raise blood pressure but also increase heart rate and oxygen demands on the heart.[151] Second, cigarette smoking damages blood vessels, rendering arteries stiffer and impairing the natural abilities of those vessels to relax.[152] When arteries are more rigid, the heart has to generate more force in order to circulate blood, which results in elevated blood pressure. Third, smoking elevates inflammatory processes in the body.[153] We've already seen how inflammation itself predisposes to hypertension. Fourth, smoking impairs blood fluidity.[154] When blood flow is compromised, blood pressure must rise to continue to circulate effectively the red blood cells and other blood elements.

This is only a partial explanation of why cigarettes raise blood pressure. After all, when you consider that scientists have isolated over 7000 chemicals from tobacco smoke,[155] multiple adverse effects on human circulation aren't at all surprising.

Is it Safe to Dip?

Scientists have known for years that other tobacco preparations also are deleterious to blood pressure control. For example, over 20 years ago Eric C. Westman, M.D., reviewed the medical literature and found:[156]

- Almost all studies demonstrated clinically significant short-term elevations in systolic blood pressure, diastolic blood pressure, and pulse. These acute blood pressure elevations can persist for up to 90 minutes after use.

- The majority of studies also linked smokeless tobacco to chronic hypertension.

- In addition to nicotine, other smokeless tobacco constituents can worsen blood pressure control—including sodium and licorice.

The Licorice Connection

An audible gasp went up from the back of the small meeting room. I had met Hilda earlier in my series of lectures, so I immediately put a name to the face that voiced such an incredulous expression.

After my presentation, I sought out Hilda, hoping to gain more insight into her shocked expression earlier that evening. Hilda, a recent immigrant from Germany, freely told me of her lifelong love for licorice. She, who had been struggling with hypertension for years, was shocked to learn that one of her favorite foods had blood-pressure-elevating properties.

Her surprise was warranted, but I hadn't made mention of

licorice in the context of desserts that raised blood pressure. Instead, licorice surfaced during a discussion about tobacco products. However, Hilda had made a valid connection. Licorice in any form, whether in smokeless tobacco or in desserts, can ramp up blood pressure.

Smokeless tobacco product recipes differ throughout the world. Even if licorice and sodium don't make the ingredient list, nicotine and other constituents invariably raise blood pressure. For example, in India, smokeless tobacco typically keeps company with fennel seeds, cinnamon, cardamom, lime, menthol, areca nuts, and betel nuts. Despite the differences in composition from European and American smokeless tobacco, Indian users of those indigenous products had significantly higher average systolic and diastolic BPs, each in the range of 3-5 mm Hg.

How You Breathe Makes a Difference

If you've eliminated tobacco smoke from your environment, you've likely done the most important thing possible for optimizing your air quality. Sure, you might be exposed to air pollutants worse than tobacco smoke but, for most of us, such scenarios are uncommon. I'm not suggesting that we stop our societal progress on the air quality front in favor of a single-minded tobacco focus; other pollutants, no question, have metabolic effects that can worsen blood pressure, or other metabolic diseases like diabetes.[157]

However, because our focus is on improving blood pressure *in 30 days*, avoiding tobacco smoke is probably the best goal most of us can reasonably accomplish when it comes to improving our inhaled air quality.

Once we've put ourselves in an environment of reasonable air quality, how we breathe can make a difference when it comes to our blood pressure. A number of studies suggest that slow deep breathing can help curb blood pressure.[158]

Some years ago, I was fascinated to learn about a patented

device, called RESPeRATE, that claimed to help individuals lower blood pressure by training them to breathe slower and deeper. This particular product, and its approach to "device-guided breathing" (DGB), has been the subject of multiple clinical trials.[159] Some of the initial data I saw claimed this particular device helped users lower their average blood pressure by 14 points systolic and 8 points diastolic. And these all-day blood pressure reductions were accomplished by using the device as little as 15 minutes daily, three to four times per week.

Armed with such good news, I began to encourage patients and seminar attendees to try out the device and give me feedback. I didn't have a lot of takers; only two or three shared their impressions with me, and none were particularly impressed. This alone doesn't incriminate DGB; after all, those few individuals may not have properly used the system. Nonetheless, reports subsequently came out in the medical literature also questioning just how effective RESPeRATE was. Was it truly more beneficial than a placebo therapy?

For example, in November 2014 a meta-analysis out of the Netherlands concluded: "Treatment with DGB did not significantly lower office blood pressure compared with a sham procedure or music therapy."[160] I share the two sides on RESPeRATE because I think the data does support deep breathing and its role in blood pressure lowering. I'm not in a position currently to endorse RESPeRATE per se. However, I think everyone with high blood pressure should look into the subject of potential benefits occurring from some type of approach that encourages deep breathing exercises.

Aromatherapy: Another Connection Between Breathing and Blood Pressure

I've highlighted what I believe are two of the most important blood pressure aids in the breathing arena, smoking cessation and deep breathing. I'd be negligent, though, if I failed to mention another promising option: aromatherapy.

Aromatherapy refers to the medicinal or otherwise therapeutic use of aromatic essential oils. Though these plant-derived compounds have been used by indigenous cultures for centuries, only recently have they generated significant research interest in the United States.

I first got interested in aromatherapy 15 years ago when running residential stop smoking programs. At that time, I learned of research suggesting greater smoking cessation success among those who inhaled the vapor from lavender oil. The connection made sense. The smoker was substituting another "inhalation behavior" for his old habit, and lavender oil had been documented to have relaxant effects.[161]

More recent research suggests aromatherapy may help lower blood pressure independent of any smoking considerations. In 2010 Korean researchers studied the cardiovascular effects of aromatherapy using a blend of three herbs (lavender, lemon, and a less familiar plant called *ylang ylang*).[162] Though studying a normotensive group, they found an impressive and statistically significant six point drop in blood pressure. They found evidence, too, of a tempering of the sympathetic nervous system, which suggested stress-relieving benefits. The results are depicted in Figure 10.7.

These Korean findings are not unique. Two years later, Thai researchers demonstrated similar results using lavender oil alone.[163] Again they recorded blood pressure lowering along with other indicators of decreased sympathetic nervous system activation.

The case for blood pressure lowering through aromatherapy is not iron-clad, however. In 2012 an exhaustive review article found evidence of "favourable effects of aromatherapy" on hypertension but argued that more data was needed.[164]

If you're an astute medical detective and actually read that 2012 review, you'll notice something interesting: they scoured the medical research literature only through 2009. So, unfortunately, they didn't include some of the apparently compelling data we've examined in this section.

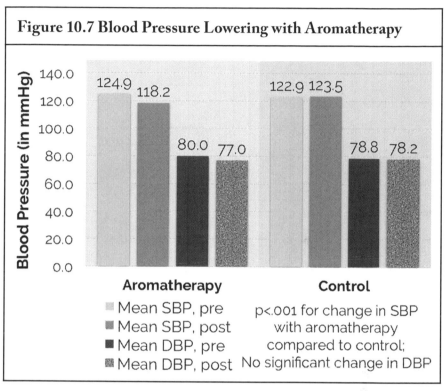

Figure 10.7 Blood Pressure Lowering with Aromatherapy

At the end of the day, the decision doesn't seem all that difficult. If you're dealing with recalcitrant blood pressure numbers, then what have you got to lose? Why not carry a small glass vial of some lavender oil in your pocket? If you take a whiff periodically throughout the day—especially when feeling stressed—you might be surprised by the results.

Connect with Nature

Gymnasiums, indoor pools, high tech libraries and well-equipped study centers all have their place. However, many have observed that children suffer when they are deprived of natural surroundings. Journalist Richard Louv coined the term "Nature-Deficit Disorder" to highlight the impact of artificial lives on our most vulnerable citizens. Louv's neologism was quickly embraced by some researchers while others summarily rejected the designation. Either way, medical data increasingly indicates a natural environment can have significant benefits on our metabolism, and specifically on our blood pressure.

Clearly, children are not the only ones who suffer when they are removed from things green and naturally beautiful. Some of the most interesting research along these lines comes from Japan. Researchers there have been studying an immersive forest experience referred to as "*shinrin-yoku.*" A number of studies indicate that such immersion in a green, forested environment can actually lower blood pressure.[165]

Though questions abound, the preliminary evidence is promising enough to encourage us to spend more time in natural settings. Whether in Central Park in New York City, a state forest in Mississippi, a swath of rural China, or a Canadian provincial park, many rural and urban dwellers alike have relatively easy access to natural settings. Why not consider walking outdoors in such a venue and see if, over time, this seems to help further improve your blood pressure?

Companion Animals and Blood Pressure

Although it is not a substitute for a walk on the beach or a hike in the woods, research suggests there may be a way to bring some of the benefits of nature into even the most sterile urban environment. It comes in the form of companion animals, commonly known as "pets."

Over two decades ago, Dr. W.P. Anderson and colleagues at the Baker Medical Research Institute in Melbourne, Australia sought to assess the impact of pet ownership on heart disease risk factors. They recruited over 5000 individuals who attended a free screening clinic. The researchers found that pet owners had significantly lower blood pressure than those who did not have pets. Cardiovascular benefits, however, were not limited to BP. Cholesterol and triglyceride readings were also lower in those who owned pets. Furthermore, other lifestyle factors did not explain the differences.[166]

Some have argued that the Baker Institute's study as well as other "cross sectional" studies (looking at people at just one point in time) are intrinsically flawed. After all, in this context they reason, "Really sick people can't care for pets— so, of course, pet owners will be the healthier ones. They're the only ones who can handle the necessary animal chores and responsibilities."

Such a charge is answered by what is called "longitudinal research." This occurs when you recruit a group of people and then follow them over time. A number of such studies have also documented benefits from pet ownership.[167] On the cardiovascular front, one of the world's major heart studies (simply referred to as CAST) found that, compared to those without dogs, individuals with canine companions had a markedly increased likelihood of surviving when assessed one year after a heart attack.[168]

The data is suggestive enough that I think non-pet owners who have high blood pressure or other chronic health risk factors should seriously ask themselves whether a companion animal might prove an asset.

However, another Australian study reminds us that pet ownership is no panacea. This time the researchers were Drs. Ruth Parslow and Anthony Jorm of the Australian National University in Canberra.[169] About a decade after Anderson's work, they reported on a similar sized population, again numbering over 5000 individuals. Although Parslow and Jorm didn't measure cholesterol or triglycerides among their adult participants, they did assess their blood pressures. Their results yielded a surprising finding: blood pressure readings were *higher* in the pet owners.

Before you throw up your hands in frustration, there was one potential explanation for the differing findings. In Parslow and Jorm's research, pet owners and pet-less individuals seemed to differ in far more than whether or not they owned a companion animal. Those with animals had lower educational levels, weighed more, and were more likely to smoke.

My take home point from this study is simple: pet ownership alone will not reverse the dangers of other unhealthy lifestyle habits.

Back to the Environment

None of the data on pet ownership proves that living with a companion animal exerts its benefits through a connection with nature. To the contrary, many believe that pets provide their greatest benefits on blood pressure and other parameters through something called "the bond."

"The bond" can be thought of as somewhat analogous to social support, only provided by animals rather than by humans. Supporting such an explanation is the following: when individuals are more socially connected, they seem to get less benefit from companion animals. Those who are lonely or disconnected from society (in various ways) seem to receive the most benefit.

Regardless of the mechanisms involved, having a pet may further aid you in your quest for natural blood pressure control. Pet ownership combined with quiet and natural surroundings, ample sunshine (accompanied by adequate levels of vitamin D), and fresh air devoid of tobacco smoke provide a powerful environmental quartet with salutary effects on blood pressure.

Chapter 10 Environment – Draft Worksheet

(Need I remind you? When you've completed the chapter and finalized your goals, transfer no more than three of them to Appendix B.)

	Week 1							Week 2						
Day #	1	2	3	4	5	6	7	8	9	10	11	12	13	14
Behavioral Goals														
Example 1: Switch the location of our bedroom and our den to capitalize on the present den's quieter location (on the side of the house away from the major road nearby)														
Example 2: Have my vitamin D level checked, and begin taking a supplement if it is too low.														
Example 3: Plan to spend at least 60 minutes each week in a natural setting.														
My Goal 10:1														
My Goal 10:2														
My Goal 10:3														
My Goal 10:4														
My Goal 10:5														

11

STRESS MANAGEMENT: A CRITICAL ALLY IN HYPERTENSION CONTROL

IN SOCIAL SITUATIONS, I tend to keep my medical practice to myself. For example, I don't wear a t-shirt with the initials "M. D." emblazoned in gold. However, there are some occasions where I just can't keep my medical training a secret.

That particular Friday was one such occasion. I had been attending a meeting focused on community health concerns. There were some clinicians in our ranks, but the greatest number were community leaders and clergy. So when I kept running into Judy, I didn't have the confidence that anyone had spoken to her about what seemed like an obvious medical malady.

Judy was a large woman, carrying probably an extra 150 pounds on her five foot, ten inch frame. But, to my medical eye, her size was not as remarkable as her proportions. Judy's weight was largely concentrated around her middle, her arms and legs being quite thin. Her face was extremely round, "moon-shaped" some of my colleagues would likely say. Add to all this an oily face with increased facial hair, and my medical mind was screaming, "Cushing's Syndrome!"

Finally, during another "chance" encounter with Judy I introduced myself and disclosed my occupation. After some disclaimer like, "I know this is really none of my business...", I broached the subject.

I breathed an internal sigh of relief as Judy appeared quite appreciative of my solicitude. She had been dealing with health issues and was due to see a physician soon. Judy also disclosed that her BP had been gradually rising and now was running 190/100. This was not surprising. Studies show a compelling connection between Cushing's and high blood pressure with as many as 74 to 87 % of those affected having full-blown hypertension.

I never heard from Judy again, but I left that conference convinced her health problems were likely due to the very syndrome named after that famous neurosurgeon, Harvey Williams Cushing.

Why the Cushing's Story?

Why would I start a chapter on stress management with a story about Cushing's syndrome? The answer may already be obvious if you have health professional training. The medical problems and physical features of Cushing's are largely due to an excess production of the stress hormone, cortisol. (Individuals with Cushing's typically have a tumor directly or indirectly producing relatively large amounts of this hormone). In fact, when a physician checks her patient's cortisol levels as part of a Cushing's syndrome evaluation, she must keep in mind the impact of chronic stress. After all, excessive psychological stress, as is seen in cases of severe depression, can elevate blood cortisol levels all by itself.

Cushing's syndrome provides a powerful reminder of a connection that has already surfaced a number of times in this book. Stress, the sympathetic nervous system, and high blood pressure are intimately connected:

- Stress activates the sympathetic nervous system

- This then ramps up hormones like cortisol and norepinephrine

- These hormones, in turn, raise blood pressure

Although this is the 11th chapter on our blood-pressure-lowering journey, some experts consider this material to be at the very heart of the essential hypertension problem. In fact, more and more researchers are embracing the position that those with high blood pressure—for various reasons—may have their sympathetic nervous systems ramped up to levels higher than optimal.[170]

This research is not saying that if you have high blood pressure, you are somehow "stressed out." It merely underscores the connection between unconscious nervous system factors and our blood pressure.

Not a New Observation

Drawing connections between stress and high blood pressure is not a recent discovery. As one example, consider the work of researchers at New York Hospital-Cornell Medical College from the early 1990s. In their study of eight worksites, the investigators found a convincing connection between a measure of job stress and higher blood pressure levels. In their study, high "job strain" (a stressful situation where one has significant job demands, but little control over his or her work environment) pushed systolic blood pressure up nearly 7 points and diastolic nearly 3 points.[171]

Whether we focus on Cushing's syndrome, the latest theories on high blood pressure causation, or research linking work stress to high blood pressure, we end up discussing the sympathetic nervous system—a system exquisitely sensitive to the effects of stress. The bottom line is clear: if you have high blood pressure, you must get serious about stress management. There's a corollary as well: if you don't have hypertension—and want to keep your BP down—you too must be invested in stress management.

Some Definitions

Although many talk about *stress* in terms of both the challenges they face and how they deal with those challenges, stress scientists are much more precise. They refer to the challenges as *stressors*. They label our reactions *the stress response*.

Anything that forces your body to adapt or cope can be classed as a stressor. Imagine the following scenario. It is a hot summer's day and you're relaxing in the relatively cool 78 degree temperature of your air-conditioned apartment. However, your brother, visiting from a research base in Antarctica, is not happy with your energy-saving 78 degrees. Without consulting you, he turns the thermostat down to 65. Prior to this you were comfortable, but now as the air conditioner continues to pump out frigid air, your body begins to face the physical stressor of cold temperature.

Fast forward to another venue. Your boss makes another demeaning comment at work. You are now facing a mental stressor. If you begin to ruminate about her consistent messaging, you may face a spiritual stressor, wondering if you have chosen the wrong lifework.

Here's the main idea: Stressors can come at us on a number of levels. These include physical, mental, emotional, social and spiritual. But because we are mentally engaged creatures, a stressor that confronts us on one level can cause a stress response that has multifaceted implications.

In the case of the thermostat reset, although you may be dealing with the physical stressor of cold, when you mentally size up the cause of your physical stress, you may also be stressed on other levels. You may find yourself dealing with mentally, socially and emotionally stressing concerns like, "Why didn't my brother ask before changing the thermostat setting?"; or, "Doesn't my brother realize finances are tight and that air conditioning is costly?"

Consequently, one of the key messages in the stressor-stress response dialogue is this: my mind has a lot to do with what stresses me out. Indeed, what generally stresses us most is not what someone or something does to us, but rather how we process what comes our way.

Figure 11.1 Reinhold Niebuhr's Serenity Prayer

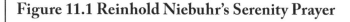

God grant me the serenity
to accept the things I cannot change;
courage to change the things I can;
and wisdom to know the difference.

Living one day at a time;
Enjoying one moment at a time;
Accepting hardships as the pathway to peace;
Taking, as He did, this sinful world
as it is, not as I would have it;
Trusting that He will make all things right
if I surrender to His Will;
That I may be reasonably happy in this life
and supremely happy with Him
Forever in the next.

Amen.

What We Can Change, What We Can't

Arguably, one of the things that has ingrained Alcoholics Anonymous into societal consciousness is their promotion of "the serenity prayer." AA's founders never claimed the prayer was original with them. Some have attributed authorship to the theologian, Reinhold Niebuhr. However, others have traced its roots centuries earlier. This history is relevant only as it speaks to the timelessness of the message, extending far beyond its current popularity with support groups worldwide.[172] In deference to Niebuhr, though, who clearly did pen the words prior to AA's adoption of them, we share in Figure 11.1, in its entirety, a version of this prayer-poem attributed to the late theologian. Whether or not you identify with Niebuhr's invocation of a God, the prayer calls for a radical approach to stress management. It reminds us of two critical issues. First, we are not always in a position to change the stressors that come our way. Second, we always have a choice, nonetheless, in deciding how to respond to a stressor. Even if we can't remove the stressor, we can "accept" it and learn to live with it.

An understanding of these basic concepts is crucial. We are not destined to be adversely affected by the difficulties that come our way.

A Lion in the Room

Over the years I have conducted many group stress management sessions. One of my favorite exercises is to paint a picture of a stressor with which my entire audience can identify. I find a large predatory feline is almost universally effective. Join me for a class, in your mind's eye, as we do this exercise together.

Imagine you're lying on your bed reading a book (like the one in front of you now). All of a sudden, you become aware you're not alone. An instant later you hear a menacing roar and quickly turn over to see a large lion—right inside your own bedroom. What do you do?

For the sake of the illustration, let me assure you, you're not imagining things. There really is a lion in your bedroom. So, how do you respond?

My audiences have come up with a number of responses. Figure 11.2 lists some of the options they've identified.

Many of us have become quite adept at utilizing the first three strategies for stress management. Whether we hide from a stressor, ignore it, or play dead, we generally haven't made any progress in dealing with the potential threat. Indeed, it's not likely any of those strategies will help us survive when faced with a ravenous lion.

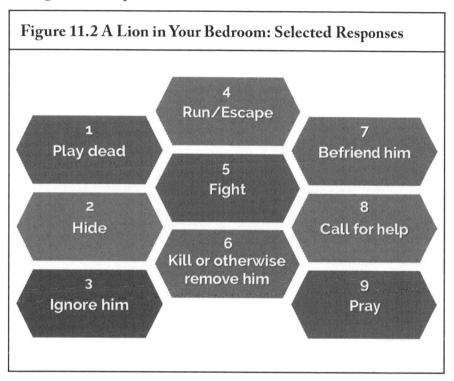

Figure 11.2 A Lion in Your Bedroom: Selected Responses

1 Play dead
2 Hide
3 Ignore him
4 Run/Escape
5 Fight
6 Kill or otherwise remove him
7 Befriend him
8 Call for help
9 Pray

Why do we think it is any different in our human relationships? For example, in that earlier workplace scenario, trying to avoid chance meetings with your boss (so as to not hear those demeaning comments), or simply ignoring her downgrading remarks, will often take a chronic toll.

When we don't face our stressors head on, we usually ramp up our anxiety levels. For example, we may fear being placed in stress-inducing situations. If that's our worry, we'll likely raise our level of vigilance in order to avoid those settings. However, regardless of whether we label it caution, vigilance, or self-preservation, we're talking about a path to anxiety and worry. And anxiety is one of our enemies when it comes to high blood pressure.

217

Anxiety: a Counterproductive Stress Management "Strategy"

Most people wouldn't label anxiety a "stress management strategy." After all, in the medical community we talk about a host of anxiety disorders. These include such diverse conditions as Generalized Anxiety Disorder, Social Anxiety Disorder, and Panic Disorder. There are also specific phobias such as Agoraphobia (literally fear of the market place—or venues where people concentrate), Acrophobia (fear of heights) and Arachnophobia (fear of spiders).

For many of us, anxiety and worry have become intimately associated with our stress management strategies. If there are stressors in your life that you *fear* dealing with—whether a family member, a co-worker, a neighbor, a dog, or any one of a hundred other things—you are already telling me something: your stress management strategy of avoidance is, in effect, a strategy that is rendering you more anxious. And this is bad news for blood pressure.

Even if you don't have an anxiety disorder, the more anxious and worried you are, the greater the likelihood that you will have high blood pressure. If you have high blood pressure, anxieties and worries increase the likelihood you will have difficulty controlling it. One window on these relationships was provided by a classic Framingham Study paper as illustrated in Figure 11.3.[173]

As illustrated by that graphic, heightened levels of anxiety put us on a path to hypertension. Similarly, elevated levels of anxiety perpetuate high blood pressure. But the corollary is equally powerful: addressing anxiety has blood-pressure-lowering effects.

The ideal way to ultimately deal with anxiety is to address the causes of your fears. Now, that very suggestion may already be making you more anxious! Although I promise you some help on that "big-picture" front, let me give you some relief right now. There are a number of very real and practical ways to tune down your level of anxiety *without* confronting your stressors.

Help For Anxiety

In this chapter, it's not my purpose to provide a *Cliff's Notes* version of any of the excellent resources on the market for stress management. However, I do want to give you some tools you can utilize *right away* to ramp down your anxiety levels. The first strategy probably comes as no surprise: exercise.

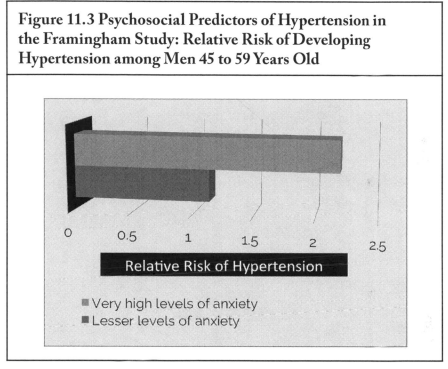

Figure 11.3 Psychosocial Predictors of Hypertension in the Framingham Study: Relative Risk of Developing Hypertension among Men 45 to 59 Years Old

Dr. Kaushadh Jayakody and colleagues in the United Kingdom recently did an extensive review of six medical research databases in order to probe the relationship between physical exercise and anxiety. Their work, complemented by hand searching through other journals, uncovered only eight randomized controlled trials that had studied exercise as a therapy in full-blown anxiety disorders. Despite the limited information available, the investigators still found evidence of an anti-anxiety effect from exercise. When dealing with a serious anxiety disorder, they noted that patients seemed to do best if exercise was combined with either medication and/or mental health interventions (such as group cognitive behavioral therapy).[174]

In looking more broadly at the research, the Anxiety and Depression Association of America (ADAA) reviewed the benefits of physical activity on stress and less intense levels of anxiety (like those experienced by individuals without formal mental health disorders).[175] They found evidence that exercise does all of the following:

- Decreases overall levels of tension
- Elevates and stabilizes mood
- Decreases the risk of developing anxiety disorders
- Enhances overall cognitive function
- Boosts alertness and concentration
- Decreases fatigue
- Improves sleep
- Improves self-esteem

Some of the best news about the ADAA's research is this: it takes only about five minutes of aerobic exercise to begin to reap anti-anxiety benefits. Furthermore, exercise seems to rapidly elevate depressed mood. A ten-minute walk may be sufficient to deliver several hours of mental relief.

Thus, you've got permission right now (as if you really needed it from me)—especially if you've been getting stressed just thinking about your stressors—to take a walk. You're reading this during a blizzard, or in the midst of a monsoon? Then get on your treadmill or stationary bike. No exercise equipment? Then walk around your apartment, or do calisthenics. Exercise is a powerful anxiety reliever. Make sure it is in your stress management tool kit.

By the way, this is a great time to make sure you're focused on the behavioral goals you should already be documenting in Appendix B. Have you been keeping up with your exercise commitments?

While we're talking about it, at any time you can refine goals from previous chapters. For example, if you get extremely stressed after the evening commute, why not revisit your exercise goals? Here's one possibility: If you had already made a commitment to daily exercise, why not move some or all of that exercise to shortly after arriving home from work? (I've taken the liberty to add this as one of the examples in the draft worksheet at the end of this chapter.) Just think about it this way: a short ten-minute walk will likely give you a lot more blood pressure benefit than will yelling at your dog.

Anxiety Relief Beyond Exercise

Granted, we can't exercise in every situation. But there's another powerful anxiety-diffusing, stress-managing tool that can often be employed in those exercise-impossible situations. That tool is music.

From the moment I set eyes on him, I could see that Louis was mentally challenged. His unkempt hair and clothes, the lack of eye contact, and the sullen look were tell-tale signs. Louis was sitting in the exam room with his mother when I entered to address the health concerns of his younger sister. Although I tried to make conversation with him, I never got more than a grunt. Perhaps that would have been the extent of my interaction with Louis were it not for three facts: it was the middle of flu season, Louis had a nasty cough, and he seemed incapable of understanding the need to cover his mouth. I enlisted Louis' mother to help her son don one of those ubiquitous surgical masks we keep on hand for just such occasions. That's when pandemonium ensued.

I'm sure more than one of the patients in that wing wondered if we were doing a study of the effects of torture that morning. No sooner was that mask on Louis' face than he began screaming and yelling as if we were trying to suffocate him. (Perhaps he really thought that would be the result!) Even after the mask was off, Louis tried to ensure I had some of the most difficult auditory circumstances imaginable in which to examine a patient.

It was only months later that I learned the results of a fascinating medical study that I would have loved to have adapted to Louis' situation. Researchers from Australia and Canada teamed up in an attempt to reduce the frequency of noise disruption produced by demented individuals in a hospital environment. They played baroque classical music to a small series of such disruptive patients. The results showed marked behavioral improvements.[176]

I know you're not dealing with issues as difficult as Louis', and I doubt you're presently generating the kind of decibels that risk a charge of "disturbing the peace." Nonetheless, anxiety may be disturbing your own peace. If so, there's good news.

A large body of research literature convincingly demonstrates the ability of music to affect our emotions.[177] Based on the characteristics of the music we listen to, we can induce anxiety-suppressing emotions like happiness and peacefulness, or we can exacerbate anxiety by stimulating emotions like sadness, anger, and fear.[178] One of the more comprehensive yet readable syntheses of this literature was recently provided by Neil Nedley, MD in his book, *The Lost Art of Thinking*. Nedley devotes a chapter to this topic, challenging readers in its title to "Choose Brain-boosting Music."[179] If you really want to begin plumbing the depths and nuances of music therapy, with a goal of improving brain performance and modulating your emotions, that chapter provides a valuable starting point.

Nonetheless, all of this may still seem a bit tangential to a discussion of high blood pressure. You may be following my logic, making the connections between anxiety and high blood pressure and then between the right kind of music and decreased stress. Yet you still may be wondering: if these connections really exist, shouldn't we then have direct evidence of the blood-pressure-lowering properties of music?

We do. Consider a recent example provided by researchers at Ramaiah Medical College in India.[180] These investigators used a three-month randomized controlled trial to look at the influence of traditional East Indian raga flute music on both blood pressure and the stress system. Their conclusion: "Passive listening to Indian music along with conventional lifestyle modifications has a role in normalizing BP through autonomic function modification and thus can be used as a complementary therapy along with other lifestyle modifications." In plain English, their research demonstrated that you could tone down the anxiety/stress arm of your nervous system and lower blood pressure by listening to music. What is especially compelling about their research was the relatively small time commitment involved: only fifteen minutes daily. Furthermore, the study demonstrates that different types of music from different cultural perspectives can favorably influence blood pressure (historically, published research on emotion-modulating music has been heavily skewed toward classical music[181]).

From this perspective, we can make a behavioral application. What music do you find calming, relaxing, or inspiring? Why not commit to fifteen minutes of listening to that music on a daily basis? Check your blood pressure before and after the activity to see if it seems to have any immediate impact. If your blood pressure consistently rises after listening to your preferred music, you may need to experiment with other musical genres. For example, as summarized by Nedley and others, baroque classical music has been associated with favorable emotional effects such as anxiety reduction. On the other hand, disharmonic rock music generally has negative effects.

Back to Our Lion

So far, we've entirely focused on the more passive stress management strategies identified in Figure 11.2; that is, hiding from a stressor, ignoring it, or playing dead. However, I promised you that we'd return to the topic of addressing our stressors, even the ones we fear the most. We're now there. Our first active strategy, however, the fourth on Figure 11.2's list, doesn't sound much better than its predecessors. Is "running or escaping" much different from hiding, ignoring a stressor, or playing dead? Yes; fundamentally it's superior, because by nature we're talking about an *active* approach. Doing something to limit your exposure to a stressor can be very healthy.

Imagine you've been dealing with an individual who is "a neighbor from hell," as articulated by one my patients, Bill. In this case, Bill was describing someone who lived on his same dirt road in rural Oklahoma. This man had the nasty habit of shooting his neighbors' pets with the slightest of provocations. But aren't there legal ways to hold someone like that accountable? Perhaps. Problem was—the nightmare neighbor was the local sheriff.

Put yourself in Bill's place. If you love your home, your community and everything about where you live, it's probably a foregone conclusion: You're staying put. If you're going to address the gun-slinging-neighbor stressor, it won't be by running. Maybe you'll call a local legislator. Or perhaps you'll do nothing, every day fearing that if one of your dogs gets out of your fenced-in yard, it will probably be the last time you see her.

However, suppose you're not all that enamored with the neighborhood; you've lived in the house only a few years, and it has appreciated considerably. Perhaps, too, you were laid off just a few weeks ago. Now, escaping from the stressor (selling your house and leaving the neighborhood) may sound like a viable and productive stress management strategy.

Do you catch the point? Sometimes running from a stressor is not cowardice but wisdom.

When Escaping Only Augments Stress

On the other hand, we sometimes try to escape from our stressors in ways that are counterproductive. The classic escape hatch has been alcohol, not a wise move. We've already seen that alcohol tends to raise blood pressure all by itself. Furthermore, alcohol works on your brain's frontal lobe, making you more likely to act impulsively, which will likely add to life's stressors.

Now, in many settings, alcohol has taken a back seat to marijuana. There is no question that cannabis has the potential to tone down anxiety.[182] So should we embrace marijuana as a viable stress management strategy? I think not, and at least for two main reasons.

The first is relatively simple. We need all our mental faculties if we want to optimally negotiate life's daily challenges. Realize those challenges involve not only the stressors that come at us but also our often counter-productive stress responses. Along these lines the medical literature has linked cannabis to a number of adverse chronic effects that can impair mental processing. In fact, authors of a 2015 review on the topic pointed out that despite cannabis' reputation as "harmless", there is now "cumulative evidence for its potentially damaging consequences."[183]

Some of the mental health problems associated with marijuana are summarized in Figure 11.4. Granted, all of the associations have not been proven causal. For example, just because rates of schizophrenia are significantly higher among cannabis users does not necessarily mean that the cannabis was the factor putting them at increased risk of that disorder. However, there is some evidence for causality in that association, as in all of the associations listed. In fact, the mental health "rap sheet" against marijuana is becoming so long that it is hard to see how any one concerned about optimal stress management—or optimal mental health in general—would touch the stuff.

The second reason is that it's simply bad for your blood pressure. The data indicates that a person who starts using marijuana increases her blood pressure and pulse, as well as increasing her risk of something called "orthostatic hypotension."[186] The latter term refers to the phenomenon of one's blood pressure dropping—often precipitously—when she stands up after lying down or sitting.

Marijuana advocates will tell you these effects tend to vanish over time with chronic use. Although this appears to be true, chronic use is setting you up for further blood pressure problems later. When a chronic cannabis user suddenly stops the behavior for any reason, he will typically see a dramatic rise in BP—on average over 22 points systolic and 12 points diastolic.[187]

Figure 11.4 Mental Health Problems Linked to Marijuana Use[184,185]

1 ▸ Memory impairments

2 ▸ Decreased attention span

3 ▸ Adverse effects on decision making

4 ▸ Impairments in complex reasoning

5 ▸ Schizophrenia and other psychotic disorders (conditions where a person loses touch with reality, typically hallucinating)

6 ▸ Atrophy of key brain regions including the thalamus, hippocampus, and amygdala

7 ▸ Increased risks of depression and suicidality

8 ▸ Perturbations of important neurotransmitters like dopamine

9 ▸ Decreased motivation and apathy

Why then all the "health" buzz about marijuana? There are some marijuana constituents that appear to have legitimate beneficial effects. One example is cannabidiol (CBD), a compound which, in isolation, may actually help certain mental health disorders.[188] Such constituents have led some educated marijuana users to believe the benefits are worth the risks. But, when it comes to optimizing blood pressure—and managing stress optimally—I would suggest that marijuana be avoided. If your health practitioner feels an isolated compound from cannabis might help you—without raising your blood pressure or adversely impacting your mental health— I'll leave that to your judgment.

Indeed, sometimes escaping from a stressor can be a sound stress management strategy; other times, it's not. I'll often give a thumbs up to leaving a psychologically destructive neighborhood, resigning from an overly stressful job, or ending a bad social relationship. However, using mind-altering substances to "escape" from stress is, usually, not a solution but a prescription for additional problems instead.

"Fighting" Your Stressors

Another active strategy for dealing with stressors is encompassed by the word "fight." Surprisingly, this is a rather common approach to stress management. Yet, if your rationale for "fighting" or "resisting" a stressor does not include a clear and rational plan to either remove the stressor or befriend it (options 6 and 7 in Figure 11.2), then that strategy is likely to be counterproductive.

Let's return to our lion. Imagine you decide to wrestle with that hungry carnivore. If you think, based on your past experience (perhaps you worked in the lion's den at a major zoo), you have a fighting chance of wrestling the lion into submission, then you might have come up with a winning strategy. But even if you do actually come out on top, you're still going to have to do something with that stressor of a lion. You'll either have to remove him from your home; or, if you're writing a movie script, the king of the jungle will become your subservient pet (since you established your dominance).

Do you get the picture? There's no value in fighting just to fight. If you beat the lion up a bit and leave him breathless in the corner, you can't just return to a leisurely reading of this book. That old lion is going to get his second wind, and you're likely to end up on his dinner plate.

As obvious as this might seem in dealing with a prowling predator, many of us completely miss this point when it comes to real life stressful situations. Ironically, one of the most common demonstrations of the "fighting" stress management strategy is seen in the display of anger or hostility.

Years ago, a common myth was perpetuated: If you feel anger, it is better to let those angry feelings out than keeping them "bottled up" inside. We now know this is not true, at least in most cases. The American Psychological Association recently crystalized the current evidence as follows: "Research has found that 'letting it rip' with anger actually escalates anger and aggression and does nothing to help you (or the person you're angry with) resolve the situation."[189]

On top of all this, hostility and the expression of anger have been linked to elevated blood pressure. Such a relationship was seen in the CARDIA Study (short for Coronary Artery Risk Development in Young Adults Study). CARDIA involved over 5000 black and white young men and women from four U.S. metropolitan areas. The subjects were between the ages of 18 and 30 when recruited in the mid-1980s. After following this population for about fifteen years, the researchers made an impressive discovery: the more hostility a person had, the greater his or her likelihood of developing high blood pressure.[190] As illustrated in Figure 11.5, when compared to those with the least hostility, individuals with the highest scores had over an 80% increased likelihood of developing hypertension.

What might all this look like in the real world? Simply put: whether or not you relate to the metaphor of fighting your stressors, we do generally want to confront them. But, remember—the goal is to either remove the stressor or change it from an enemy to a friend.

Let's go back to Bill and the animal-terrorizing sheriff in his neighborhood. Again, put yourself in Bill's place. Let's say you've decided not to move. We've already seen that ignoring the sheriff's behavior or trying to hide yourself (or your animals) from him will not really diffuse the stressor. Those solutions are just putting you on a path to chronic stress and anxiety.

Figure 11.5 Hostility and the Development of Hypertension in the CARDIA Study

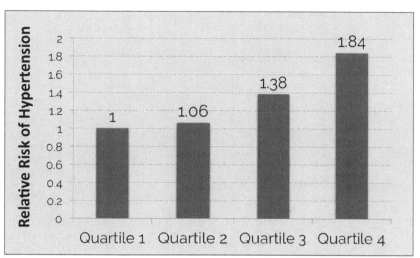

Study population stratified based on amount of hostility, with Quartile 1 representing the ¼ of the population with the lowest hostility scores.

However, there are some ways of "fighting" or "wrestling with" the stressor that may have a favorable outcome. For example, you could take legal action against the sheriff. Such a course may actually increase the tension in the neighborhood before it does anything to relieve it. Still, it is an example of trying to deal with the stressor in a way to mitigate it.

On the other hand, a poor example of fighting the stressor would be to literally get into a physical altercation. A shouting match may sound more civil, but whether a war of fists or a war of words, it is likely only to escalate emotions—and the stress. The physical option may well end you up in jail for assault; that is, if you don't end up in the hospital or someplace worse (after all, he *is* armed).

Removing a Stressor

Drip. Drip. Drip. The incessant drip of the master bedroom faucet was enough of a stressor to keep me from dozing off that night. I must have been awfully tired because I remember actually debating whether or not I should get up and remove the stressor. Finally I had enough. I rolled out of bed, stumbled into the bathroom, and turned the faucet a bit more in the clockwise direction. Now don't you wish all life's stressors were that easy to remove?

This point is of great importance. Many of our stressors are more amenable to removal than we realize.

Consider another scenario. Let's say you live in an apartment and just had a new neighbor move in. Although you haven't yet met, it becomes clear you're on different schedules. For the past week, every single morning you've been awakened two hours before your normal arising time by your neighbor's TV blaring CNN's Headline News.

Although this may offer you the excuse to move out of an apartment complex you really don't like, you may also have an opportunity to remove the stressor. True, you may dread confronting your neighbor, but just a friendly introduction may go a long way. Once you get talking you might make an observation that you've noticed he's on an early schedule. There's a real chance that, once he knows you can hear his TV, he'll actually turn the volume down enough so that you won't be bothered.

The message here is simple: don't avoid confronting stressors. Some can be removed more easily than we think.

Befriending Your Stressors

Because most stressors are perceived negatively, why would anyone want to make peace with, let alone befriend, them? Let's look at a practical example of a stressor that none of us can avoid, the clock.

We all relate to time pressures differently. However, some of us live under constant stress that we attribute to the clock. If you have a high sense of time urgency (a euphemistic term for "impatience"), then you're probably ramping up your blood pressure. Such an implication emerged from the aforementioned CARDIA study. The researchers administered a simple four-question quiz to participants as a means of measuring their sense of time urgency.[191] In Figure 11.6 I've adapted that quiz so you can take it right now.

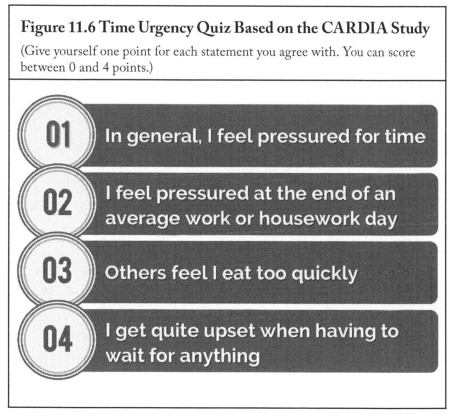

Figure 11.6 Time Urgency Quiz Based on the CARDIA Study
(Give yourself one point for each statement you agree with. You can score between 0 and 4 points.)

01 In general, I feel pressured for time

02 I feel pressured at the end of an average work or housework day

03 Others feel I eat too quickly

04 I get quite upset when having to wait for anything

Once you've determined your score, look at Figure 11.7. That graphic documents what the CARDIA researchers learned after following those young adults for over fifteen years. The long-term blood-pressure-raising effects of time urgency were unmistakable.

Imagine you're in a grocery store, waiting in a very slow moving line. If you tend to view such delays as stressors, is there any way you could look at this stressor in a different way, one in which it emerges as your friend?

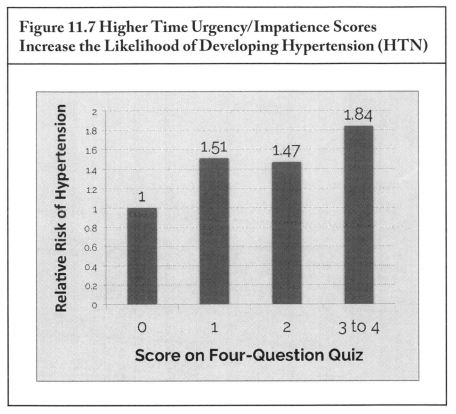

Figure 11.7 Higher Time Urgency/Impatience Scores Increase the Likelihood of Developing Hypertension (HTN)

For example, let's say you always wanted to learn Spanish. While in that grocery store line, you could pull out your Spanish phrase book (or, more likely, open the Spanish app on your smart phone) and begin learning. Your perception of waiting changes from a stress-inducing nuisance to an opportunity.

We can even befriend the sources of interpersonal stress. Years ago I had accepted a new position (and, for any of my colleagues reading this, it's not a setting where I now work). I found myself in a medical clinic where one of the medical assistants, who we'll call Herb, seemed to have a less than positive attitude toward my style of practice. Although Herb didn't directly report to me, and I didn't have hiring and firing authority over his position, he was working under me. Though in theory he was there to make my job easier, it seemed as if Herb served more to frustrate than to help me.

At the end of one busy clinic day, I had had enough. Although I could have lobbied the clinic manager to remove my stressor, I drove to a fairly secluded forest nearby and began walking and talking to God.

If that sounds strange, it would have sounded strange to me, as well, years ago. I didn't grow up thinking prayer had any special stress-relieving power. Over the years, however, prayer and meditation have become crucial tools in my stress management kit. (I'll talk more about spiritual strategies in this book's final chapter. The insights there should be of relevance, even if you label yourself an atheist or agnostic.)

But back to my story: a strange thing happened in that process of walking and praying. I don't know how it occurred, but somehow my attitude toward Herb began to change. I began to put myself in Herb's situation. Herb seemed like a person who liked to be in control. Now here I was, asking him to take on some new responsibilities that he probably didn't feel all that capable of dealing with.

As I thought more about Herb and his behavior, I started to wonder about his family life and how he ended up where he was today. I began to have more compassion for him, even though my cogitations were based largely on conjecture.

At the end of my walk, I vividly remember concluding, "God has put Herb in my life to be a special blessing." Don't ask me all I meant by that verdict. Perhaps I was reflecting on how dealing with Herb and his idiosyncrasies was going to build my character. Or, perhaps, I had decided our interaction was going to help me be more patient and kind to those who seemed to be asking only for retaliation!

Nevertheless, that was a turning point in our relationship. As I continued to work with Herb, we actually did become friends, close enough that he ultimately disclosed a number of very dark chapters in his past.

I relate that story for two reasons. First, we can actually befriend our stressors. But second, sometimes we're not changing the stressor so much as simply changing the way we relate to it.

The Serenity Prayer Revisited

Together we've taken a bit of a foray into the world of stressors and stress management. We've seen that failing to address life's stressors can be a major factor perpetuating anxiety and high blood pressure. At the same time, we've recognized that maladaptive ways of dealing with stressors like anger and hostility can also keep our BP numbers too high.

On the other hand, we've seen that constructively addressing our stressors may be more in the realm of possibility than we initially imagined. In essence we've really come back to the serenity prayer:

God grant me the serenity
to accept the things I cannot change;
courage to change the things I can;
and wisdom to know the difference.

There's one additional dimension to that prayer that we haven't addressed: the value of reaching out beyond ourselves. In essence, that serenity prayer points us to the last two options back in Figure 11.2: calling for help and praying.

Whether or not you can pray with the confidence of a Reinhold Niebuhr, knowing Someone is listening and will answer, you still can call out to other people for help. This is an incredibly important point. Stress and the problems that accompany it are some of the most difficult things we face. If this chapter has only brought things to the surface that you don't know how to address, consider talking with your physician, a mental health professional, or the leader of your faith community. If the hurdles seem too high to talk with a professional, share your concerns with a close friend or family member. And, by all means, if things look really bleak and you are thinking of harming yourself or someone else, pick up the phone and make a quick, toll-free call to the National Suicide Prevention Lifeline at 1-800-273-TALK (8255).

Your Turn

Yes, it's that time again. Have you already begun to formulate some behavioral goals as we navigated the troubled waters of stressors and stress? If not, now is the time to articulate what stressors you need to change. If you've identified some problem areas, but still don't know where to start, let me recommend David Allen's *Getting Things Done*. That book can provide insights, complementary to this chapter, that can—through better organization and time management—help you decrease your stress load and make progress toward stress-related goals.

Behavioral goals for stress management don't, necessarily, take the form of things you do on a daily basis. Therefore, let's take a few minutes to look at the examples on the draft worksheet. First, consider *Example 1*. Talking to your boss about a specific work-related issue may require only a one-time discussion, and your boss may actually remove that stressor. By the way, this is often the case with interpersonal stressors you have heretofore failed to address. If your goal is something that a single discussion solves, then just put a check under the day when you actually addressed the issue and draw a horizontal line through all the subsequent boxes. However, there are other interpersonal issues where you will have to repeatedly address the issue. It may not be appropriate to resurrect the topic on a daily basis. Nonetheless, on any day when you are thinking or praying about how and when to introduce (or reintroduce) the subject, then check the respective box.

Now let's look at *Example 2*. This is similar to a scenario I painted in discussing the general stressor of time. This example is straightforward. Simply check off any day that you are either making or using the flashcards.

Finally, move to *Example 3*. In this case, you could check a box on any day you don't complain about your current residence and/or state positive affirmations about it. One example of a positive affirmation could be: "I am so glad to be living in a quiet place outside of the city" (even if you're tempted to complain about your long commute). An affirmation on the other end of the spectrum might be: "I'm so glad that I can walk to work—it's saving me money and I'm getting exercise" (particularly if you are tempted to complain about how you live in such a noisy and busy venue in close proximity to so much industry).

Chapter 11 Stress – Draft Worksheet

		Week 1							Week 2						
Day #	1	2	3	4	5	6	7	8	9	10	11	12	13	14
Behavioral Goals														
Example 1: Talk to my boss about _____ _____ (Something in your workplace— be specific— that is stressing you and seems to be impairing your productivity.)														
Example 2: Make and carry German vocabulary flash cards with me, so I can resurrect a language I studied in college during times when I would normally be impatiently waiting (e.g., long lines at a stop light or at a grocery store checkout).														
Example 3: Realizing I can't move from my present residence at this time, I choose to make the best of it by stating positive affirmations rather than complaining about it. I'll take five minutes daily to write down five things about my present situation for which I'm thankful.														
My Goal 11:1														
My Goal 11:2														
My Goal 11:3														
My Goal 11:4														
My Goal 11:5														

12

USE OF NATURAL ADJUNCTS: HERBS AND SUPPLEMENTS AS BP AIDS

ON THAT PARTICULAR SUNDAY, large numbers from the community showed up at the school gymnasium. No one seemed particularly surprised by the impressive turnout. After all, how many times has a major teaching hospital sent a cadre of health professionals to conduct a health screening in your local elementary school?

A senior medical student at the time, I was in attendance both to assist and to observe. It was the latter role that left the only lasting impression from the event. It was the heart screening station that provided the backdrop for the most fascinating drama of the day.

Physicians were actually performing cardiac stress testing. I know that terminology is familiar to most of you. But, for the uninitiated, imagine people lining up to walk on a treadmill. Participants are wired up so their hearts' electrical activity can be monitored as the treadmill incrementally increases in speed and grade every three minutes.

Since I've mentioned drama, perhaps you are already anticipating a cardiac catastrophe? However, nothing like that occurred. What captured my attention was George, a man in his early 40s who looked quite fit. That was, until he climbed onto the treadmill.

George was clearly the worst performer of the day. He couldn't tolerate that treadmill for long at all. I was especially struck because a woman in her 70s had turned in an impressive performance shortly before he did the test.

Despite all that, none of these details are what engrained the experience in my mind. It was George's reaction to the doctor's evaluation of his poor test. George sat there in disbelief. He was shaking his head saying, "But I take so many nutritional supplements. How could I not be in good health?"

The Ultimate Natural Blood Pressure Therapy?

There's little question: most patients seem to think the ultimate *natural* blood pressure strategy must involve popping pills obtained from a health food store or an on-line vendor. This is a false assumption, according to both the research literature and my years of medical experience.

Over the years I've witnessed many individuals trying to cut corners. Lifestyle therapies seem so cumbersome compared to resorting to a "natural" pill. Yet I've not seen a single supplement—or group of them—that has even a fraction of the power to reverse disease as do the lifestyle strategies that we've covered so far. Furthermore, "natural" pills are not necessarily superior to medications. In other words, if you're really serious about natural control of your blood pressure, don't think you can chuck the rest of this book and merely add a few of the supplements advocated in this chapter.

With that disclaimer, I admit that I have prescribed many supplements over the years. However, in light of what I just noted, it's worth relating principles to aid you in choosing supplements.

240

Figure 12.1 lists characteristics of the best supplements. These guidelines help identify compounds that not only offer intrinsic benefit but also make it *more* likely you will take lifestyle changes seriously.

Figure 12.1 Characteristics of an Ideal Supplement

- Directly impacts the pathophysiology of the disease process (i.e., in the case of high blood pressure, the supplement would have a known mechanism of action that addresses one or more blood-pressure-raising factors).
- Offers adjunctive effects that further enhance health (a supplement that also lowers cholesterol and blood sugar, for example, in addition to providing blood pressure benefits).
- Has other beneficial "side effects" that enhance the likelihood of achieving lifestyle goals (e.g., a supplement that has an additional effect of helping curb appetite, if you are an overweight overeater).
- Is non-toxic and doesn't interact with other medications you're using.
- Actually contains the product that it claims to contain.
- Is free of harmful contaminants such as lead or arsenic.

The details in Figure 12.1 may seem but an articulation of common sense. However, many of these points are lost on the supplement-seeking public. Two of the latter points are particularly challenging ones for many people. It's hard to believe that something natural could be harmful. However, even "natural therapies" can have potentially serious side-effects.

Some of the most dangerous side-effects relate to how

certain natural therapies may interact with prescribed medications. Researchers Izzo and Ernst found significant interactions between prescribed drugs and five of what were then the seven top-selling herbal medicines (ginkgo, St John's wort, ginseng, garlic, and kava).[192] Such interactions can be especially dangerous if you are taking drugs with a "narrow therapeutic window."

"The Therapeutic Window"?

This designation applies to the window or opening where a drug has desirable effects. Taking a dose below that open window renders the drug ineffective; taking a larger dose above the window renders it toxic where actual damage occurs. Medications with a narrow therapeutic window thus have relatively little space between their range of effectiveness and toxicity.

Figure 12.2 graphically illustrates the concept of the therapeutic window. You will notice that the "clear" or white area in both illustrations represents the "open window." In Figure 12.2A that open window is very narrow. In other words, any perturbation of the metabolism or dose of that medication could easily push drug levels into the range of ineffectiveness, or even toxicity. Taking any supplement—especially if you are unaware of its interactions with all your prescription drugs—could be dangerous. On the other hand, Figure 12.2B shows a different medication, this time with a very wide therapeutic window. In this case, major changes would have to occur in a person's metabolism or the dose ingested before the drug levels became either toxic or ineffective. Therefore, it is unlikely in scenario B that a supplement would push a prescription drug out of the acceptable range.

This is important because the addition of herbal preparations or other supplements can affect the metabolism of, or otherwise interact with, prescribed medications. For a drug with a narrow therapeutic window like warfarin (a common blood thinner), problems can occur quickly. For example, take a supplement that slows the metabolism of warfarin, and the warfarin will have a longer and more powerful effect on your body, potentially putting you at risk for serious bleeding problems. On the other hand, if your supplement stimulates metabolic processes that degrade immunosuppressive drugs, your blood level of those protective medications may plummet. As a result, if you are living with a transplanted kidney, your body may reject the organ.

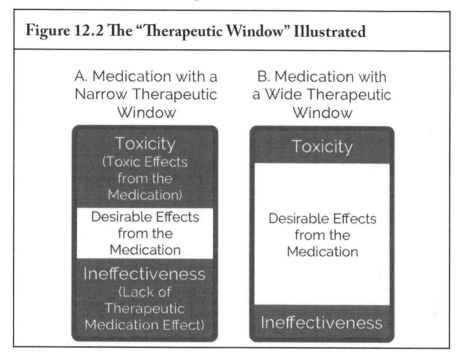

Figure 12.2 The "Therapeutic Window" Illustrated

A. Medication with a Narrow Therapeutic Window

B. Medication with a Wide Therapeutic Window

Toxicity (Toxic Effects from the Medication)

Desirable Effects from the Medication

Ineffectiveness (Lack of Therapeutic Medication Effect)

Toxicity

Desirable Effects from the Medication

Ineffectiveness

Another example of a class of drugs with a narrow therapeutic window is those used to fight AIDS or HIV infection. Innocently popping some supplements can interfere with the actions of these medications and allow HIV infection to gain the upper hand.

These are not mere theoretical considerations. The medical literature has documented cases just like the ones I've presented. Thus, if on any prescription medication, check with your doctor to ensure one or more supplements will not move you onto dangerous ground.

Assessing Blood-Pressure-Lowering Supplements

So let's assume you're not on any medications, or that your doctor and/or pharmacist has given you the green light to at least consider one or more supplements in light of the other medications you're using. (No doubt they'll want to know exactly what supplements you ultimately hope to utilize; that way they can check for any specific interactions with medications you've been prescribed). The question remains: How do you sleuth out the best supplements for you *personally*? Who is going to help you decide whether or not the criteria presented in Figure 12.1 are fulfilled by any specific supplement?

You're not likely to find the answer in the average health food store or internet site that caters to the "naturally minded." Those venues and the resources they provide will generally bombard you with information promoting their supplements. The supplement bottles and boxes that hold them will typically contain carefully worded statements, like "helps support healthy blood pressure," to keep them out of the FDA's purview.

Let me suggest a different strategy. Why not gain some insight into optimal hypertension-relieving supplements by looking first at the ones that serious medicine practitioners are employing?

Top Hypertension Supplements Used By Natural Practitioners

In 2011, Dr. Ryan Bradley and colleagues looked at the prescribing practices of doctors at one of our nation's premier naturopathic institutions, Seattle's Bastyr University.[193] A number of supplements were frequently recommended for hypertension. Figure 12.3 illustrates what they were.

Several years earlier, Richard Nahas, MD had reviewed the medical literature looking for promising complementary and alternative therapies for hypertension. He also was impressed with one of the Seattle-based naturopathic physicians' most frequently prescribed agents, Coenzyme Q10. In addition, Nahas found support for the blood-pressure-lowering properties of vitamin D (in those who are deficient) as well as melatonin.[194]

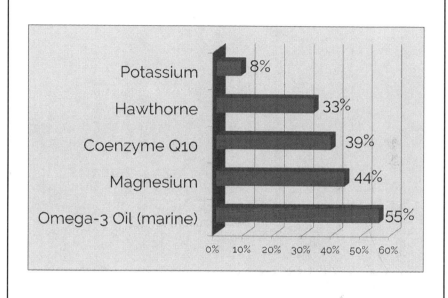

Figure 12.3 Bastyr Center for Natural Health, Prescribing Practices: Percent of Patients Recommended Various Supplements for Hypertension

Potassium — 8%
Hawthorne — 33%
Coenzyme Q10 — 39%
Magnesium — 44%
Omega-3 Oil (marine) — 55%

0% 10% 20% 30% 40% 50% 60%

More recently, Cesare R. Sirtori, MD, PhD and his colleagues published an article entitled "Nutraceuticals for blood pressure control."[195] This Italian team generated a list of supplements where "a very large body of evidence supports" their use in blood pressure lowering. That list contains a number of, by now, familiar agents: potassium, vitamin D, coenzyme Q10, and controlled-release melatonin. Their list also contained other agents that we haven't yet mentioned. Among the most promising from my vantage point: beetroot juice, some probiotics, and aged garlic extract.

What is remarkable is many of these agents have already surfaced on our journey to that goal of drug-free blood pressure control. Interestingly, we've seen that we can optimize our intake of many of these "supplements" without taking a single pill. We can get an abundance of potassium and magnesium from a whole plant foods diet. Vitamin D can be obtained from adequate sun exposure. And if we follow the simple natural practices, like those recommended by Dr. Nedley in Chapter 9, our bodies can make their own melatonin. Perhaps this gives you some further insight into why I said earlier that "I've not seen a single supplement—or group of them—that has even a fraction of the power to reverse disease as do the lifestyle strategies we've covered up to this point." At best, many of these supplements are supplying only a portion of the benefits that the lifestyle practices afford.

In the U.S., supplements are designated legally as GRAS (Generally Regarded As Safe) and have no regulatory oversight to verify the legitimacy of their constituents. As a result, despite the presence of numerous high-quality supplement companies, a number of charlatans have arisen, peddling placebos bearing the name of any number of well-known supplements. To combat this problem, independent laboratories have taken on a necessary oversight role. One such entity is Consumer Lab (at www.consumerlab.com) who, for a reasonably-priced subscription service, provides evaluation and testing of product potency, label accuracy and contaminant presence on a variety of the most common supplements. They also issue stamps of approval on products that consumers can use to verify quality. If you're considering a particular brand of supplement but are unsure of its quality, consider looking up the brand at an independent laboratory such as consumerlab.com.

A Rational Approach to Blood Pressure Supplements?

Several years ago I was giving a lecture series on natural strategies for hypertension. I was working my way through the *No Pressure* acronym over the course of three evenings. After the first evening a gentleman, whom I'll call Tyler, said this: "Doc, I'm doing all the stuff you're recommending but my blood pressure is still too high." Perhaps he really was already following all my recommendations on diet, beverages, and physical exercise (I'm not sure we had covered much more than those three topics at the time of his query). However, Tyler was quite interested in what supplements could be used to give his blood pressure a further nudge downward. Those sentiments are normal, and I applaud them.

Yet I want to emphasize something. Don't get overly enamored about what is to follow unless you've been quite serious about all the other elements I've presented to this point. Even natural compounds have side-effects, and in general supplements don't come close to the power of comprehensive lifestyle changes.

With that caveat, I do admit that there is some encouraging evidence with regard to some supplements. Yet one other problem remains. Every list I've mentioned—and there are plenty of other lists generated by other authors—is different. What should we do? Should we attempt to come up with the top 25 supplements and begin taking each one tomorrow, or would we be better off focusing on one or two supplements and going from there?

I cast my vote, decidedly, with the latter option. The more supplements you start with, the more difficult the process will be down the road. For example, let's say you add ten supplements tomorrow. (Whether you chose ten different supplements all packaged in separate pills or whether some entrepreneur bundled them into a single capsule or two is immaterial, as you'll soon see.) If within a month, your BP drops ten points systolic and eight points diastolic, you'll likely be elated. However, before long you'll be asking: "How long do I have to continue all these supplements?" If you asked me, "Can I eliminate one or more of these agents and still retain the benefits?" I would tell you frankly: "The answer very likely is 'yes,' but because you started them all at the same time, there's no telling which are the efficacious ones."

Worse, let's say within a week of starting the ten supplements you develop an itchy skin rash. That's right, you've come down with an allergic reaction. Now, you've got real problems. You have no idea to what you're allergic. It could be due to any one (or more) of those ten agents, not to mention any fillers or ingredients that they might be packaged with. Safety will argue for avoiding all ten agents when, odds are, only one is the culprit. In other words, you'll likely have crossed nine perfectly good supplements off your list for initial consideration.

For similar reasons I recommend avoiding multiple-agent proprietary supplements. They usually have names like "Dr. Elias Jones' Amazing Ultra High Potency Formulation." They'll skirt the law by *not* claiming on the pill bottle that it's a "blood pressure remedy," but there will be plenty of easily accessible information telling you how the twenty nutrients in each pill were specially selected by this amazing researcher. (And don't be a bit surprised if some conspiracy innuendos find their way into print, something like: *The FDA and pharmaceutical industry ordered a hit man to kill Dr. Jones, knowing that if his remedy got out to the public, all sales of antihypertensive medications would come to a screeching halt.*)

Maybe this sounds cynical, but I've had enough patients get bamboozled over the years that it's easy for me to get pretty impassioned about this topic. In fairness, some reputable scientists and companies do put multiple agents into one pill. However, remember, take multiple agents—whether they're in one pill or in multiple pills—and you've got at least two big problems: First, if the supplement works, you don't know which agents in the pill were helping you; second, if you experience a side effect, then you've lost ground in your quest for effective natural agents. Let me add a couple other concerns with those proprietary formulations: they typically cost a lot more than taking a single nutrient or two; and, even if the supplement gives you benefits, you may have received even more benefit from taking the one or two agents in that proprietary blend that are really helping you, and not diluting them with eight other compounds that aren't benefitting you a whit.

Where Then Do We Start?

If you're going to choose a supplement or two to add to your lifestyle regimen, which should you choose? A reasonable place to start is with supplements that keep surfacing in multiple independent reviews. This makes our starting point quite easy. After all, only one agent found its way onto all three lists we've looked at thus far (those compiled by Drs. Sirtori, Nahas and the Bastyr practitioners). That agent is Coenzyme Q10. So if you're already thinking this agent probably has some legitimate blood-pressure-lowering power, then you're exactly right, as we'll see momentarily.

The Blood Pressure Lowering Promise of Coenzyme Q10

Coenzyme Q10 (often abbreviated CoQ10) is an important molecule in cellular energy processes. It is also called ubiquinone, because it belongs to a family of organic molecules known as quinones and it is *ubi*quitous (found virtually everywhere) in biological systems. For some time, CoQ10 has been the subject of interest along blood pressure lines. This interest has resulted in a number of scientific studies, some of which were collectively reviewed in 2007.[196] A meta-analysis (pooling of studies) at that time encompassed 12 clinical trials with 362 patients. As illustrated by Figure 12.4, the data was impressive, even in the most carefully designed studies.

Randomized controlled trials (RCTs) are considered the "gold standard" in clinical research studies. In these experiments, typically neither the subjects nor those doing the study are aware of who is getting the active treatment and who is getting a placebo (the so-called "double blind" study). Note in Figure 12.4 the results in the RCTs are almost identical to the open label studies (where both patients and investigators know who is getting the treatment, in this case, CoQ10). The numbers are remarkable, with drops in the range of 15 points systolic and 8-10 points diastolic.

In the face of such promising data, other questions typically arise. One has to do with safety of the supplement. The investigators looked at the twelve studies to answer this question. They found either no or minimal side effects. However, eight of the studies made no remarks about side effects. In the four that did comment on side effects, two reported them to be absent. The other two raised concerns about intestinal issues such as nausea or flatulence, in a minority of patients.

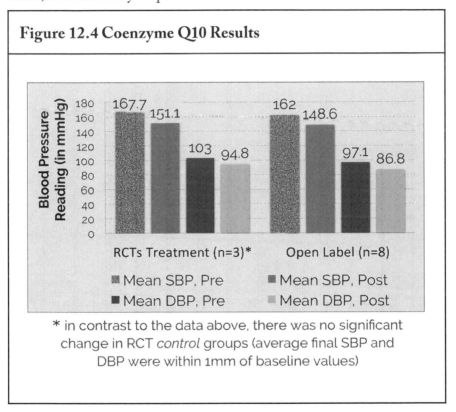

Figure 12.4 Coenzyme Q10 Results

* in contrast to the data above, there was no significant change in RCT *control* groups (average final SBP and DBP were within 1mm of baseline values)

Based on data like this, CoQ10 seems to be quite safe and potentially helpful when it comes to lowering blood pressure. It is one of the supplements that I recommend patients consider.

Yet there's one other important question to answer before rushing out to your nearest drugstore or health food store: How much CoQ10 should I take? That's a bit more difficult to answer. In the twelve studies mentioned, dosages ranged from 34 mg/day to 225 mg per day. Based on their extensive review of CoQ10 (over 600 scientific references cited), the well-respected *Natural Medicines Comprehensive Database* recommends a dosage of between 60 and 100 mg taken twice per day (for a total daily dosage of 120 to 200 mg).[197] Yet, there's one other wrinkle to this discussion: Coenzyme Q10 is not well absorbed. The well-absorbed version of CoQ10 is called ubiquinol. In my experience 60 to 100 mg of ubiquinol is an adequate daily dose for most patients whereas 300 to 400 mg of Coenzyme Q10 is often needed due to its poorer absorption.

More Options from Drug Stores and Health Food Stores

As we look for some other candidates to add to a blood pressure-lowering regimen, let's revisit Figure 12.1. The second and third points in that figure are related. They stress the value of choosing supplements that have additive benefits. Look at it this way: Why not choose something that will help you on other fronts even if it doesn't deliver on its pressure-lowering promises?

With that in mind, I'd like to move two rather humble candidates to the fore: magnesium and omega-3 fats. Both agents have an impressive resume when it comes to health benefits in addition to having a good track record for safety (except in some unusual contexts that I'll mention later).

The Magnesium Story

Figure 12.5 summarizes insights about magnesium gleaned from the U.S. Department of Health and Human Services' Office of Dietary Supplements.[198]

Blood pressure lowering has also been documented in research on magnesium (chemically abbreviated simply Mg). In 2012, Lindsy Kass and colleagues at the University of Hertfordshire, United Kingdom, published an exhaustive review of all the studies to date exploring magnesium supplementation and blood pressure.[199] They found evidence that supplementation decreased systolic blood pressure an average of

3-4 points and diastolic BP 2-3 points. Results appeared best when individuals were taking at least 370 mg of elemental Mg daily.

Figure 12.5 Selected Aspects of Magnesium's Health Resume

1. Necessary for more than 300 enzyme systems in the human body.

2. Can help prevent migraine headaches.

3. Higher intake associated with lower risk of heart disease and sudden death.

4. Increased consumption appears to decrease risk of developing diabetes.

5. May decrease risk of osteoporosis.

6. Plays a key role in nerve conduction, muscle contraction and heart rhythm control.

More recently, Kass teamed up with Filipe Poeira to demonstrate that magnesium supplementation even exerted blood-pressure-lowering effects among healthy, fit individuals who were ingesting adequate amounts of dietary magnesium.[200] An additional finding of their research was evidence for increased athletic strength performance.

Based on the data available, I recommend individuals seeking to lower their blood pressure give consideration to magnesium supplementation. I generally recommend a goal of at least 300 mg of elemental magnesium daily.

Since I'm mentioning dosages, some explanations are in order. You will notice I keep prefixing magnesium dosages with the term "elemental." The reason for this is that Mg always comes "partnered" with another compound, just as the sodium we ingest typically is linked to chloride. Consequently, when you see a "per capsule" dosage on a magnesium oxide supplement, you are looking at the contribution not only from magnesium but also from the oxide component. For example, in this case, 500 mg of magnesium oxide equals 300 mg of elemental magnesium.[201] There are many readily accessible sources of magnesium. For example, one tablespoon of Phillips' Milk of Magnesia® delivers 500 mg of elemental magnesium (in the form of magnesium hydroxide).

The mention of Milk of Magnesia highlights another one of magnesium's uses: It is a reliable laxative. In fact, unless you have kidney problems, there is little danger of serious magnesium toxicity. If you get too much magnesium, you'll have looser stools, with the excess Mg exiting your system. Hardly reassuring? Well, for most people, an extra 300 mg daily will not likely have significant intestinal ramifications.

Special Magnesium Considerations

Individuals who take diuretics for their blood pressure already may be dealing with magnesium deficiency. Diuretics tend to cause the loss of both potassium and magnesium. Another class of medications linked to Mg deficits are the powerful acid blocking drugs known as PPIs (proton pump inhibitors). If you use an "industrial strength" acid-blocking drug like omeprazole, or one of its cousins (their generic names typically end in "prazole"), then you are at risk for magnesium deficiency. In cases like this, Mg supplementation may be particularly valuable.

There are potential dangers on the magnesium front. The worst occur in individuals with impaired kidney function. In these cases, magnesium can build up to dangerous levels, causing weakness, fatigue and even death. Never take a magnesium supplement on your own unless you are sure you have normal kidney function.

You can also get into trouble if you take supplemental Mg in close proximity to certain prescription medications. Magnesium can interfere with the absorption of drugs, including certain anti-biotics, and medications used to treat osteoporosis (e.g., alendro-nate sold as Fosamax®). Most of these problems can be avoided by taking the prescription drug at least two hours before ingesting the Mg. The safest course, however, is to check with your pharmacist.

Before you begin supplementing with magnesium or any of the agents in this chapter, I recommend consulting with your phy-sician. Prior to that visit, you may want to review the previously cited *Magnesium Fact Sheet for Health Professionals*, prepared by the Office of Dietary Supplements. For example, it includes a more comprehensive review of the special magnesium considerations I've covered in this section. An easy-reading fact sheet is also available on the referenced website.

Omega-3 Fats for Blood Pressure Relief?

We've all heard the aphorism, "You are what you eat." However, does that succinct statement really ring true? The answer, at least in many respects is, "Yes." After all, other than the time you spent in your mother's womb, every cell in your body is directly composed of nutrients and other compounds that you ate, drank, or breathed. So, in a very real sense, our dietary choices affect the structure of our bodies.

Perhaps nowhere is this seen as clearly as when we look at the membrane surrounding each cell. Those cell membranes are com-posed largely of fat. And, if you're following my logic, the type and kinds of fat you eat directly affect those cell membranes. Part of the reason for this hinges on a simple biochemistry fact: The more flex-ible your cell membranes, the healthier you tend to be. For exam-ple, when membranes are more flexible, cells respond better to vital chemical messengers like insulin, dopamine, and serotonin.[202]

Some fats predispose to rigid cell membranes; others help those membranes remain more flexible. Which fats foster healthy, flexible cell membranes?

High fat foods that come directly or indirectly from animals tend to be solid at room temperature. Butter, cheese, the marbleized fat in meat, all tend to be solid at the prevailing temperatures in grocery stores, homes, and—for that matter—our bodies. These fats typically are made of predominantly saturated fats. On a microscopic structural level, saturated fats are largely straight molecules that stack very tightly. It is this characteristic that renders them more solid at room temperature, and contributes to more rigid cell membranes in your body. To give a crude illustration, think of stacking up 1000 wooden Popsicle sticks. Those straight pieces of wood will tend to form a quite stable or rigid structure.

On the other hand, if you isolate the fats from plant sources of nutrition, such as extracting the fat from an olive (olive oil) or the fat found in corn kernels (corn oil), you typically end up with a liquid fat. These unsaturated fats are made of fatty acids that don't stack well, rendering them more liquid at body and room temperatures. If saturated fats could be thought of as straight Popsicle sticks, polyunsaturated fats could be envisioned as branching tree twigs. Stack up 1000 such twigs and—even if each one has the same volume as a Popsicle stick—you're going to end up with a far less rigid structure. (If you're wondering, the villainous "trans" fats, made when polyunsaturated fats are partially hydrogenated, tend to resemble the saturated fats. They too predispose to rigid cell membranes.)

I've taken some time to try to give you a visual picture of the difference between the largely straight saturated fats and the more kinked polyunsaturated fats. My motive is simple: I want those of you who don't have much chemistry background to better understand a major reason *why* saturated fats tend to be unhealthy and unsaturated fats healthy.

The so-called omega-3 fats are a special type of unsaturated fat. Don't let the "omega-3" confuse you. It is simply a chemical designation as to where the first molecular kink in these non-rigid fats occurs. Omega-3 fats appear to have unique benefits. Some of those benefits have been appreciated by the medical community for many years; others are only now emerging. Figure 12.6 lists some of their documented benefits.[203,204]

Figure 12.6 Selected Health Advantages of Consuming More Omega-3 Fats

1. Decreased risk of heart-related death and cardiac events including heart attacks.

2. Lower levels of blood triglycerides (a harmful blood fat).

3. Decreased blood pressure.

4. Reduced joint pain and decreased need for anti-inflammatory medications in individuals with rheumatoid arthritis.

5. Possible decreased risk of Alzheimer's and other dementias.

6. Improvements in mood and decreased risk of depression.

Research Supporting Omega-3 Fats for Hypertension

The research on omega-3 fats and blood pressure lowering is similar to that seen with other natural therapies. Namely, eating more of these polyunsaturated fats may have a small to moderate benefit when it comes to blood pressure. However, emerging research suggests some individuals may stand to gain much more than others when it comes to such dietary- or supplement-based interventions.

Consider a recently published study from Sweden. Researchers based at Lund University and the University Hospital of Malmö found that individuals with certain genetic profiles appeared to benefit significantly from increasing omega-3 fat consumption, while others with different genetics did not.[205]

The practical applications emerging from the literature when it comes to omega-3 fats thus transcend the subject of dietary fat intake. However, the bottom line brings us back to the potential value of omega-3 fats as dietary supplements:

1. Certain natural strategies that may not appear all that promising in general may have profound benefits in specific individuals.

2. Until genetic testing—and an understanding of various variants—is widely available, trying an intervention like increasing omega-3 fat intake may make sense for many individuals with high blood pressure, even if that intervention only ends up significantly benefitting a percentage of people.

My Recommendations

Ample evidence argues for each of us optimizing his or her omega-3 fat intake. The big question remains, though: What is the best way to accomplish this goal? I've provided some recommendations in Figure 12.7.

Let me explain why I've come to the conclusions articulated in Figure 12.7. First, in my estimation, dietary sources of any nutrient are always ideal. When you eat a whole food rich in a particular constituent, you generally obtain benefits that transcend any individual constituent. For example, some of the most recent data suggest heart preventive benefits accrue only from food sources of omega-3 fat, not supplements.[206]

Second, when it comes to choosing a source for your omega-3 fat intake, fish don't rise to the top of my list. More and more studies are raising concerns about toxic exposures linked to fish consumption. Although special concerns are usually voiced regarding the most vulnerable populations, like pregnant women and young children, who needs more exposure to toxins like mercury or PCBs?[207,208] No fish on the planet make omega-3 fats. These valuable polyunsaturated fats are produced only by land plants and related sea-dwelling "plants," such as phytoplankton.[209] Therefore, why not get your omega-3 fats from plants?

Figure 12.7 Recommendations Regarding Omega-3 Fat Intake

1. Prioritize dietary sources of omega-3 fats over supplements.

2. De-emphasize fish consumption; globally we don't have enough fish to sustainably meet the omega-3 requirements of the world population.

3. Also beware of toxin exposure associated with fish consumption.

4. Keep omega-3 fat sources refrigerated.

5. If you must take a supplement, consider a liquid source rather than an encapsulated one.

Some of you may have heard that the omega-3 fats from land plant sources are "short chain" and those from marine sources are "long chain." If you don't have much of a chemistry background, you may not realize how small the differences really are. Would you call a train a "short train" if it only had 18 cars? Perhaps. If so, I doubt you would call trains with 20 and 22 cars "long." However, this is exactly the amount of difference we are talking about. The main plant omega-3 fat is called alpha linolenic acid (ALA). It is made up of a chain of 18 carbon molecules. The fish omega-3 fats, eicosapentaenoic acid (EPA) and docosahexaenoic acid (DHA), are made of chains with 20 and 22 carbons respectively. Furthermore, your body can convert ALA into EPA. Although the conversion is often criticized as not being very "efficient," a diet abundant in omega-3-rich plants can significantly raise your body's levels of longer chain omega-3 fats. The data indicate this plant-driven rise of EPA and DHA can even exceed that obtained by eating many fish species. Figure 12.8 provides data on the relationships between plant and fish omega-3 fat sources.

Let's interact with Figure 12.8 by drawing some comparisons. If you eat three times daily and have either one tablespoon of flaxseed oil or 1.5 ounces of chia seeds with each meal, you would be eating over 20,000 mg of ALA each day. Even with only a 5% conversion to long chain omega-3 fats,[211] this would still give you 1000 mg daily or 7000 mg per week. This compares favorably with the roughly 5000 mg of long chain fatty acids obtained by eating fish twice weekly (a common recommendation). However, even this favorable comparison does not fully address the issue. Because many experts now believe that some of the cardiovascular benefits of ALA may be similar to those offered by EPA and DHA, you may be getting far more benefit from the flax and chia than if you were eating fish occasionally.

One study suggesting benefits from ALA (without direct consideration of DHA or EPA) was published in 2011 by a Netherlands research team. The Dutch researchers identified low alpha linolenic acid intake as a significant risk factor for stroke, with those in the lowest 20% of intake increasing their stroke risk between 50 and 100%.[212] Data like this led a recent review team to conclude: "The epidemiologic evidence suggests comparable benefits of plant-based and marine-derived n-3 (omega-3) PUFAs... the evidence suggests many comparable CVD [cardiovascular disease] benefits of ALA vs. EPA + DHA."[213]

Figure 12.8 Top Plant and Fish Omega-3 Fat Sources[210]

FOOD	SERVING SIZE	ALA**	EPA	DHA
Flaxseed oil	1 Tablespoon	7258 mg	0 mg	0 mg
Chia seeds, dried	1 ounce (28.35 grams)	5055 mg	0 mg	0 mg
Black walnuts, dried	1 cup	3346 mg	0 mg	0 mg
Flaxseed, ground	1 Tablespoon	1597 mg	0 mg	0 mg
Salted mackerel*†	100 grams (approx. 3.5 oz)	159 mg	1619 mg	2965 mg
Pacific herring* (cooked with dry heat)	100 grams (approx. ¾ cup)	73 mg	1242 mg	883 mg
Alaskan Native Sockeye salmon† (smoked filets with skin)	100 grams	130 mg	905 mg	1520 mg
Most other fish	100 grams	< 60 mg	< 1000 mg	<1500 mg

* the two highest fish sources of EPA in the USDA database (excluding fish oil and caviar/roe)
† the two highest fish sources of DHA in the USDA database (excluding fish oil and caviar/roe)
** Content of ALA in the fish sources and in the ground flax may be falsely elevated by the inclusion of polyunsaturated fats with 18 carbons that are not in the omega-3 family

Fishing for Trouble?

I'm very supportive of fish consumption by maritime subsistence economies. Some of the most ecological, sustainable cultures have been based on fish, whether they be coastal Native Americans, Native Alaskans, Coastal Mediterranean Europeans, Pacific Islanders or members of a variety of other cultures.

However, recommendations to eat more fish can threaten such robust ecological cultures by depleting world fish stocks. For example, approximately 30% of the world's fish stocks are being fished at biologically unsustainable levels.[214] Put simply, if consumption even continues at present levels, many species are on a path to extinction. The fish on the depleted stocks list include Atlantic cod, Atlantic salmon, Haddock, Southern Bluefin Tuna and over two dozen other varieties.[215] Clearly, we cannot continue to depend on fish to meet our omega-3 fat requirements.

Unstable Omega-3s

The same chemical characteristics of omega-3 fats that render them ideal for your cell membranes also predispose them to oxidation. Expressed another way, omega-3 fats are prone to go rancid, especially if exposed to air and left at room temperature. For this reason, I make two recommendations. First, refrigerate any omega-3 supplements or sources; second, take your omega-3 fats in liquid form.

The rationale for this last recommendation includes the following: Rancid omega-3 fats have a distinctive taste. Therefore, ingesting, for example, plain flax seed oil (rather than flaxseed oil in a capsule) will allow you to taste whether or not rancidity has set in. Theoretically this may sound like a great idea, but many of you are likely saying: "This doesn't help me; I don't know how to identify that distinctive taste of rancid omega-3 fat."

Actually, I bet you do. Rancid omega-3 fat is what imparts that "fishy" taste to fish. That's right. A really fresh fish with no appreciable rancid omega-3 fats will not have a fishy taste. (By the way, liquid omega-3 sources should also cost you less than the encapsulated forms.)

So How Much Omega-3 Fat Should I Use?

Organizations like the American Heart Association (AHA)

have seen the benefits of ingesting more omega-3 fats. However, many have not yet incorporated recommendations that transcend fish consumption. For example, the AHA currently recommends "eating fish (particularly fatty fish) at least two times (two servings) a week."[216] They explain that the serving size that they're talking about is the same one we used in Figure 12.8—3.5 ounces cooked (equivalent to approximately 100 grams or ¾ cup of flaked fish). As illustrated earlier, such a recommendation is tantamount to setting a goal eating of at least 5000 mg of long chain fatty acids per week.

The 5000 mg figure is reasonable. In a "worst case scenario," where ALA has absolutely no benefits itself and we're forced to rely entirely on conversion from ALA to either EPA or DHA to reap benefits, then we would need to consume about 15,000 mg of ALA daily. (This presupposes a conversion rate of only 5% from ALA to the longer chain omega-3 fats,[217] although more recent animal models suggest that figure may be closer to 10% for most tissues.[218]) This goal can easily be accomplished by adding some ALA to two or three meals daily. One tablespoon of flaxseed oil twice daily would do it. A quarter cup of walnuts, two tablespoons of ground flax, and a couple ounces of chia seeds would also put you in that same 15,000 mg daily ballpark.

Although in certain situations, groups like the AHA recommend daily supplementation with anywhere from 1000 to 4000 mg of long chain omega-3 fats (i.e., EPA and DHA), I generally don't recommend higher ALA intake than 15,000 to 20,000 mg daily. Research suggests, however, that it may take daily doses as high as 3000 mg of long chain omega-3 fats to most effectively lower blood pressure.[219] If conversion of ALA to EPA and DHA is as inefficient as the most pessimistic commentators suggest, what other options do we have?

Fish-Free Long Chain Omega-3 Fat Supplementation

Because of concerns with toxins in fish, and with sustainability of fish supplies, researchers and corporations alike have been looking for ways to isolate EPA and DHA directly from plant sources. An example is provided by Martek Biosciences Corporation who has been effectively harvesting EPA and DHA from microalgae. Their website claims that they provide the DHA for "99% of infant formulas used in the U.S."[220] Martek's omega-3 product, branded "life's DHA" is also found in a myriad of over-the-counter supplements.

Omega-3 Fat Cautions[221]

As mentioned earlier in this chapter, if you are taking medications with a narrow therapeutic window, you need to make sure you and your prescribing practitioner are on the same page before taking supplemental omega-3 fat or anything else, for that matter. An interesting example is provided by an anti-rejection drug sometimes used by transplant recipients. If you are taking cyclosporine (Sandimmune®), some evidence exists of a possibly beneficial interaction where the omega-3 supplementation may actually decrease your risk of blood pressure elevation and kidney problems. Although this interaction appears to be favorable, any interaction is reason for consultation with your medical providers.

On the other hand, adding more omega-3 fats could be particularly dangerous for individuals on blood thinners such as aspirin, warfarin (Coumadin®), and clopidogrel (Plavix ®). This is due to the blood thinning that results from liberal intake of these fats. By worsening blood sugar control, omega-3 supplementation can also pose problems for individuals with diabetes.

Safety of Selected Supplements for Cardiovascular Disease Generally

In a fascinating compilation of research, experts collaborated with the U.S. Agency for Healthcare Research and Quality (AHRQ) to look in detail at a number of supplements with potential benefits on high blood pressure and other heart-related issues.[222] They looked very carefully at many of the supplements I've mentioned to this point, including magnesium, coenzyme Q10, vitamin D and omega-3 fats. Despite their meticulous work, the investigators admitted that we still don't have enough data to fully evaluate the risks and benefits of these supplements, especially when they are being consumed by individuals already taking multiple other medications.

Nonetheless, two observations are noteworthy. First, no serious complications or side-effects have emerged with the supplements we've just examined. Second, perhaps the most encouraging aspect of their research—and the work of similarly focused investigators—is that many of these supplements offer other desirable benefits, even if your blood pressure never drops a single point. For example: omega-3 fats may help lower triglycerides (a potentially dangerous blood fat) in those with the highest values; CoQ10 may help with muscle-related pain stemming from cholesterol-lowering statin medications; and magnesium can both help combat constipation as well as helping ward off certain electrolyte problems that stem from diuretics ("water pills"), commonly prescribed for high blood pressure. Incidentally, less constipation decreases the risk of excessively high blood pressures that are generated when straining with a bowel movement.

A "New" Supplement Enters the Blood Pressure Arena

Another class of supplements that may offer special help for hypertension has eluded many recent review articles on the topic. However, emerging data suggests that probiotics—the so-called "good germs" that are growing in consumer popularity—may also offer blood-pressure-lowering benefits.

Just What Are Probiotics?

Probiotics are supplements made up of living microorganisms

that appear to provide health benefits when consumed orally. The rationale for their use stems from the realization that our gut is colonized with thousands of billions of microbes. Research has linked certain of these microorganisms with better health and others with poorer health and disease. A glaring case of the latter occurs when you are exposed to nasty germs that leave you with a bad case of diarrhea.

Although probiotics have been used for years to address a host of intestinal conditions,[223] a growing literature base suggests we should include them as potential anti-hypertensive agents. In 2014, Saman Khalesi and colleagues from Griffith University and Gold Coast Health in Australia performed a systematic review of all studies to date looking at the use of probiotics for hypertension.[224] The Australian team found an impressive blood-pressure-lowering effect from these "good bacteria" supplements as illustrated in Figure 12.9.

According to the data, greater benefit came from the probiotics if individual users met the following three criteria:

- They consumed multiple species of probiotics
- They used them for eight weeks or longer
- They ingested at least 100 billion colony-forming units per day

Consequently, when I recommend probiotic supplementation for hypertension, I recommend you take a supplement that meets all these criteria. I realize some of you are looking for a particular brand. There are expensive medical-grade probiotics, but I'm not convinced these are necessary for every individual. I take a more pragmatic approach.

Why Do Probiotics Work?

Over the years, I've found patients are much more likely to follow a new recommendation if it makes sense to them. However, even I'm constrained to admit, the connection between probiotics and blood pressure isn't immediately intuitive. Therefore, look with me at a number of documented scientific explanations as to how probiotics might help lower blood pressure. These include:

Figure 12.9 Probiotic Supplementation and Blood Pressure Improvement: Blood pressure decreases (in mmHg) among 543 adults in nine studies

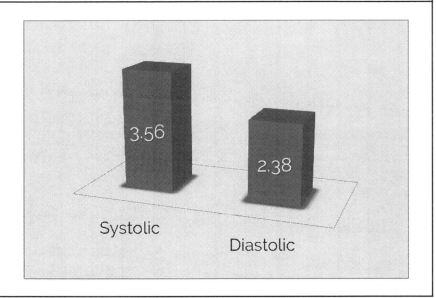

- The good bacteria in probiotics may directly or indirectly produce blood-pressure-lowering ACE inhibitory peptides.

- Probiotics may stimulate the production of gamma aminobutyric acid (GABA), another blood-pressure-lowering compound.[225]

- Fragments of the good bacteria themselves may directly lower blood pressure.[226]

- Certain probiotics may improve insulin resistance and blood sugar levels, possibly through metabolizing sugar in the gut or otherwise decreasing sugar absorption.[227]

The first of these points is not new to this book. Certain microbes have been shown to produce small protein-like molecules called tripeptides, which have angiotensin converting enzyme (ACE) blocking properties. These tripeptides may be produced in foods (as in the case of cultured milk products like yogurt);[228] they probably also can be produced in our intestinal tracts from ingested foodstuffs, so long as these good bacteria are present. If you don't remember ACE from earlier in the book, ACE inhibitors or blockers are blood-pressure-lowering compounds that have been marketed as pharmaceutical agents. We now know they are found abundantly in plant foods. They are also present in cultured dairy products. (If you think this is an endorsement for liberal yogurt intake, think again. As I presented in chapter 5, the closer you move to a total vegetarian diet the better. This is especially true from the blood pressure perspective. And, yes, you should be able to get all the natural ACE inhibitory compounds you need from plant foods without resorting to dairy consumption. Furthermore, dairy products—yogurt included—are common vehicles for exposure to persistent organic pollutants.[229])

The last bullet point in my four-point list of probiotic's blood-pressure-lowering mechanisms also deserves a bit more explanation. I've not yet mentioned the important connection between your blood pressure and insulin metabolism. "Insulin resistance" means that one's tissues are not responding to insulin optimally. In this condition, blood pressure tends to rise. Risk of cholesterol abnormalities, female infertility and even cancer also occur. With such powerful connections, you might ask "Why are we hearing about this only now?" As important as insulin resistance is, the strategies to address it are the very ones we've been discussing on hypertension's grounds alone. That's right; if you're worried about insulin resistance, your ideal lifestyle will feature a nutrient-dense vegetarian diet, regular exercise, and weight loss (if you are overweight). Furthermore, we can now add another insulin resistance preventive to the list: a daily dose of probiotics featuring multiple bacteria and at least 100 billion colony-forming units daily.

Can We Get the Benefits of Probiotics Without Taking Supplements?

For years researchers have been demonstrating that following an excellent whole-food, plant-based diet results in favorable changes in the bowel flora and its activities. Studies revealed, for example, that those eating a plant-rich diet had both greater positive attributes in the stool (prebiotics, resistant starch and non-starch polysaccharides in dietary fiber, increased fecal flora diversity, and increased anti-inflammatory gut bacteria) as well as fewer harmful elements (cancer-causing "mutagens" such as nitrosamines, pro-inflammatory gut bacteria such as *Bacteroides*-enterotype and *Clostridium* species, pro-inflammatory toxins such as lipopolysaccharides, putrefying protein, and reduced fecal flora diversity). Don't let all those technical details obscure the key point: Medical data indicate a connection between diet, healthier flora and less disease—including less cancer.[230, 231]

More recently, researchers have been describing how "prebiotics" in plant foods can favorably alter the colon microbiome. Experts have put forth the following definition as to what constitutes such a prebiotic effect: "The selective stimulation of growth and/or activity(ies) of one or a limited number of microbial genus(era)/species in the gut microbiota that confer(s) health benefits to the host."[232] More simply, prebiotics can be thought of as "fertilizers" for the good germs in our bowels.

For example, research indicates that the lowly peanut, when skinned (the way it is typically eaten), has constituents that favor the growth of good bacteria like those in the *Lactobacillus* family and suppress the growth of bad "germs" like toxin-producing *E. coli*.[233] Interestingly, compounds in peanut skin may offset some of these beneficial effects. Similarly research on lowbush blueberries revealed this fruit tends to favorably impact flora by suppressing more aggressively bad germs (like toxin-producing *E. coli* and *Salmonella*) compared to good germs, like those in the *Lactobacillus* family.[234] I could give a multitude of other examples as diverse as apples,[235] chicory,[236,237] and other inulin-rich foods like garlic[238,239] (inulin is one of many soluble fibers found in plant foods).

In short, if you have been on an excellent diet for years—and haven't recently used antibiotics (known to disrupt intestinal flora) then you may not have any need for a probiotic supplement. However, relatively few Americans meet these two criteria. Denizens of many other nations often don't fare much better.

Probiotics rank among the simplest and safest of blood-pressure-lowering supplements. As we look back on this chapter, I recommend giving special consideration to probiotics as a first line supplement in your goal of natural blood pressure control.

A Special Supplement for Individuals with Multiple Cardiovascular Risk Factors

I was finishing up this chapter when I got an e-mail from a health professional colleague who I'll call Brett. The day before, Brett watched his patient, Gwen, storm out of his office, "fed up with this whole medication business." He was convinced Gwen was headed home to flush her statin drugs down the toilet.

Since I've been advocating non-drug approaches in this book, you might wonder if my first reaction was to celebrate Gwen's bold decision. It wasn't. Although I'm also an advocate of more natural approaches to dealing with cholesterol, abruptly stopping statin drugs can be dangerous, just as we saw earlier with high blood pressure medications.

For those not familiar with the terminology, "statins" are the popular name for a class of drugs with powerful cholesterol-lowering effects. More technically referred to as HMG-CoA reductase inhibitors, the generic names for these drugs all end in "statin" as illustrated by atorvastatin, fluvastatin, lovastatin, pitavastatin, pravastatin, rosuvastatin, and simvastatin. However, statins affect more than cholesterol. They suppress inflammation and help blood vessels relax, reducing stress on your heart. Consequently, when statins are abruptly stopped, susceptible patients can face a host of metabolic consequences that can dramatically increase their risk of heart attack or stroke.[240]

Although this information is not proven by rigorous studies, I shared with Brett some strategies that might decrease the risks of statin discontinuation. First is gradually tapering the drugs rather than stopping them abruptly. Second is the addition of a supplement known as L-arginine.

L-arginine is a fascinating substance. It is categorized as an amino acid, which you may recall is one of the constituents or building blocks of body proteins. Every protein in our bodies can be broken down into a string of amino acids.

However, L-arginine is far more than a boring molecule holding interest only to biochemists. This compound is also used by your blood vessels to make nitric oxide (NO), a natural blood vessel relaxant.

Now, when individuals abruptly stop their statin drugs, one of the substances that tanks is NO. So, if we can boost nitric oxide levels with supplemental L-arginine, we may be able to stave off some of the alleged dangers associated with stopping—or even never starting—statin drugs. Tuck that information away if you're looking to embark on other strategies to decrease medication dependence after our current 30-day journey. However, for now, we must return to our hypertension focus.

As you might have guessed, the connection between L-arginine and nitric oxide can be a boon for blood pressure lowering. A stunning example of this was recently provided by an Iranian team led by Arash Dashtabi.[241] Dashtabi and colleagues randomized 90 volunteers to take either one of two doses of L-arginine or a placebo for eight weeks. The impressive blood pressure findings are documented in Figure 12.10. Of note, the research team also documented improvements in blood sugar, cholesterol, and triglycerides in those who used the L-arginine supplements. As with blood pressure, the greatest improvements were logged by those taking 2 grams of L-arginine three times daily or a total of 6 grams per day.

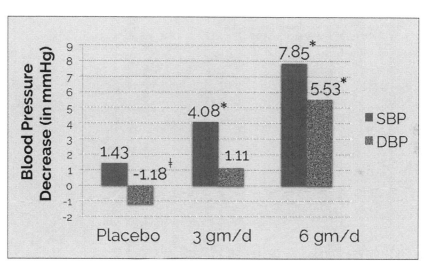

Figure 12.10 Decreases in BP with L-Arginine Supplementation: A Clinical Trial in 83 Overweight Adults

* Statistically significant at p<.001; all other results not significant
‡ This negative number indicates an average *increase* in blood pressure, albeit not statistically significant

So, is L-arginine for you? It depends. You probably guessed there was a reason why Dashtabi chose overweight patients. It turns out that L-arginine supplementation seems to benefit primarily those who have other heart disease risk factors.[242] The biochemistry is complex but involves a rogue chemical called asymmetric dimethylarginine (ADMA).[243] ADMA partially blocks the uptake of L-arginine by your blood vessels and thus decreases your body's ability to make that vital nitric oxide. On the other hand, taking more L-arginine can help your body compete with these enemy combatants, and boost NO production. The bottom line: The higher your ADMA levels, the more likely L-arginine will help lower your blood pressure.

Are you ready for me to sell you a blood test? Sure, it would be nice to know where you stood on the ADMA front, but for most of us it's not necessary. High blood pressure alone tends to raise levels, but the worst ADMA values tend to occur in the face of multiple cardiovascular risk factors like elevated cholesterol, kidney failure, atherosclerosis, and chronic heart failure. [244] If it sounds like I'm talking about you, supplemental L-arginine may be worth considering.

I would particularly recommend a serious look at L-arginine, if you're like Gwen and have stopped, or otherwise avoided, pre-scribed medication for elevated cholesterol or other heart-related conditions. Of course, the L-arginine is not a substitute for fol-lowing your doctor's advice. However, it may theoretically give you some benefits between now and the time you and your health care provider can agree on a long-term strategy.

A Final Natural Remedy for Your Consideration

One final supplement of promise, that seems to elude many of the lists of blood-pressure-lowering herbs, is hibiscus. I really like hibiscus tea as it is a "whole plant" option, has been used for centuries in many cultures without known adverse effects, and has demonstrated its effectiveness in a number of my patients.

In 2015 researchers combed the literature for studies examining the impact of hibiscus tea on high blood pressure.[245] The investiga-tors uncovered five randomized controlled trials (the gold-standard in clinical research studies) that included a total of 225 subjects in the hibiscus tea supplementation groups and 165 in the control groups. The pooled data revealed impressive benefits from hibiscus tea consumption as illustrated in Figure 12.11.

Another recent study, this time from Africa, explored the mechanisms by which hibiscus lowers blood pressure.[246] They found hibiscus was similar to the popular blood pressure drug, lisinopril, in its effects on the renin-angiotensin-aldosterone system. Both hibiscus and lisinopril equally lowered pressure-raising compounds in this system (specifically, plasma renin and serum angiotensin-converting enzyme).

Ready to try a beverage besides water? A typical blood pressure recommendation is to drink three cups of hibiscus tea daily.

Figure 12.11 Hibiscus Tea Supplementation Improves Blood Pressure: Blood pressure decreases (in mmHg) among 225 subjects in five studies

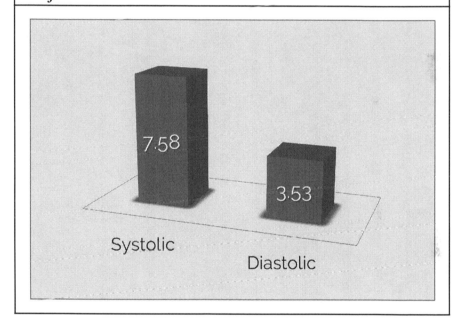

Your Turn

As you've worked your way through this chapter, I hope that you've come up with some ideas of how to further enhance your natural blood pressure regimen. In light of our initial conversation about therapeutic windows, however, those of you already on prescription drugs will probably want to commit to Example 1 in the Draft Worksheet before going much further. Once you've ensured that one or more of the supplements in this chapter are likely safe for you, you can make a decision about which one(s) to add to your daily program. That decision, of course, can be aided by a knowledgeable health professional. Far too many health care providers have a knee-jerk response to supplements, simply telling their patients to avoid them. This is neither helpful nor practical. If a provider cannot give you concrete reasons to refrain from a given supplement, I would suggest you find a professional who can give you more balanced guidance.

Chapter 12 Natural Adjuncts – Draft Worksheet

	Week 1							Week 2						
Day #	1	2	3	4	5	6	7	8	9	10	11	12	13	14
Behavioral Goals														
Example 1: Check with my doctor and/or pharmacist to see if some of the supplements in this chapter may be safe for me in light of my current prescriptions.														
Example 2: Add daily probiotic supplement with at least 100 billion colony-forming units.														
My Goal 12:1														
My Goal 12:2														
My Goal 12:3														
My Goal 12:4														
My Goal 12:5														

13

REFRAINING FROM PRESSORS AND EXCESSES: AVOID THESE "FALSE FRIENDS"

IN NOVEMBER 1874, THE efforts of many progressive women culminated in the formation of the Women's Christian Temperance Union (WCTU). That organization quickly became the largest women's organization in the U.S. and, ultimately, the world.[247] Although the cause that rallied those women, concern for the destructive powers of alcohol on families and communities, may seem passé, their movement—and the word at the heart of it, *temperance*—still speaks to us today. Among the lessons, two are especially important on our journey toward medication-free blood pressure control.

First, the WCTU reminds us that even the disenfranchised can powerfully impact dialogue in a democratic nation. Realize that women were not even allowed to vote in the U.S. until 1920. Consequently, at a time when those of the female gender were still debarred from one of the fundamental rights of a democratic society, the WCTU members were determined to make their voices heard in matters of social policy. This example of empowerment clearly speaks to us today. In fact, I've been arguing for a form of it throughout this book. Although you may not have a medical degree, be proactive. No one can take better care of your blood pressure than can you.

I've often told my patients: "When it comes to your body, you're the expert, I'm just a consultant." Although there's some hyperbole involved, my point is simple: No matter how much I know about hypertension (or any other condition), regardless of how thoroughly I examine you and how carefully I order diagnostic tests, I can't fully evaluate all that is impacting your health. For example, I can't feel what is going on in your body. And I can't readily assess all that is impacting you on a social level. Consequently, in certain realms, a well-educated patient can often make better decisions about their own health than can the most revered clinician. This is not license to scrap your physician's advice. But it is a call to expect that your health care providers will treat your concerns with respect. As it relates to this book and its themes of personal empowerment, your health care team, if unbiased, will accept that you may have learned some things they didn't study in professional school, and should be open to explore natural therapies unless they know of valid contraindications.

However, the WCTU presents us with a second lesson, one particularly germane to our quest for natural high blood pressure strategies: Those women (a handful of whom still fly the WCTU flag) focused their energies around a cause labeled "temperance"— not "moderation."

To this day, the WCTU embraces a definition put forward by the Greek philosopher Xenophon. He used the term temperance to connote "moderation in all things healthful; total abstinence from all things harmful."[248]

Although the WCTU and other organizations seemed to use the term "temperance" synonymously with abstinence from alcohol, that misses the power of the term "temperance." Western culture today has become enamored with "moderation," a narrow-minded focus that has undermined our health and, at the same time, increased our blood pressure.

What Are Pressors?

Broadly speaking, a pressor is anything that raises blood pressure. Classically, the term was used for things that constricted blood vessels and, in this way, raised BP. For the sake of our discussion, however, we'll look at pressors in their broadest sense: anything that can boost your systolic or diastolic numbers.

This chapter calls our attention to the importance of avoiding pressors and "excesses." As such it is calling us to embrace the concept of temperance. By now, it involves no great leap of logic to endorse avoiding pressors like alcohol and tobacco. However, I'm not shelving the need for moderation in that which is good. Though we talked about the blood-pressure-lowering power of whole plant foods, one can still eat too much of even ACE inhibitor-laden plant foods and end up with the blood-pressure-raising scourge of obesity.

Consequently, this chapter first calls on us to review areas where we may need to either eliminate things or cut back on their use. A quick look at Appendix B reveals a number of pressors to which, on a personal level, you have already said good bye. Total abstinence is a decision you have already made. Appendix B probably also features some items you have decided to moderate. Such excesses you have committed to curb represent the other arm of temperance. However, at this first decision point, I want to ask you: Have any of your changes been commitments to moderation, when total abstinence is really warranted?

As I've shared with audiences for years in my popular lecture and DVD entitled "Changing Bad Habits for Good," moderation is especially dangerous when it comes to addictive behaviors. That's right: If you're addicted to something, moderation is not a viable long-term option. You must make a clean break with the practice if you want to be free. For example, you're a slave to tobacco whether you smoke three packs or a "mere" four cigarettes per day.

My goal in this chapter, however, involves far more than inspiring you to raise the bar when it comes to areas you've already highlighted. We must now turn our attention to additional pressors that may not even have registered in your consciousness.

NSAIDs and Blood Pressure

Even a few years ago, when lecturing on blood pressure, I seem to recall gasps from my audiences when I described the dangers of nonsteroidal anti-inflammatory drugs (NSAIDs). Many no doubt wondered how such popular agents, many of them over-the-counter, could be harmful. Yet recent research developments have been widely publicized, and so the luster surrounding these once apparently innocuous drugs has largely faded, even if many people are still oblivious to their direct impact on high blood pressure, and the fact that these drugs are not good for your heart. Before looking at the literature in more detail, let's ensure everyone knows how varied the NSAID family truly is. Figure 13.1 provides a list of some of the drugs in this category.

In 2015, the Food and Drug Administration strengthened their warnings about the vascular risks of the NSAIDs. However, because of the heart-protective effects of low-dose aspirin in some populations, they excluded aspirin from their condemnation. Specifically, the agency linked the non-aspirin NSAIDs to heart failure, heart attack and stroke.[249] Some of those increased risks occurred "as early as the first weeks of NSAID use." The longer and heavier usage seemed to confer greater risk.

Despite such messaging, the blood pressure effects of these drugs are not as widely appreciated. Nonetheless, warnings have been coming out in the medical literature for some time about the hypertension dangers associated with these drugs. In 2011, researchers at the University of New Mexico Hospital in Albuquerque published a telling review. They revealed that individuals without the "high blood pressure" label experienced, on average, only a small elevation in their blood pressure from NSAIDs. These same drugs, however, could raise systolic BP up to 14 points in those with hypertension.[250] Consequently, the authors concluded: "If possible, patients who have hypertension should avoid taking NSAIDs." I heartily agree. NSAIDs may not make the "total avoidance" list when it comes to temperance, but they surely come close.

Figure 13.1 Generic Names of Various Non-steroidal Anti-inflammatory Drugs, NSAIDs (Brand names indicated in parentheses)

✔ Popular NSAIDs

- Aspirin (Anacin, Ascriptin, Bayer, Bufferin, Ecotrin, Excedrin)
- Ibuprofen (Advil, Midol, Motrin, Nuprin)
- Naproxen (Naprosyn, Naprelan)
- Naproxen sodium (Aleve, Anaprox)

✔ Other NSAIDs

- Choline and magnesium salicylates (Tricosal, Trilisate)
- Choline salicylate (Arthropan)
- Celecoxib (Celebrex)
- Diclofenac (Arthrotec, Cataflam, Voltaren)
- Diflunisal (Dolobid)
- Etodolac (Lodine, Lodine XL)
- Fenoprofen calcium (Nalfon)
- Flurbiprofen (Ansaid)
- Indomethacin (Indocin)
- Ketoprofen (Actron, Orudis, Oruvail)
- Magnesium salicylate (Arthritab, Bayer Select, Doan's Pills, Magan, Mobidin, Mobogesic)
- Meclofenamate sodium (Meclomen)
- Mefenamic acid (Ponstel)
- Meloxicam (Mobic)
- Nabumetone (Relafen)
- Oxaprozin (Daypro)
- Piroxicam (Feldene)
- Salsalate (Amigesic, Anaflex 750, Disalcid, Marthritic, Mono-Gesic, Salflex, Salsitab)
- Sodium salicylate (various generics)
- Sulindac (Clinoril)
- Tolmetin sodium (Tolectin)
- Valdecoxib (Bextra)

What then Can We Do for Mild to Moderate Pain?

For years, NSAIDs have been the mainstay for dealing with modest levels of pain. What can we use in their place? Don't be too quick to resort to aspirin. Although low-dose aspirin may have heart benefits for some, pain-relieving dosages of aspirin have not been exonerated when it comes to the blood-pressure-raising effects of this large drug family.[251]

From my vantage point, the best pain control options seem to be natural ones. Two of my favorites are omega-3 fats[252] and turmeric.[253,254] We've already seen that omega-3 fats tend to be blood pressure lowering. So using them for pain would seem to usher in a win-win situation. However, one caveat is in order. Omega-3 fats don't work as quickly as NSAIDs.

My favorite analogy is with a car manufacturing plant. If you start bringing aluminum into the plant for car bodies instead of steel, will you end up with a different end product? Definitely. But it will take a while before you see that difference at the end of the assembly line. When you change the raw materials, the world sees those changes only after the new products are fully assembled. The same is true with the omega-3 fats. Fats are the building blocks or raw materials that your body uses to construct inflammatory compounds like leukotrienes (LTs) and prostaglandins (PGs). Eating omega-3 fat right now will not change those compounds instantaneously. However, once your body processes those omega-3s and makes those LTs and PGs, they will actually be less inflammatory than if they had been made, say, from pork fat (lard). The end result is less inflammation and pain, but it takes a while. The longer you use an omega-3-fat-rich diet the longer and greater the benefits.

Furthermore, more recent research is extending the pain-relieving properties of omega-3 fats beyond the LTs and PGs, which decades of health professional students have studied. New classes of anti-inflammatory compounds like resolvins, protectins, and maresins actually endow these fats with some unique advantages over the NSAIDs.[255,256]

As we saw in the previous chapter—and we'll see in another light shortly—be careful not to equate an omega-3-rich diet with one that puts fish front and center. Not only can we get long chain omega-3s from sources other than fish, fish are often laden with other blood-pressure-raising toxins.

Turmeric to the Rescue

Back on the subject of NSAID alternatives, turmeric, that orange-yellow East Indian spice, is also an inflammation- and pain-fighting powerhouse. Although the herb can be purchased in bulk (or in the spice section of your grocery store), it is also available in capsules. A typical starting dose is 500 mg three times daily, although many people work up to taking much more. However, safety argues for not taking more than 2000 mg daily, due to risk of adverse effects such as diarrhea, indigestion, nausea, theoretical risk of liver toxicity, and lack of evidence for further benefit with higher doses. Be careful, even at prescribed dosages, some find the herb gastro-intestinally irritating, especially on an empty stomach. And of course, if you're taking other prescription medications, talk with your health care provider or pharmacist to ensure you're not setting yourself up for drug interactions. Those with gallbladder disease should avoid turmeric as it may worsen that condition.[257]

Now, if turmeric fights pain, might it also have the blood-pressure-raising side effects that accompany the NSAIDs? The answer appears to be "No." Turmeric and curcumin—one of the biologically active compounds in the herb—actually have properties that address more than pain. For example, turmeric appears to directly lower blood pressure.[258] Mechanisms involved include curcumin's ability to enhance blood vessel health,[259] thus promoting a key contributor to normal blood pressure. (Review: unhealthy blood vessels are more prone to spasm or constriction; when this happens, BP rises.)

Boswellia (frankincense) appears to be quite helpful for pain control as well. I had a patient who had good pain relief taking turmeric and Boswellia, instead of Norco (a popular narcotic), for her post-traumatic knee osteoarthritis. She was continuing to tolerate the combination well past the age of 80 without adverse consequences. A typical dose is 200 mg to 600 mg twice daily of Boswellia extract. Boswellia is usually well tolerated without side effects. Occasional minor gastro-intestinal effects have been noted.[260]

Tired of Popping Pills?

If supplementing with omega-3 fats, turmeric, or Boswellia doesn't seem to be a desirable option, why not consider some other analgesic (anti-pain) strategies. For example, exercise (if not overdone) can help relieve pain. Then there's always hydrotherapy, water treatments.

Warm water and heat in general can ease muscle spasm, a common cause of pain. On the other hand, ice and cold applications have direct analgesic and anti-inflammatory properties. Most everyone has put an ice pack on an acute injury. But ice can be skillfully employed in other settings. One great strategy is to fill a paper cup with water and freeze it. Then you can give an ice massage to a given area, gradually peeling the paper away from the block of ice as you massage an area with gentle circular strokes. I generally recommend limiting such treatments to 15 minutes.

The contrast treatment features alternating warm and cold exposure. One of the areas where I have had a lot of experience with this is in the treatment of diabetic nerve pain (commonly called neuropathy).

Begin a contrast treatment by placing the affected area in warm water. If there is impaired sensation, the water temperature should be kept below 104 degrees F (40 degrees C). For the sake of our example, let's say you're treating an ankle afflicted with osteoarthritis.

After soaking the ankle for three minutes in the warm water, move it into a basin with cold water. Most people are safe immersing their foot or ankle in very cold water, even with ice added. However, if you have a serious heart condition or very high, uncontrolled blood pressure, you'll want to keep the contrast mild. (Cold water can trigger an abrupt rise in blood pressure, called the "cold pressor" response.)

The ankle stays in the cold for only 30 to 60 seconds before going back to the warm water for another three minutes. Do four to five complete cycles (exposure to both cold and hot). This should take 20 minutes or less. Contrast treatments are generally done up to twice daily.

Pain and High Blood Pressure

Pain itself can raise blood pressure. When a pain stimulus is relayed by one or more of our sensory nerves, our sympathetic nervous system is activated and we are stimulated. The adrenaline that pours into our blood stream combines with the heightened nerve stimulation to raise blood pressure, among other things.

Interestingly, those with chronically high blood pressure tend to have a decreased sensitivity to acute pain (also known as hypalgesia).[261] In fact, the higher the blood pressure, the more pronounced the hypalgesia tends to be. Put another way, the pain stimulus has to be stronger for a person with hypertension to feel it. Thus, having a high pain tolerance is not, necessarily, a good thing if it means your blood pressures are running higher.

Normalizing blood pressure doesn't seem to be the answer. Hypalgesia often continues even when one's blood pressure is brought into the normal range with medication. This has led some researchers to suggest that an underlying pain/stress stimulus is activating the sympathetic nervous system. This in turn reduces pain sensitivity. The reduction in pain sensitivity may be an attempt to help the body reduce its sympathetic nervous system activation. This is why hypalgesia often precedes the onset of hypertension. It may also explain why those with a family history of hypertension tend to have a higher pain tolerance, and why pain sensitivity ratings in teenagers were able to predict their blood pressure levels years later.

A particularly interesting example of hypalgesia relates to blood pressure and headaches. While most think of high blood pressure as a cause of headaches, in actuality, headaches tend to occur only in those with severely elevated blood pressures. Headaches were, actually, less common in those with moderately elevated blood pressures than in those with lower pressures (systolic BP <140). Hypalgesia is the likely explanation.

The mechanism of hypalgesia in hypertensive patients appears to involve several factors. One has to do with baroreceptors, blood pressure monitors which are located in blood vessels throughout the body. The baroreceptors in blood vessels going to muscles seem to be especially important. Pain stimulates these receptors to clamp down the diameter of arteries, thus raising blood pressure. Perhaps as a protective mechanism against excessively high blood pressures, when BPs are elevated, the baroreceptors appear to send out signals reducing pain sensitivity, thus reducing the corresponding rise in pressure with painful stimuli.

Brain endorphins may also contribute to hypalgesia in those with high blood pressure. These endorphins play a role in suppressing pain signals. Medications that block endorphin production appear to make hypertensive rats more pain sensitive. This may or may not be the case in humans.

Hypalgesia is not just a novel observation, but a significant phenomenon especially important when it comes to heart problems. Silent heart attacks occur when the heart, on a cellular level, is screaming out in pain but the patient, often due to hypalgesia, fails to notice it. Unfortunately, pain may be the only sign of a problem; thus, failing to sense that pain may have life or death implications.

Studies are clear. Silent cardiac ischemia (unperceived deficient blood supply to the heart muscle) is more common in those with both hypalgesia and high blood pressure. The lesson is, of course, just because you feel fine doesn't mean all is well!

Those with long-term chronic pain and high blood pressure did not exhibit hypalgesia. In one study of chronic low back pain patients, those with more recent onset of pain (less than a year) retained the hypalgesia; however, those with pain for more than two years exhibited higher blood pressure responses when exposed to acute pain.[262]

Can anything be done to lessen hypalgesia? We don't yet have a clear answer. Daily exercise appears to improve pain sensitivity in those with long-term chronic pain. It may also help in hypertension. The collection of techniques discussed in this book would tend to improve inflammation, reduce activation of our sympathetic nervous system, and lower blood pressure levels, which presumably would lessen hypalgesia. Further research is needed to understand better how to reverse this process.

Other Medications and High Blood Pressure

NSAIDs are not the only bad guys in the pharmacology department. Unfortunately, a number of commonly prescribed medications have blood-pressure-raising properties. Figure 13.2 highlights some common ones.[263,264,265]

Other Pain Relievers and Hypertension

Over the years, many patients have been surprised to learn that medications used to address headache pain frequently contain caffeine. As already noted, pain itself can raise blood pressure, so the BP-boosting effects of caffeine may not be readily apparent in this context. However, if you can find an effective headache medicine that is caffeine-free, then your blood pressure will likely fare better in both the short- and long-term.

Figure 13.2 Some Drugs in the Following Categories May Raise Blood Pressure

- NSAIDs
- Non-NSAID Pain Relievers
- Steroids (e.g., dexamethasone, Medrol, prednisone)
- Birth Control Pills
- Diet Pills
- Decongestants (e.g., phenylephrine, pseudoephedrine, Sudafed)
- Migraine Headache Medications
- Antidepressants (e.g., bupropion, monoamine oxidase inhibitors, tricyclic antidepressants, and venlafaxine)
- Immunosuppressive Drugs (e.g., cyclosporine A, tacrolimus)
- Erythropoietin
- Anti-HIV Medications

Another common pain reliever is acetaminophen. Popularized by the Tylenol® brand, this medication avoids some of the dangers associated with the NSAIDS. Consequently, in limited amounts, acetaminophen is often a better choice even if it is not entirely off the hook in the blood pressure arena. More recent data is pointing toward this compound also being a pressor.[266] Before you throw your hands up in despair and decide to pop a handful of ibuprofen for your looming headache, acetaminophen still seems to be the better choice.[267] However, some of the evidence suggests the more you use this pain reliever the more likely you may experience BP elevation. So, when it comes to acetaminophen, temperance in the form of moderation is clearly warranted.

Steroid compounds also have blood pressure-raising effects. This includes male and female hormones (the latter are used in birth control pills). Corticosteroids also can raise blood pressure. These drugs are sometimes given by injection to help with localized pain issues. I'm not trying to kick out all the crutches from those of you with chronic pain; I just want you to be aware that those nerve blocks (pain injections), which are commonly observed to raise blood sugar, may also raise blood pressure.

Stimulants and High Blood Pressure

Whether you're using an illicit drug like cocaine or methamphetamine or a prescription drug like Ritalin, anything with stimulant properties can boost blood pressure. This same general class of drugs often finds its way into decongestants and diet pills.

For those troubled by severe allergies—or even fighting a cold—a decongestant may seem to be just what you need. But have you ever thought about how such drugs work? They constrict small blood vessels. Although this may be desirable to help your runny nose and reddened eyes, it is not necessarily desirable in other parts of your body. Remember, when we constrict blood vessels, blood pressure rises. Tightened blood vessels increase resistance to blood flow. If resistance is up, pressure in the pipes must be increased to keep the blood circulating—and, of course, that "pipe pressure" is blood pressure.

A number of prescription and over-the-counter cold, flu, and allergy medications contain decongestants. Read ingredient labels. If you find either of the following, the medication contains these potentially blood-pressure-raising compounds: pseudoephedrine (Sudafed) or phenylephrine (Neo-Synephrine).

Diet pills (even "natural" ones) often rely on stimulants (e.g., caffeine, ephedrine, phentermine, benzphetamine, diethylpropion, or mazindol). Those stimulants seem to do the trick by revving up metabolism and suppressing appetite, but the price they exact is an elevation in blood pressure, not to mention the abuse potential. Why not recommit to sensible eating and regular exercise to trim down? They'll not only help you shed pounds but will help you lower your BP.

Migraine medications represent another common class of drugs that operate by constricting blood vessels, often with caffeine. But even a caffeine-free migraine pill can cause a significant BP rise. Why? Classic migraine headaches involve dilated (or overly relaxed) blood vessels in the brain. Those dilated vessels result in more blood flow and increased pressure within the skull, one of the contributors to migraine pain.[268] Consequently, migraine drugs often target those relaxed blood vessels. Although they have desirable effects on headaches, they can elevate blood pressure through constricting blood vessels throughout the body.

Antidepressants Can Pose Dangers

Medications prescribed for depression can also cause blood pressure elevation. Among the more commonly prescribed newer medications are venlafaxine (Effexor®) and bupropion (Wellbutrin® or Zyban®). These medications may be prescribed for conditions other than depression. Venlafaxine, like its cousin duloxetine (Cymbalta®) is sometimes used in chronic pain states. Bupropion is often used to help individuals stop smoking.

Other older anti-depressants can also cause a rise in blood pressure. The monoamine oxidase inhibitors are rarely prescribed today. However, the tricyclic antidepressants (TCAs) are still commonly used, especially for conditions other than depression. These drugs, like amitriptyline, nortriptyline, and desipramine are prescribed for conditions as diffuse as insomnia, chronic pain, and migraine headache prevention.

More Danger from Supplements

The Mayo Clinic recently highlighted a number of supplements that can adversely affect blood pressure.[269] I've added a few other common potentially BP-boosting herbs to round out the list found in Figure 13.3.

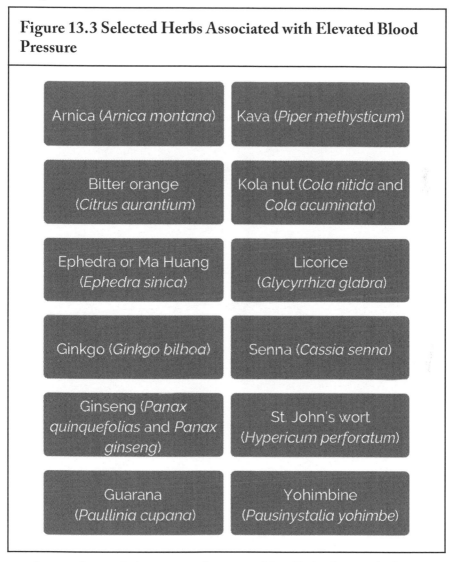

Figure 13.3 Selected Herbs Associated with Elevated Blood Pressure

Arnica (*Arnica montana*)

Kava (*Piper methysticum*)

Bitter orange (*Citrus aurantium*)

Kola nut (*Cola nitida* and *Cola acuminata*)

Ephedra or Ma Huang (*Ephedra sinica*)

Licorice (*Glycyrrhiza glabra*)

Ginkgo (*Ginkgo bilboa*)

Senna (*Cassia senna*)

Ginseng (*Panax quinquefolias* and *Panax ginseng*)

St. John's wort (*Hypericum perforatum*)

Guarana (*Paullinia cupana*)

Yohimbine (*Pausinystalia yohimbe*)

A number of these supplements like Ephedra and Guarana have historically been found in natural supplements for weight loss. Others are used for conditions as diverse as diabetes, depression, and anxiety. From my perspective, some of these herbs have legitimate uses in natural medical care. However, it is important to recognize that these and other supplements have the potential to raise blood pressure. Thus, I tell people that "unless you know for sure otherwise, any supplement should be viewed as a potential contributor to elevated blood pressure."

Toxins as Pressors

OK, you've sworn off the NSAIDs and the hypertension-predisposing herbs, can we finally put the subject of pressors to rest? Unfortunately, no. I have to include one final major class of blood pressure-raising compounds: environmental toxins.

Emerging data suggests a number of toxins can raise blood pressure, sometimes significantly. Figure 13.4 provides some examples of BP-raising contaminants.

Figure 13.4 Examples from Two Major Categories of Hypertensive Toxins

✔ Heavy Metals

- Mercury
- Lead
- Arsenic
- Cadmium

✔ Persistent Organic Pollutants (POPs)

- Bisphenol A (BPA)
- Dioxins
- Furans
  - polychlorinated dibenzo-p-dioxins (PCDDs)
  - polychlorinated dibenzofurans (PCDFs)
- Polychlorinated biphenyls (PCBs)
- Hexachlorobenzene (HCB)
- Certain organochlorine pesticides (OCs)

Heavy Metals, Higher Blood Pressures

In the year 2000, physicians from Michigan State University reported on a shocking case of high blood pressure. A four-year-old boy was found to be running BPs as high as 171/123. An exhaustive search for the cause revealed he had been exposed to toxic levels of mercury.[270] Looking for similar connections, the authors of the report then reviewed the medical literature. They found six reports of patients ranging from 11 months to 17 years old, all of whom had both mercury poisoning and high blood pressure. The most common cause of exposure? Contact with mercury from a broken thermometer.

All of these youthful patients had dramatic presentations. Subsequent diagnosis and treatment with chelating agents (*chelation* refers to a compound's ability to actually bind up heavy metals and help the body eliminate them) helped rid their bodies of the excess mercury, normalized blood pressures, and removed other potential toxic effects. Many other individuals are not so fortunate because, unless strategies are employed to eliminate toxic metals from the body, these compounds can gradually accumulate in a person's tissues throughout life. Also, when it comes to compounds like mercury, we have far more than broken thermometers to worry about. For example, over time, smaller amounts of mercury contaminating our food can have devastating consequences. The most common cause of long term exposure is fish consumption. Another common cause is amalgam fillings, which is why many dentists now use mercury-free composites.[271]

A number of other toxic metals increase our risk for high blood pressure. Figure 13.5 provides a list of these metals as well as common sources of exposure.[272,273]

Some of the data in Figure 13.5 is probably common knowledge; other details are, likely, surprising. Many lay people have long heard concerns about mercury contamination of certain fish. (It's probably now no surprise that long-lived, larger, and carnivorous fishes would be the most prone to accumulate large amounts of mercury in their tissues.) More surprising may be the connection between tobacco smoke and cadmium. The connection here is that tobacco leaves contain cadmium, which is found in the soil, air and water. Due to the large life-time exposure to tobacco among those addicted to nicotine, relatively large amounts of cadmium can accumulate. As a result, cigarette smokers have roughly double the cadmium stores of non-smokers.

Figure 13.5 Selected Toxic Heavy Metals Associated With High Blood Pressure	
Metal	**Common Sources of Exposure Worldwide**
Mercury	Occupational exposures, dental amalgam fillings, fish species (e.g., long-lived predatory fish, fatty fish, certain shellfish), thimerosal in vaccines, gold-ore extraction, magical-religious and ethnomedical mercury capsule intake
Lead	Gasoline additives leading to lead contaminated soil, food-can soldering, lead-based paints, ceramic glazes, drinking water pipe systems, and folk remedies (e.g., certain "natural" remedies sold in the U.S. have been contaminated with lead)
Arsenic	Marine fish, contaminated drinking water (beware of untested home wells)
Cadmium	Occupational exposures, contaminated food (highest levels are found in shellfish, liver, and kidney meats), contaminated drinking water, polluted air, tobacco smoke

For children, the number one food source of arsenic is poultry, but for parents it is tuna. For preschoolers the number one source of lead is dairy.[274]

The messages from the heavy metal connection are at least two-fold. First, be aware that your blood pressure could be elevated from contaminants in your workplace, your main water source (such as a home well), your foods, and the air you breathe. Second, if you needed any more reasons to move to a less polluted environment, eat more vegetarian foods, and stop smoking, perhaps you've just found them.

Other Persistent Environmental Toxins

Environmental health researchers talk about "persistent organic pollutants" (POPs). These long-lived compounds can exist in the environment for decades. Furthermore, they are typically stored in the fat cells of mammalian creatures. Consequently, they share something in common with heavy metals: Once ingested, they generally reside in the body for years, creating an enduring toxic burden. And that burden is not limited to the parents. Breastfeeding the first infant is known to unload half of the mother's toxic burden into the child.

Population data analysis has pointed to a connection between these compounds and cardiovascular disease.[275,276] Continuing research, like that from the U.S. National Health and Nutrition Examination Survey (NHANES), has linked many of these compounds to elevated blood pressure.[277]

In this NHANES data set, researchers found that over 60% of a representative sample of the U.S. population had detectable levels of one or more of the 21 POPs studied. Worldwide, urban dwellers in certain developing nations have the highest rates of POP exposure. However, Americans in general are now among those experiencing some effects from these compounds.

The reason for shining the spotlight on the POPs is because

most people are unaware of these stealthy robbers of health. We can all work to decrease continued exposure. In general, the main source of exposure comes from the consumption of animal products. Think about it. Because these toxins are stored in fat, creatures bioaccumulate these toxins. In other words, they steadily accrue them throughout the course of their lifespan. When compared to vegetables and grains that typically live for a few months and then are harvested, fish, chickens, pigs, and myriad other animal species have much longer to concentrate these toxins in their tissues.[278] Fish are among the most POP-laden foods consumed in many cultures.[279]

Furthermore, we can also fortify ourselves against the effects of inadvertent exposure. Scientific literature increasingly indicates the practices advocated in this book, like a diet abundant in omega-3 fats and phytochemicals, can mitigate the effects of toxin exposure.[280] For example, a 2014 study conducted by toxicologists at the University of Kentucky suggested that a plant-rich diet that is also liberally endowed with omega-3 fats can help protect the body from the cardiovascular damage caused by PCBs.[281]

Help for Toxin-Laden Bodies

Speaking about environmental toxins might sound a bit depressing. After all, we've all been living on a polluted planet for our entire lives. Depending on where we lived, the source of our water, the quality of the air, and the foods we chose (or had chosen for us), we are all presently carrying toxin burdens of varying degrees.

I highlight this area for three very important reasons. First, as I've already emphasized, if you and your doctors are baffled by your high blood pressure—especially if you are largely following the practices outlined in this book—you probably deserve to have some type of detailed toxin assessment. Start with your health care provider. If there is a reasonable suspicion of a connection, then they may end up having you consult with a medical toxicologist or a local poison control center. Second, if you are found to be harboring unhealthy levels of selected toxins, there are a variety of remediation strategies. At this point, specialty consultation is typically warranted.

Third, we're finding that some of the strategies recommended in this book for blood pressure may actually work, in part, by ridding the body of toxins. Two examples are provided by probiotics and turmeric.

Probiotics and Turmeric to the Rescue

If you've already started on a probiotic regimen based on our earlier discussions, good for you. New data is suggesting that your new-found practice may also be helping you in the area of decreasing your body's toxin levels. The gut microbiome may also help us to avoid some of the ravages of toxin exposure.

For example, Belgian researchers reported that probiotics may be able to prevent certain toxic exposures. They employed an animal model to assess protective effects of probiotics in the face of bisphenol A (BPA) exposure. When rats were concomitantly given Bifidobacterium and Lactobacillus probiotics, they found that they absorbed far less BPA when it contaminated their food.[282]

Turmeric (and one of its main functional chemicals, curcumin) also offers help dealing with environmental toxins. Research suggests those using turmeric on a regular basis may be protected from some of the hypertensive effects of heavy metals like cadmium.[283] This protection seems mediated, in part, by curcumin's chelating properties. Additionally, curcumin appears to help keep blood vessels healthy in the face of heavy metal exposure.

Your Turn

We've looked at a number of other factors that can affect your blood pressure. We began with me attempting to help you better appreciate the power of true temperance, as opposed to merely chanting the mantra of moderation. Have you identified places where a complete break is warranted? Some of those would be great behavioral goals to add to the Chapter 13 worksheet.

Other topics we've touched on in this chapter are not amenable to complete avoidance. As much as I would like to make a clean break with all heavy metals and POPs, it's simply not possible. Moderation, however, comes into play here when it comes to strategizing ways to decrease my exposure to blood-pressure-raising compounds, whether in the form of dietary contaminants or prescription drugs.

Chapter 13 Temperance (Avoiding Pressors and Excesses) – Draft Worksheet

		Week 1							Week 2						
Day #	1	2	3	4	5	6	7	8	9	10	11	12	13	14
Behavioral Goals														
Example 1: Check with my doctor to see if I can get off of the _____ medication that may be associated with blood pressure elevation.														
Example 2: Talk with my health care provider about screening for heavy metal or other toxic exposures that may be contributing to my high blood pressure.														
Example 3: Make a clean break with eating fish; get my omega-3 fats from plant sources like ground flaxseed and walnuts.														
My Goal 13:1														
My Goal 13:2														
My Goal 13:3														
My Goal 13:4														
My Goal 13:5														

14

EXERCISING FAITH IN GOD? SPIRITUAL CONNECTIONS TO HIGH BLOOD PRESSURE

CONGRATULATIONS. YOU'VE MADE IT to the end, almost. You're either essentially at the end of your 30-day journey, or just beginning a final, arduous ascent. How could you be staring at such disparate paths?

The topic of spirituality, and its impact on blood pressure, is complex and powerful, but the link is undeniably there, and so it must be addressed. In fact, the analogy of the 30-day journey provides the solution to the question above about the two disparate paths. After all, any lengthy trip usually offers more than one way to get to your final destination. So you can *take the full journey,* and go through this chapter as rigorously as you've gone through the rest of the book; or you can *take the shortcut,* and simply skim through the material.

If you're inclined to choose the latter, then commit about 60 minutes to it. Have a pencil as you quickly read through the high points of the chapter (paying special attention to headings, tables, and graphs). Don't get bogged down. If interested in one section, don't stop there. Simply make a notation in the margin, then continue at your rapid pace. (You can always return to topics that caught your interest.) This way you'll get a reasonable overview of the chapter and recognize whether or not it's vital to your personal journey. But do spend at least 60 minutes. If nothing connects, skip the goal setting exercise at the end of the chapter. However, even if you think a chapter on spirituality has nothing to offer, even a "shortcut" through this material will uncover some oft-neglected, non-drug keys to high blood pressure control.

How Long Does It Take to Develop a New Habit?

Whenever I talk to patients or groups about lifestyle change, one question invariably arises: *How long will it take for this new lifestyle to really become a habit?* In other words, when will all these changes become virtually automatic and less of a discipline?

Even if you haven't been asking that question from the first chapter, there's a good chance it's now high on your list. After all, for those of you who have been following the program to this point—setting behavioral goals and implementing them—it's likely you have been logging significant blood pressure improvements. Therefore, it's not unusual to be reasoning: Yes, this program works, but do I really have to do *all* this for the rest of my life?

For starters, you definitely *don't* have to follow *for the rest of your life* every one of your behavioral goals. Our deal was that you do this for thirty days and, then, re-evaluate. However, if you have seen significant improvements in your BP, I suggest you stick with as many elements as you can *for as long as you can.*

Back to the Original Question

So how long does it take to develop a new habit? Conventional wisdom used to assert the magic period was somewhere around twenty-one days. However, it's likely some of you haven't developed firm new habits even after thirty days. That reality may help what I say next to resonate with you.

Over the years I have come up with a better answer for the precise amount of time it takes to develop a new habit, and that is—"It depends." After my helping thousands change their lifestyles over the past thirty-plus years, it's the only honest answer I can give.

Two Stories Help Illustrate My Point

I met "Susan" some years ago when I was running residential lifestyle change programs outside of New York City. In spite of a deeply ingrained cigarette smoking habit, she knew she had to quit and, so, she simply threw away all her cigarettes. The next day Susan was sitting in the back seat of a car surrounded by smoking friends. Instead of inhaling as deeply as she could to "benefit" from the second-hand smoke, Susan was overwhelmed by an aversion to the tobacco smoke. Fortunately, she was sitting beside the window. She rolled it down and stuck her head out. Susan had already developed a new nonsmoking habit! Her desires for tobacco were gone—never to return again.

In contrast there was "Julie," who I also dealt with while working at that same New York facility. Her electronic communication detailed a very sad story.

Approximately two years before she contacted me, Julie was dealing with at least a couple of problems. First, she had been smoking for many years; second, she needed an automobile. Now, Julie had a helpful boyfriend, Ralph, who stepped into the narrative, determined to help Julie on both fronts. He agreed to buy her a brand new car, provided Julie stopped smoking.

Julie took him up on the offer. She said goodbye to the cigarettes and found herself with the keys to a new automobile.

Fast forward now, two years, to the time when I received Julie's e-mail. There she disclosed an additional, sad detail: she was miserable. Every day Julie struggled with strong desires to smoke, but a deal was a deal, and so despite the misery, she hadn't touched a cigarette for two years. Besides, there was one more incentive, too:

if she returned to smoking she'd owe him for the vehicle. And she still didn't have the money.

This story illustrates a sobering reality: you can be physically free of a behavior, but still, even years later, be attached to it on a mental level.

"Spiritual Guidance" and Behavior Change

What made the difference between these two ladies' stories? Well, I deliberately left out one critical detail in Susan's narrative. It was what moved her to the point of knowing "she had to quit." That missing ingredient was a spiritual experience. Susan told me she was "convinced by God" that her cigarettes had to go.

At this point some of you might be saying "Amen," or something equivalent; others may be less enthusiastic. If you are among the latter, and don't now relate to the world from any religious tradition, listen to this simple point. Without debating whether or not there is a God who can help people make lifestyle changes, similar benefits to those Susan reaped could *possibly* come from other spiritual experiences. For example, one of my Christianity-eschewing Native American colleagues might have a similar experience following a vision quest. If he came back from his time of solitude convinced he was called to lead his tribe to lives free from "addictive commercial tobacco" use, he might quickly have given up as much as a three-pack-per-day habit—even if he had no belief in a personal Creator or "Great Spirit."

The point is, spirituality has a profound effect on issues relating to the natural therapy of blood pressure, or any other lifestyle-associated disease process. I'm not going argue about evidence for a Great Spirit or God (I think there is one); nor am I going to talk primarily about whether such a higher power might give you special help in your lifestyle endeavors (I think He does).

Instead, I want to look at three aspects of spirituality.

First, whether or not we regard ourselves as religious, we all are spiritual beings. That spiritual dimension of our humanity has to do with meaning and purpose in life, among other things. In fact, even agnostic neuroscientists now argue our brain structures are wired for the spiritual.[284] No wonder, meaning and purpose have a huge bearing on our motivation when it comes to making and adhering to lifestyle changes. The examples of Susan and Julie have already illustrated this.

Second, spirituality plays a major role in a key blood pressure determinant: how we deal with stress. As we already saw in Chapter 11, spirituality is an important filter through which we pass many of our stress-related experiences.

Third, spirituality has other connections with health and improved blood pressure that might be difficult to quantitate mechanistically. In other words, we can measure benefits even though we don't know how those benefits accrue.

Underscoring aspects of all three of these areas, the medical community has, with growing interest over the past several decades, looked at connections between spirituality and health. Studies have often indicated connections between spiritual beliefs and/or practices and better health outcomes. For example, even a decade ago, researchers could honestly summarize the literature as shown in Figure 14.1.[285]

Of particular interest to us, of course, are the connections between spirituality and lower blood pressure. A number of studies have examined these relationships, and all have come to similar conclusions: religious practice and beliefs appear to have blood-pressure-lowering properties. For example, as early as the 1970s, researchers were documenting better blood pressures among those attending church regularly. These benefits were not explained by differences in age, obesity, cigarette smoking rates, or socioeconomic status.[286] A subsequent study on a different population found that an individual's assessment of the personal importance of religion appeared to result in lower blood pressures, even more than church attendance did.[287] Along similar lines, researchers studied nearly 4000 men and women over 64 years of age and found consistently better blood pressure readings among those who prayed and/or studied the Bible daily. Blood pressure improvements were generally modest, similar to many other lifestyle factors, with the religiously active individuals logging improvements of up to 4 points in systolic and diastolic pressures.[288]

Despite all the favorable evidence, spirituality is not always good when it comes to health—or blood pressure. In an extensive review of some 3200 studies on spirituality and health, Drs. Fernando Lucchese and Harold Koenig found 63 papers that examined connections between religiosity and blood pressure. Of these 63 studies, 57% showed that increased religion/spirituality resulted in lower BP or less hypertension. However, 11% showed an inverse connection, with greater spirituality being linked to higher BPs.[289]

Under what circumstances could religion and spirituality raise blood pressure or, otherwise, be deleterious? At least a partial answer came from Koenig's group at Duke University, this time in collaboration with Bowling Green State University. The researchers recruited nearly 600 men and women, 55 years or older, who were dealing with significant illness. As they followed these individuals for two short years, they found that those who had a "religious struggle with illness" experienced an increased risk of death.[290] Such a religious struggle was reflected by affirmative answers to one or more of the following:

- "Wondered whether God had abandoned me"

- "Questioned God's love for me"

- "Decided the devil made this happen"

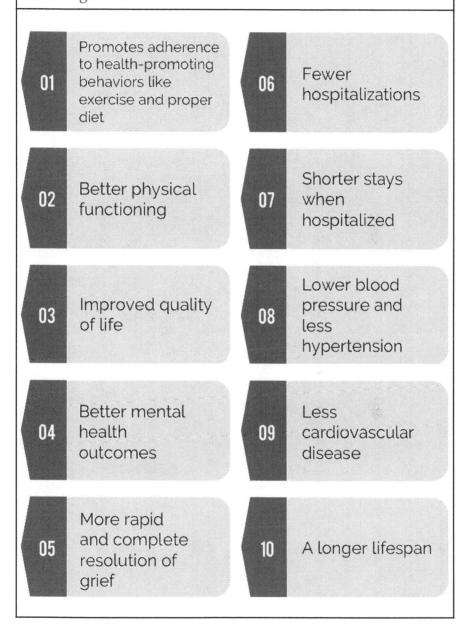

Figure 14.1 Spirituality and Health: Medical research has linked religious involvement and spirituality to each of the following benefits

01 Promotes adherence to health-promoting behaviors like exercise and proper diet

02 Better physical functioning

03 Improved quality of life

04 Better mental health outcomes

05 More rapid and complete resolution of grief

06 Fewer hospitalizations

07 Shorter stays when hospitalized

08 Lower blood pressure and less hypertension

09 Less cardiovascular disease

10 A longer lifespan

Personally believing even one of those questions increased their risk of death over those 24 months by about 20-30%. It is likely that similar negative attitudes connected with spirituality and religion would also adversely affect other parameters, like blood pressure.

Although some might interpret this result as a compelling health rationale for atheism, the Duke team was not finished with their observations. A couple of years later the same authors reminded us that these negative connections did not invalidate the benefits of spirituality. They wrote: "positive methods of religious coping... were associated with improvements in health."[291]

So, there's clearly help available in the spiritual realm, but also liabilities. How can I help you navigate those treacherous waters? The bottom line is this: I feel constrained to give you material on spirituality and health that can help you, regardless of your spiritual persuasion. At the same time, I want to give you concrete examples and evidence to bolster my claims—just as I've done throughout this book. However, I can really guide you only to places where I've been. And I can accurately describe only what I've seen. So, although as a young adult I embraced an agnostic worldview, I now view the world from a settled Christian perspective.

Thus, I'm going to share the material that follows from a Judeo-Christian framework. If you come from another orientation, I encourage you to read what follows from your own spiritual perspective. The underlying principles that follow are, truly, timeless and transcend specific religious affiliations. Finally, I think you'll share my conviction that the examples and explanations I give make this chapter much more valuable than if I merely referenced some kind of "generic" spirituality.

Acknowledged Dangers of Using "Christian" Illustrations: The Framework for the Rest of This Chapter

The name *Christian* evokes the warmest sentiments among many; nonetheless, throngs turn with disgust from that moniker. Although those who proclaim to be followers of Christ may be met with sentiments anywhere across this vast continuum of reactions,

Jesus himself is largely respected across most cultural traditions, and much of his broad appeal can be found in his widely acclaimed *Sermon on the Mount.*

The message proclaimed from this unnamed mount in Galilee transcends denominational identities, illuminating life principles to monotheists, polytheists and atheists alike. We have already touched on the research evidence showing the two-edged nature of spirituality: how it can both heal and destroy. From that perspective, I believe the introduction to Jesus' Sermon on the Mount, known as *The Beatitudes*, provides a roadmap to a health-giving spirituality.

Thus, it seems fitting to close the practical content of this book with the eight foundational insights that constitute *The Beatitudes*. If you're a bit skeptical about the connections, please, read on anyway. I think you'll see that the heart of that sermon provides a fitting recap for our entire journey, for it calls us to fully embrace the principles we've explored together—as well as providing some additional help and motivation for change. Figure 14.2 summarizes some of the reasons why studying *The Beatitudes* is likely to be a worthwhile investment, regardless of your spiritual persuasion.

"Virtues": Part of the Christian Tradition, Now Embraced by Secularists

Holding seemingly absolute power over the spiritual interests of Medieval Europe was the papacy. Royalty, clerics, and peasants alike feared to cross the will of the sometimes mercurial pontiffs. Even many modern Roman Catholics repudiate the behavior of past leaders, commonly regarded as infallible, like those chronicled in E. R. Chamberlin's 1969 book, *The Bad Popes.*

Atheists and agnostics will often point with disdain to such chapters in the history of the Christian church (and, yes, I would remind Protestant readers that the Church of Rome forms part of their ecclesiastical history as well). However, despite the undeniable abuses in the Dark Ages, some noble teachings were espoused, such as the seven heavenly virtues: chastity (purity), temperance, charity, diligence, patience, kindness, and humility. What is truly remarkable about this list is that it has largely been supported by modern psychologists, many of whom disavow any religious connections. For example, the American Psychological Association's 2004 publication of *Character Strengths and Virtues: A Handbook and Classification,* provided empirical research attesting to the mental health benefits of cultivating virtues like those embraced by the Medieval Church.

Figure 14.2 Health Blessings from the Beatitudes

The Beatitudes, the introduction to Jesus' famous Sermon on the Mount, pronounces a set of blessings that highlight the foundations of a health-enhancing spirituality—regardless of one's spiritual orientation. Some of the reasons why *The Beatitudes* are especially fitting for our study include:

- ✔ They are consistent with virtues espoused by many faith traditions.

- ✔ They are an area of spirituality that the author has personal experience with.

- ✔ They highlight widely accepted spiritual methods for coping with stress.

- ✔ Rather than presenting rules, they feature blessings which the human spirit finds much more attractive.

- ✔ They are brief and thus both easy to conceptualize and remember.

The Roots of Valuing Virtues in the Modern Era?

Both the medieval valuing of virtues and the modern secular interest in the same have roots, dating at least as far back as Jesus' *Beatitudes*. I believe that the eight virtues, or values, found in *The Beatitudes* provide a spiritual foundation—regardless of your religious orientation (or lack thereof)—that can greatly facilitate your *No Pressure* journey.

It may seem strange to some that I would speak about spiritual values aiding a *No Pressure* journey. After all, many of us come from spiritual backgrounds where burdensome religious exactions only made our life difficult. But rather than presenting a list of burdensome, pressure-filled "do's and don'ts"—the virtues espoused in *The Beatitudes* are given in the context of *blessing*. That is, correctly understood, these words serve as a set of prescriptions for happiness and freedom, even in the midst of adversity, regardless of your religious persuasion.[292]

Because I've been making a case for the cross-cultural relevance of these principles, I'll take a specific approach to each of these eight moral imperatives. First, I'll simply state the principle in a concise, action-oriented word or phrase. Then I'll quote Jesus' actual words from a modern translation of the Bible (*The English Standard Version*) and provide an overview of the principle. Next, in order for you to more fully appreciate the nature of the counsel in its original context, I'll illustrate how that prescription fit contextually into the Judeo-Christian worldview in which Jesus lived. Finally, I'll unpack the Beatitude as far as its practical significance for us today—across spiritual and cultural lines. By the time you finish this chapter, I think you'll agree that each of these eight prescriptions offers tangible help as you continue on your *No Pressure* journey. Figure 14.3 summarizes the eight timeless prescriptions and thus provides a road map for what will follow.

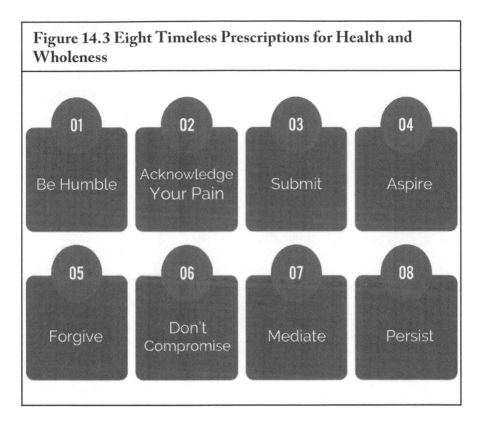

Figure 14.3 Eight Timeless Prescriptions for Health and Wholeness

01 Be Humble

02 Acknowledge Your Pain

03 Submit

04 Aspire

05 Forgive

06 Don't Compromise

07 Mediate

08 Persist

Timeless Prescription #1: Be Humble

Blessed are the poor in spirit, for theirs is the kingdom of heaven. Matthew 5:3

In many sectors of contemporary culture, humility is not valued as a virtue. For athletes, performers, and politicians, unbridled confidence often seems to be rewarded. Furthermore, in today's culture, the arrogance of some who claim to be "Christians" is one of the most compelling arguments in favor of agnosticism and atheism.

I've often said, "The people I try to run away from the fastest are those who are convinced they have all the answers." Unfortunately, some of those individuals wave the Christian flag. However, a know-it-all posture where one presumes to judge others based on a personal understanding of "Bible teaching" was never advocated by the Scriptures themselves.

What is humility? Is humility just another form of cowardice or timidity? Is it lacking a back bone and letting others walk all over you? Authors Rick Howard and Jamie Lash put it this way, "Real humility is not thinking less of ourselves but thinking of ourselves less."[293] It is "the art of self-forgetfulness," as one blogger put it.[294] Expressed another way, humility involves an accurate assessment of myself, lacking conceit, with an attitude toward benefitting others no matter what their position is in life.

In the medical community, humility is now being viewed as an important characteristic of the most effective healers. Jack Coulehan, MD, MPH, recently went on record: "The new professionalism movement in medical education takes seriously the old medical virtues. Perhaps the most difficult virtue to understand and practice is humility, which seems out of place in a medical culture characterized by arrogance, assertiveness, and a sense of entitlement. Countercultural though it is, humility need not suggest weakness or lack of self-confidence. On the contrary, humility requires toughness and emotional resilience. Humility in medicine manifests itself as unflinching self-awareness; empathic openness to others; and a keen appreciation of, and gratitude for, the privilege of caring for sick persons."[295]

However, humility is a prerequisite not only for optimally effective health professionals. It is important for each of us as we become engaged in our own personal healing process. One of our greatest dangers is feeling we know best how to care for ourselves. Along these lines, one of my mentors once reminded me of the adage: "The doctor who treats himself has a fool for a patient and a fool for a doctor."

Humility in the Biblical World

Jesus was a Jew. The only Scripture he had access to is the one

Christians today refer to as the *Old Testament*. Consequently, it is germane to our dialogue to realize that many scholars believe a single verse in those Scriptures summarized the whole duty of man. It is found in the words of the prophet Micah:

> He has told you, O man, what is good;
> and what does the Lord require of you
> but to do justice, and to love kindness,
> and to walk humbly with your God?[296]

Jesus himself illustrated humility in a story that should give contemporary religionists cause for concern. The master teacher provided his listeners with a countercultural illustration. In the Judaic worldview of Jesus' day, the Pharisees were held in high spiritual esteem. Rather than commending a religious leader of this class, however, the story's hero emerges as one whom mainstream society labeled as spiritually bankrupt.

> He [Jesus] also told this parable to some who trusted in themselves that they were righteous, and treated others with contempt: "Two men went up into the temple to pray, one a Pharisee and the other a tax collector. The Pharisee, standing by himself, prayed thus: 'God, I thank you that I am not like other men, extortioners, unjust, adulterers, or even like this tax collector. I fast twice a week; I give tithes of all that I get.' But the tax collector, standing far off, would not even lift up his eyes to heaven, but beat his breast, saying, 'God, be merciful to me, a sinner!' I tell you, this man went down to his house justified, rather than the other. For everyone who exalts himself will be humbled, but the one who humbles himself will be exalted."[297]

In its historical context, this story reminds us that most of us find ourselves in one of two spiritual camps. On one hand, many of us are proud of our own spiritual position whether we're

314

an atheist, agnostic, or an adherent of an organized religion. We look down on those who don't seem to have our level of "spiritual maturity" and practice. On the other hand, some of us occupy a humbler place. That latter position, although it may reek of self-deprecation, embodies the commended virtue.

No matter which spiritual perspective you hold, embrace with me the virtue of humility. We can learn a lot from listening to each other—and then passing things through our own spiritual filters. Although I'm doing all the talking now, I'm available for dialogue, because I give public lectures, host a nationally-syndicated radio show, and dialogue via the web.[298]

This common tendency of pride in our own opinions, to the exclusion of all other philosophies, once characterized acclaimed Massachusetts Institute of Technology Professor Rosalind W. Picard, Sc.D. In these words, she shared her own journey:

> I grew up thinking that all religious people had basically thrown their brains out the window. I thought they had concocted their faith out of some kind of intellectual weakness. Or, perhaps they liked ritual for its own sake, or believed what they believed to please their parents. Perhaps religion was some kind of comforting deception. I prided myself on being tolerant of their beliefs, but I was not interested in religion for me. Who needed it? I thought "I am doing quite fine in life without it."
>
> Although I might have attended a talk on religion I would probably not have been a good listener. Because of my closed-mindedness against religion, it would be hard to be objective. I thought my atheism was scientific, and therefore the best way to be. What it took me a while to realize was that my belief that there was no God was as unprovable as

the religious beliefs I assumed were wrong. I had to face up to the fact that I really had not carefully considered the issues.[299]

Don't make the same mistake Picard once made, concluding that anything with religious trappings (or trappings not directly aligned with your own religion) isn't worthy of consideration.

Let me point out, as well, one other relevant insight from the Holy Scripture's vantage point. In contrast to the way many religionists have behaved throughout history, the Scriptures paint a very different picture of how someone will act when aware of God's presence. During and before Jesus' ministry, those writings illustrated a common response to encountering the Divine: humility.

For example, when the Old Testament prophet Isaiah was given a vision of God, Isaiah exclaimed, "Woe is me! For I am lost; for I am a man of unclean lips, and I dwell in the midst of a people of unclean lips; for my eyes have seen the King, the LORD of hosts!"[300] When Peter perceived that Jesus was more than human, he fell down at his master's feet and cried out, "Depart from me, for I am a sinful man, O Lord."[301] Jesus himself illustrated a similar attitude of humility during his entire ministry. He did not boast about who he was, what he knew, or what he had experienced. Instead he stepped down to serve others—at his own expense. Indeed, as the Scriptures describe it, Jesus, despite his exalted pedigree, "emptied himself, by taking the form of a servant... he humbled himself by becoming obedient to the point of death, even death on a cross."[302]

Consequently, from the perspective of the biblical worldview, a true Christian will follow this first inspired prescription and will seek to embrace humility. He will not give you overt or covert messages about how much better he is than you are—or how greatly superior his values are to yours. He will have a truly humble opinion of himself.

The Practical Healing Significance of Humility

We've already noted Dr. Jack Coulehan's observations about the importance of humility for health professionals. He is not a lone voice. Many are concerned that medicine has become too impersonal and, as a result, medical encounters are not optimally healing.

What is being debated among doctors is also of great importance when it comes to the social relations among lay people. This is especially relevant when it comes to the two "S"s in our *No Pressure* mnemonic. For example, if you want to reap the greatest benefits in the area of social support, then you must be willing to support others in their own health journeys. And those healing social relationships are optimized if we come alongside others, humbly, as equals, and not with an air of superiority.

Humility can also play a major role in ameliorating interpersonal stress. We've all heard of heated arguments that turned out badly. Occasionally the person that "wins an argument" ends up lying in a pool of his own blood, literally or figuratively. In such emotionally-charged contexts the wise man of Scripture described the value of humility: "A soft answer turns away wrath, but a harsh word stirs up anger."[303]

Humility is foundational to much of what I've written in this book. For example, when you encountered concepts here that challenged a current practice or enjoyment, did your heart harden or soften toward those ideas? Have you been willing to try some new things that nudged (or pushed) you from your comfort zone? If not, consider whether pride—rather than humility—has been operative, holding you back from reaping the full benefits of the *No Pressure* program.

Dr. Coulehan presented four aspects of humility that he posited were essential for "good doctoring": unpretentious openness, honest self-disclosure, avoidance of arrogance, and modulation of self-interest.[304] For example, Dr. Coulehan wrote in an earlier article how humility included "a keen appreciation of, and gratitude for, the privilege of caring for sick persons." Do you count it a privilege when needy people find their way into your life, or do you begrudge those with difficulties, whether it be in your neighborhood, your work place or even in your own home? You may object that you're not called to be a physician or a healer. However, I would suggest a posture of true humility helps us cultivate an attitude of service.

When it comes to behavior change, the research literature indicates that this spirit of service—which often springs from humility—increases your own likelihood of success. For example, over a decade ago, researchers from Johns Hopkins University followed some 500 individuals with drug and alcohol addiction who were enrolled in so-called "12-step" programs like Narcotics Anonymous (NA) and Alcoholics Anonymous (AA). After only a year, the investigators found that those who helped others, serving as "sponsors," had significantly better abstinence rates.[305]

Indeed, the path to healing often lies alongside the humble path of self-forgetfulness in helping others. Don't be surprised if embracing humility in all its multiple facets provides an added boost in your journey toward an ever more natural antihypertensive regimen.

Timeless Prescription #2: Acknowledge Your Pain

Blessed are those who mourn, for they shall be comforted. Matthew 5:4

We live in a society that seems overly preoccupied with bolstering our own egos. We should realize something is amiss when we give every child athlete a "participation" trophy, or when every grade school student leaves the science fair with either a first, second, or third place ribbon.

For some reason, we look at loss, shortcomings, or even outright failures as tragedy, whereas this second great moral principle suggests our success in life may actually be dependent on learning from our missteps.

Consider this timeless prescription through other lenses: those of the medical community. Any physician knows you often can't help a patient who conceals his true medical history. The patient who refuses to disclose he's suffering with abdominal distress is unlikely to get prompt treatment for appendicitis. Similarly, the woman who dismisses chest pain as "nothing" is the one most likely to die of a heart attack.

Many commentators believe that the *mourning* spotlighted in this verse especially includes sorrow for sin. Consequently these words are talking about a concept—*repentance*—that largely has been shelved in a culture primarily focused on protecting our egos and promoting moral relativism.

This is far from a tangential point for, after all, in this thirty-day journey we've been talking about lifestyle and lifestyle change. Remember what we learned from Susan and Julie: those most likely to efficiently develop new and lasting good habits are those who sense some type of moral imperative to change. By acknowledging our pain, we become open to availing ourselves of healing remedies, addressing underlying causes, and growing in ways we never otherwise could.

Certainly, it is unlikely we would ever make any lifestyle changes unless we acknowledge the pain stemming from undesirable behaviors that, for example, might be elevating our blood pressure. More than merely an acknowledgment, our mourning stimulates change. We take an honest self-assessment and decide we don't like the road we're on. We make a sharp turn and take another route. The act of turning around in the setting of mourning is called repentance.

Mourning and Repentance in the Biblical World

Repentance was a key word throughout the Scriptures of Jesus' day. Dozens of times in multiple books of the Old Testament the concept recurs. In Jesus' ministry, repentance played a key role. When Mark begins his biography of Jesus (*The Gospel of Mark*), he first introduces John the Baptist. John's message was founded on repentance. "John appeared, baptizing in the wilderness and proclaiming a baptism of repentance for the forgiveness of sins."[306] Jesus' first words in the *Gospel of Mark* are also centered on repentance: "The time is fulfilled, and the kingdom of God is at hand; repent and believe in the gospel."[307]

From a contemporary vantage point, many individuals find discussions about sin and repentance move them into a mental state that is far from health-giving. However, rightly understood, the concept of biblical repentance is, in reality, shining a spotlight on our shortcomings for just one reason: so that we might ultimately overcome them. In a very real sense, the Holy Scriptures paint God as a divine physician who points out the potentially deadly diagnoses that need to be addressed if we want to maintain or regain health. Sure, sand may feel good on our feet, but if we choose to keep our head in it after learning what is best for our health, significant harm is sure to come.

However, the Bible is not a self-help book. In the biblical worldview, God as diagnostician is followed by God as divine surgeon. So long as we provide informed consent, he takes responsibility for removing the disease of sin or shortcoming from our lives. Furthermore, when it comes to God's hospital or clinic (which is not limited by time and space), finances are never an issue. He offers free diagnosis and treatment to any who come to him. From the spiritual perspective of the Bible, we approach him simply by asking (praying) for his help wherever we are. Furthermore, no matter how "bad" a person feels his or her life has been, anyone can come to God for forgiveness. Jesus himself said: "whoever comes to me I will never cast out."[308] Of the Savior, the apostle John affirmed, "If we confess our sins, he is faithful and just to forgive us our sins and to cleanse us from all unrighteousness."[309]

This view of God as divine surgeon, who only wounds to heal, is crystallized in the book of Job:

> Behold, blessed is the one whom God reproves;
> therefore despise not the discipline of the Almighty.
> For he wounds, but he binds up;
> he shatters, but his hands heal.[310]

However, even if the great teacher's words don't connect with you on that level, listen to this very important principle: Most of us never experience full healing because we hide our wounds. Let me make this practical. In our chapter on stress we talked about dealing with your stressors. Do you remember the danger of ignoring your stressors? Embracing stoicism in the face of your (or a loved one's) health issues doesn't mitigate the pain, and it will never help you arrive at a solution.

The biblical world calls out to each of us: admit your need, recognize your shortcomings, acknowledge your weakness, and begin to make a turn for the better. God will help you. It is only in this context that full healing comes.

The Practical Significance of Acknowledging Pain and Repentance

Twelve-step groups are among the most popular outpatient approaches for dealing with addiction. Some research suggests the social support afforded by such groups may be their most important asset.[311] However, other studies indicate "working through" the 12 steps themselves is particularly efficacious.[312] If you're not familiar with what constitutes those 12 steps, at least a quick look is warranted. Figure 14.4 provides an overview.[313]

What should be immediately apparent from Figure 14.4 is just how central repentance and reformation are. The essence of repentance is encapsulated in an admission of powerlessness (Step 1), admitting our wrongs (Step 5), turning from them (Steps 6-7), and making restitution (Steps 8-9). If addictive behaviors are interfering with our lifestyle success in controlling our blood pressure, this data suggests we need to examine ourselves for areas where we may need to repent.

No, for many people in our culture, a call to repent often doesn't resonate. However, think about it this way: When it comes to those who've wronged us, most of us actually expect the wrongdoers to repent and make appropriate restitution. If they don't, we may even take legal action. Why, then, is it so hard for us to see *our own need* to repent?

Perhaps we have tried too hard to convince ourselves that there is no right or wrong, even though on some fundamental level we know that's nonsense. The reason for my strong language is this: as a physician, I have had numerous patients over the years talk with me about being wronged or victimized. I don't ever recall such a victim telling me she was fine with the outcome because the perpetrator obviously was doing what was "right for him." Atheist or devout religionist, all of us know some things are just plain wrong. And so we expect some type of repentance—and restitution—from those who have wronged *us*. Why can't we then be open to following AA's recommendation and turning that spotlight on ourselves?

OK, some may say that, perhaps, addicts need to worry about this second beatitude. But what if I don't have any major addictions? Is there any other evidence that mourning—acknowledging our pain and repenting—may more generally have efficacy in addressing hypertension? Interestingly, many indigenous people groups have systems of healing that include the concept of repentance and/ or making things right. For example, traditional Hawaiians have a problem-solving approach known as "ho'oponopono," which literally means "to correct or to make right." One form of ho'oponopono therapy has actually been subjected to scientific scrutiny and found to hold promise for dealing with both high blood pressure and the stress that often contributes to it. [314,315]

Figure 14.4 The Twelve Steps of Alcoholics Anonymous

1 We admitted we were powerless over alcohol – that our lives had become unmanageable.

2 Came to believe that a Power greater than ourselves could restore us to sanity.

3 Made a decision to turn our will and our lives over to the care of God as we understood Him.

4 Made a searching and fearless moral inventory of ourselves.

5 Admitted to God, to ourselves and to another human being the exact nature of our wrongs.

6 Were entirely ready to have God remove all these defects of character.

7 Humbly asked Him to remove our shortcomings.

8 Made a list of all persons we had harmed and became willing to make amends to them all.

9 Made direct amends to such people wherever possible, except when to do so would injure them or others.

10 Continued to take personal inventory and when we were wrong promptly admitted it.

11 Sought through prayer and meditation to improve our conscious contact with God as we understood Him, praying only for knowledge of His will for us and the power to carry that out.

12 Having had a spiritual awakening as the result of these steps, we tried to carry this message to alcoholics and to practice these principles in all our affairs.

Additional Applications

When we allow ourselves to feel the pain—and acknowledge our wounds—then we can do something about it. Thus, don't push under the carpet those things that are calling for change. Your blood pressure and your health will be the ultimate benefactors. If it's the coffee cup, the red meat or the salt calling you to cut back, embrace the call. Listen to that chronic cough and quit smoking. Heed your growing girth and make the dietary changes you know you need to make.

Finally, if Jesus' words resonate on a spiritual level, consider setting a goal of consulting a faith community leader. If you embrace an atheistic or agnostic perspective, you can seek spiritual, emotional, or mental healing outside of religious channels. Contact a mental health professional or physician if you are struggling with pain in your life—especially pain resulting from your own poor choices or, dare I say it, *sins*.

Timeless Prescription #3: Submit

Blessed are the meek, for they shall inherit the earth. Matthew 5:5

Meekness and humility are related, but not synonymous. While humility especially calls us to confront any exaggerated ideas of our self-importance, meekness summons us to put humility into practice. Consequently, typical dictionary definitions of meekness include the concepts of submission and gentleness—especially in the face of injury.

In the 1960s and 70s, Nabisco launched a series of cartoons and TV commercials that featured "Mort Meek," a common and apparently weak man preoccupied with counting chocolate chips in their branded cookies. When assailed by villains, Mort's only recourse was to change into his alter-ego, "Cookie Man," to defend himself. One not-so-subtle message behind the advertising campaign was that meekness was tantamount to weakness.

324

In contrast to such common associations, meekness and submission are most eloquently expressed when they are embraced by someone who has great strength or power. This is clearly seen in the biblical world. Indeed, regardless of our spiritual persuasion, this dimension of meekness offers special insights for each of us on our *No Pressure* journey.

Submission in the Biblical World

Jesus not only preached meekness and submission in *The Beatitudes*, he lived it. If we take the Scripture's claims at face value, Jesus pre-existed before his birth in Bethlehem. From a biblical perspective, Jesus was the active agent in creating this earth (although God the Father and the Holy Spirit were also involved).[316] However, he set aside his divine prerogatives and came to live on this earth as a man and to die on man's behalf.[317]

Such a perspective is difficult to mesh with secular theories regarding the origins of our universe. However, don't get bogged down by this now. Also difficult for those with a secular vantage point is the idea of Christ's death as a sacrifice. Again, let's try to see through the eyes of the Bible's penmen. From their perspective, sin (or lack of conformity to God's will as expressed through natural and divine law), results in eternal death.[318] This is depicted as a natural consequence, rather than some arbitrary exaction. Consider the words of Jesus in *The Gospel of John*, Chapter 15. There he compares believers to branches who must remain attached to him as the vine if they want to have spiritual life and productivity.

What Jesus is saying is: I am the creating and sustaining God; if you want to have life and wholeness you must remain connected to me. Such a connection necessitates a harmonious relationship. Consequently, John 14 and 15 both include statements about the importance of following God's counsel or "keeping his commandments."[319] If you reject those commandments, you are, in essence, embracing that which separates you from God. As a result, you are breaking the divine connection and will ultimately die, just as surely as a tree branch dies when severed from the parent stock. Our human nature loves the idea of a warm, close connection but, unfortunately, we often bristle when asked to break beloved habits we know aren't good for us. And that's one reason why submission is a virtue worth nurturing.

Consider submission in relation to one of the natural laws expressed in Scripture. Centuries ago the book of Proverbs stated emphatically, "Wine is a mocker, strong drink a brawler, and whoever is led astray by it is not wise."[320] If we've been enjoying our interactions with alcohol, we may initially shrink from such an axiom. But medical research repeatedly and convincingly asserts alcohol consumption is associated with nearly all forms of violence, including higher rates of suicide, assault, domestic violence, rape, child abuse, homicide, gang violence, and catastrophic injury, as well as fatal and nonfatal motor vehicle crashes, drownings, and death. [321,322,323,324] From a modern perspective the acute physiologic effects of alcohol intoxication are obvious: euphoria, impaired coordination, poor judgment, labile mood, slurred speech, nausea, vomiting, memory lapses, coma, respiratory failure, and eventually death.[325] The conclusion is simple. Drink plenty of alcohol and experience grave mental, social, and relational consequences, perhaps even death. Avoid alcohol and avoid the risks.

Submission to the proverb above offers the potential for improved health and longevity. It provides but one example of the far-reaching biblical "commandments" or counsels that seem calculated to enhance our health.[326] These same Scriptures underscore other health principles we have already encountered during our 30-day journey. For example, the initial lifestyle advocated in the Bible consisted of a whole plant-based diet[327] with later counsel calling for the avoidance of some forms of saturated fat.[328]

Other biblical topics corroborated by contemporary public health science may also help address high blood pressure. These include the importance of cleanliness,[329] avoiding water and food contamination,[330] mold remediation of buildings,[331] proper sewage disposal,[332] avoiding inbreeding,[333] and infectious disease prevention.[334] If the Holy Scriptures were able to accurately identify such health and wellness connections long before the scientific method confirmed those relationships, wouldn't it be wise to consider enlarging your commitment to any spiritual connections that make sense? After all, if it makes sense and it's good for my health and blood pressure, why not?

Learning from a Light bulb

Let's look at a more contemporary illustration linking the ideas of spiritual connection, submission, and choices. Consider the light bulb. That bulb has no intrinsic ability to "live" and carry out its purpose without being connected to a power source. Disconnected from the electricity, the light bulb dies, in a sense. No legislation is needed to declare, "Light bulbs disconnected to electricity shall not shine." It just happens. Police powers are not necessary to ensure disconnected light bulbs don't shine. We can't shine (i.e., make good, wise, daily choices) when disconnected either.

These dynamics are illuminated by Jesus' dying words on the cross: "My God, my God, why have you forsaken me?"[335] (Note: Jesus didn't ask, "God why are you killing me?") In those moments of agony, he may not have fully understood why he felt alone. However, his submission was based on God's counsel, as found in the Scriptures. Up until that point, Jesus knew and experienced God's approval of his life and decisions.[336] However, in the anguish of pain, loneliness, and humiliation, his feelings did not align with his choices. But he followed through on his decisions regardless.

We often experience something similar when we choose to change our lifestyles. A choice for what's right may not align with our feelings and emotions. We may feel discomfort, loneliness, even humiliation. At first, things may look grim. Mercifully, this experience doesn't have to be long and, usually, isn't.

Jesus died very soon after questioning why God forsook him. His struggles were over. At the risk of stretching the analogy too far, I say that we may go through a kind of death too that signals an end to our lifestyle battles on any given front. As we learn to love our new lifestyle choices, knowing they are right for us, the old feelings (love for our bad habits) die. For Jesus, he was bearing the separation that sin creates between God and man. He died as the sacrifice for our sins.[337] For us, we submit to right choices, and as love grows for those new and better choices, we experience a death of the old feelings, actions, and even identity (perhaps?). During this difficult process, we often long for connection—just as Jesus, in anguish, longed for connection with his father, as he cried out, "Why have you forsaken me?" To maximize our success in lifestyle change, we will exercise submission in relationship with supportive people, and, as AA puts it, "God as we understand him."

White-knuckling it to force good choices by ourselves often doesn't work.[338] It's a set-up for failure. The "white-knucklers" are many and include the quitters who keep smoking, the dieters who keep overeating, the exercisers who keep sitting on the couch, just to name a few. Instead, our most entrenched habits often require assistance from a power outside of ourselves.

Power for better choices and a better life can come. As the old feelings and old choices die, the new feelings and new choices can come to life. So, compare your experience to the resurrection of Christ. How could Jesus rise again?" By using the same creative power that ordered the world, he rose again.[339] Jesus did not die for his own sins.[340] Based on his own behavior he was not separated from God the Father. Therefore, he still had a measure of divine life in himself that could respond to the father's call, even from the grave.[341] In the same way, God gives us power to allow old choices and feelings to die.[342] And through his creative power he helps our good choices come to life.[343]

The God revealed in the Bible is interested not only in our life, in the here and now, but even more so for eternity. Contrary to popular belief, the Bible does not describe an eternal burning hell where sinners are being punished forever. Instead, Scripture talks about an eternal death[344]—where those who are not connected with God die, never again to live. This is what is referred to by the end-time lake of fire.[345] In contrast, those who accept God's gift of forgiveness receive eternal life.[346]

The Submission of Jesus

Hold on for a bit longer, because we're coming to some more practical points. However, I realize by now, you readers are probably stratified into at least three groups. Some think I've done a reasonable job of depicting the biblical world and are thinking about what Jesus sacrificed on our behalf. Others of you think I've done an inadequate job (or worse) in trying to distill the biblical background. You're ready to write me an angry letter. A third group is completely befuddled by my attempted explanations. What I've said makes absolutely no sense and has only confirmed you in your disrespect for anyone who would take the Bible literally.

If you're in either of the last two groups—or in any similar place in your thinking—let me, first, apologize. For, from my study, the Bible presents the world's most accurate picture of human nature, as well as the most compelling foundation for meaning and purpose in life. However, regardless of whether you're following along with what I'm calling the biblical worldview or not, wouldn't we all agree that Jesus was at least a remarkable personage and, as alluded to above, he viewed his own life as one of submission? In the hours before his crucifixion, he found himself in a garden called Gethsemane. There he prayed to his father, asking for deliverance from the mocking, scourging and death that awaited him.

However, at the heart of his prayer are these words, "nevertheless, not as I will, but as you will."[347]

Here's the point: Whether or not we understand what was going on in Jesus' mind, his death was an act of submission. And this really is the essential point in understanding this beatitude. For throughout the Scriptures, the Bible writers struggled with the same issues that have influenced others to embrace atheism and agnosticism. One of those issues is the apparent injustice of God. Habakkuk wrestled with this concern. As the book bearing his name opens up, the prophet agonizes over why God seemingly does not hear his prayer for justice:

> O Lord, how long shall I cry for help,
> and you will not hear?
> Or cry to you "Violence!"
> and you will not save?[348]

However, when God does answer, Habakkuk is astounded by the explanation. God is going to use Babylon, a nation which the prophet considers unjust, to accomplish his purposes. Throughout the book, Habakkuk is really struggling with the greatest of human concerns as it relates to the divine. Has he seen enough evidence to believe that God exists and trust him with the events of his life and those around him? The book largely deals with Habakkuk's own challenges in submitting to God. He continues to be tempted to think that his view of the world is better than God's.

Because I had been an agnostic, these issues resonate with me. I saw many inconsistencies in what religionists told me were the ways of God. However, when I actually read and studied the Scriptures for myself, I found that, despite many of the popular teachings of my Christian and Jewish friends and their faith communities, the Bible answered life's questions in a most compelling—and logically consistent—manner. I saw enough evidence that God could be trusted. And I've been inspired to embrace a posture of submission (although, admittedly, I sometimes still try to wrest control out of God's hands). Habakkuk had this same experience. He finally realized that no matter what was happening around him, God was trustworthy. Habakkuk concludes his book speaking about what looks like utter failure; this is especially evident when you realize he's writing from an agrarian perspective. In the face of a world crashing down around him, he still chooses to trust in an all-wise God who has demonstrated to him his love and justice, despite how things appear:

> Though the fig tree should not blossom,
> nor fruit be on the vines,
> the produce of the olive fail
> and the fields yield no food,
> the flock be cut off from the fold
> and there be no herd in the stalls,
> yet I will rejoice in the Lord;
> I will take joy in the God of my salvation.[349]

The Practical Significance of Submission

Any health education resource is really based on submission. Medical experts share their conclusions and recommendations with the hope that the reader will submit his or her own opinions to their medical research and experience, and therefore make life changes. If you're like many of my patients over the years, you can be your own worst enemy. The areas where you most need to change you stubbornly resist. Excuses like: "This bad habit is too important for me," or "If I give that up, I'll be miserable," or "Everyone's got to have a little fun" are common justifications for holding on to poor lifestyle choices.

I want to challenge you, then, to take five or ten minutes right now. Scan your collective Behavioral Goals in Appendix B. As you go through each chapter's goals reflect on whether there are some areas where you have been resisting full submission to an optimal lifestyle program. If you come up with something you're willing to change, then put that under your behavioral goals for this chapter.

Beyond Submitting to Medical Authority

What we're really talking about here is the topic of medical compliance. Non-compliance or failure to follow medical advice is often cited as a major cause of poor health outcomes. Interestingly, in one of the studies cited earlier, individuals who were more religiously active were more likely to take their blood pressure medication as prescribed.[350]

However, physicians—myself included—are not always right. In light of *The Beatitudes*, to demand patients always follow my instructions would display something far different from humility! Furthermore, even a doctor's medically sound advice may sometimes result in harm to a patient. That's right, even a medically indicated treatment might, for selected patients, not be the right thing to do at a specific time. Over the years I've learned to listen to my patients' concerns and respect their sense of spiritual direction, even if it resulted in their following a course different from the one I advocated.

Some of my colleagues, no doubt, rolled their eyes when they read that last paragraph. I share their sentiments. The last thing I want to do in this book is to tell you that any whim or impression you have should trump a doctor's advice. However, I have seen evidence in my own life of a higher source of guidance to which submission is my best response. This is not a unique perspective among physicians.

John Shin, MD, a second-year Internal Medicine Resident, spoke to a gathering of Christian physicians and dentists during the fall of 2015. Dr. Shin directly credited his acceptance into medical school and his entering residency at the Mayo Clinic to submission.[351] Shin's premise was that a divine hand guided him throughout his educational pursuits. However, that supernatural guidance often demanded he submit his own judgment to the guidance of providence.

Some who do not embrace a faith background may want to argue that, despite Dr. Shin's educational achievements, he is displaying a naiveté that is hardly exemplary. However, I think Shin's journey speaks to us on a very deep level (and, yes, the free audio recording of his presentation is worth listening to). You see, his story is set against an early life history characterized by disdain for the entire medical profession. Only something outside himself could have changed John Shin's direction—in a way that has already had profound influences for himself and hundreds of others.

At the same time Shin was speaking to a small gathering of health professionals, another more prominent physician was grabbing headlines. Dr. Ben Carson, formerly Johns Hopkins' Chief of Pediatric Neurosurgery was on the presidential campaign trail. Even a cursory reading of Carson's biography, *Gifted Hands*, will reveal that Dr. Carson also heard—and heeded—multiple calls to submit to a power beyond himself throughout his formative years and during his accomplished medical career.

Still another physician, Dr. Larry Dossey, embraces more of a New Age spirituality rather than identifying with a single religious philosophy. Nonetheless, over the past three decades, Dossey has become a vocal advocate of prayer and spiritual guidance. In books like *Prayer is Good Medicine* and *Healing Words*, he has illuminated the scientific underpinnings of practices like prayer. In fact, Dossey's website offers us a fitting conclusion to the third beatitude:

> I used to believe that we must choose between science and reason on one hand, and spirituality on the other, in how we lead our lives. Now I consider this a false choice. We can

recover the sense of sacredness, not just in science, but in perhaps every area of life.[352]

Indeed, if you've not been open to spiritual guidance in your own life, Drs. Shin, Carson, and Dossey appear poised to cosign a prescription of mine: Take time to reflect, meditate, pray or otherwise seek to tap into divine guidance. It may be the missing ingredient for ultimate success on your *No Pressure* journey to medication-free blood pressure control.

Timeless Prescription #4: Aspire

Blessed are those who hunger and thirst for righteousness, for they shall be satisfied. Matthew 5:6

We *do* tend to accomplish no more than that which we attempt. Sure, things can happen serendipitously, like the Northern California couple who stumbled on a cache of gold coins buried on their property. They didn't have a studied goal of amassing great wealth but such did fall into their laps.

Similarly, you've only arrived this far on our *No Pressure* journey because you had some aspirations to really make a difference with your blood pressure. I commend you for your diligence to this point. However, the aspiration called for in the fourth beatitude has a particular goal in mind: righteousness, sometimes simply equated with right doing.

Aspiring for Righteousness in the Biblical World

Christianity embraces what seem like paradoxical virtues. On one hand, believers are called to be content with whatever they have, regardless of how little. On the other hand, they are encouraged to strive for more, especially in the sphere of moral development. Even on the Sermon on the Mount, Jesus called believers to be content with whatever they had. Years later, Paul reechoed those same sentiments.

Let's first examine how Jesus prescribed contentment—regardless of life's circumstances. During his immortalized sermon the master teacher said:

> Do not be anxious about your life, what you will eat or what you will drink, nor about your body, what you will put on. Is not life more than food, and the body more than clothing? Look at the birds of the air: they neither sow nor reap nor gather into barns, and yet your heavenly Father feeds them. Are you not of more value than they? And which of you by being anxious can add a single hour to his span of life? And why are you anxious about clothing? Consider the lilies of the field, how they grow: they neither toil nor spin, yet I tell you, even Solomon in all his glory was not arrayed like one of these. But if God so clothes the grass of the field, which today is alive and tomorrow is thrown into the oven, will he not much more clothe you, O you of little faith? Therefore do not be anxious, saying, 'What shall we eat?' or 'What shall we drink?' or 'What shall we wear?' For the Gentiles seek after all these things, and your heavenly Father knows that you need them all. But seek first the kingdom of God and his righteousness, and all these things will be added to you.
>
> Therefore do not be anxious about tomorrow, for tomorrow will be anxious for itself. Sufficient for the day is its own trouble.[353]

Paul's crystallization of the same principle was articulated in a letter to the early Christian church of Philippi, a city located in modern day Greece. His words are remarkable, considering he was unjustly incarcerated at the time: "I have learned in whatever situation I am to be content. I know how to be brought low, and I know how to abound. In any and every circumstance, I have learned the secret of facing plenty and hunger, abundance and need."[354]

On the other hand, in that same Sermon on the Mount, Jesus

called his followers *not* to be content with their own moral attainments. His goal was for them to be ever striving to be more like their heavenly Father: "Let your light shine before others, so that they may see your good works and give glory to your Father who is in heaven."[355] Note, however, Jesus' rationale for moral excellence was not to win public accolades but, rather, to be more like a God who serves others. He made this clear a while later in that famous sermon:

Beware of practicing your righteousness before other people in order to be seen by them, for then you will have no reward from your Father who is in heaven.

Thus, when you give to the needy, sound no trumpet before you, as the hypocrites do in the synagogues and in the streets, that they may be praised by others. Truly, I say to you, they have received their reward. But when you give to the needy, do not let your left hand know what your right hand is doing, so that your giving may be in secret. And your Father who sees in secret will reward you.

And when you pray, you must not be like the hypocrites. For they love to stand and pray in the synagogues and at the street corners, that they may be seen by others. Truly, I say to you, they have received their reward. But when you pray, go into your room and shut the door and pray to your Father who is in secret. And your Father who sees in secret will reward you.

And when you pray, do not heap up empty phrases as the Gentiles do, for they think that they will be heard for their many words. Do not be like them, for your Father knows what you need before you ask him.[356]

The Practical Significance of Longing for a More Righteous Character

Whether religious or not, don't you think our world would be a better place if all of us valued more highly "righteous virtues" like integrity, kindness, and humility?

Even scientists who look at human behavior from a totally secular perspective talk about the concept of righteousness as helping perpetuate collective societies. In their models they typically look for evolutionary explanations (rather than those motivated by religiosity or spirituality) for righteous behaviors, which include the punishment of societal members who don't work cooperatively.[357] Yet no matter where people fall on the spirituality continuum, there is something called *righteousness* that is advantageous for societies, if not for individuals themselves.

"Righteousness" in Health Lines

Does right doing and striving to be like a loving Creator help foster a greater commitment to self-care? Some of the medical literature suggests this. Consider research from Norway. There investigators found significantly lower blood pressures and cholesterol values among Seventh-day Adventists. The data suggested the differences were due to healthier lifestyles—long advocated by that Christian denomination.[358]

This Beatitude's emphasis on righteousness calls us to treat others right, but it also urges us to take proper care of our own bodies. This ethic brings us back to one of my key points as we began this chapter: if you have spiritual underpinnings for your lifestyle commitments, you are more likely to accomplish them.

However, righteousness and related values like justice have other powerful connections in the blood pressure arena. Some of these connections rely on neurochemistry. When we behave in a loving, consistent manner, our relationships tend to be characterized by trust. And those trusting relationships tend to foster the production of an important brain chemical known as oxytocin. This compound was once thought to be of importance only for nursing mothers; we now know that this small protein, made in the brain's hypothalamus, is vital to optimal societal living.

What is so fascinating about oxytocin is its *feedforward* effects. Specifically, when you are involved in trusting relationships, you produce more oxytocin, but that very oxytocin boost helps you actually trust others more.[359] Experimental research has shown that giving someone oxytocin through a nasal spray will render them more generous, for example.[360]

This research has profound implications for high blood pressure. Being a trustworthy, righteous person actually fosters healthy relationships. Stress signals are suppressed under the influence of oxytocin and relational tensions can be more quickly resolved.

Perhaps this provides some further insight into the connection between faith community attendance and better blood pressures. It also begs the question as to whether a trusting relationship with a divine personage might not have similar benefits, even if you never set foot in a temple, mosque, church, or synagogue.

Regardless of whether or not you are comfortable in a place of worship, find ways to enlarge your circle of trusted friends and relatives. Trust-filled, righteous relationships appear to be powerful allies in our quest for better blood pressure. Why not set a goal of prioritizing more trusting relationships—and, if warranted, improving your own trustworthiness as well.

Timeless Prescription #5: Forgive

Blessed are the merciful, for they shall receive mercy. Matthew 5:7

Richard had a terrible case of rheumatoid arthritis; it was refractory to all we had to offer. He also was bitter about his past. Edie, even in her 70s or 80s, seemed the picture of health. She was one of the most positive, effervescent people I have ever met. These two individuals shared a common experience: both were Jews who had survived the horrors of Nazi concentration camps. However, their attitudes toward that terrible history differed markedly. Richard still lived in a world of resentment and anger. Edie had moved beyond the injustices of the past and had extended forgiveness to those who had so terribly wronged her, her family, and her people.

We may be tempted to attribute health outcomes to our ability to forgive. However, the connection is not so simple. In any individual's life, be it Richard's or Edie's, far more is at play than even the worst injustices of the past. However, what does the research show? Can a spirit of mercy and forgiveness benefit the forgiver?

Forgiveness in the Biblical World

Forgiveness, on its deepest level, is about healed relationships. It is, therefore, foundational for healthy social interactions, whether they occur in the family, the tribe, the community, or the workplace. Consequently, Jesus' attitude toward forgiveness transcends the simple clichés bantered about even by Christians. Forgiveness is not merely something we choose to do on a personal level. Full forgiveness is a two-way street, where the one wronged first chooses to forgive, and then the wrongdoer actually accepts that forgiveness. Genuine acceptance of forgiveness occurs only when the perpetrator recognizes and admits to his wrongdoing and repents.

On the cross, Jesus modeled the first step in the process of forgiveness: choosing to forgive, even before his wrongdoers displayed any remorse. While nailed to that instrument of torture and death, the Messiah articulated his classic expression of forgiveness: "Father, forgive them, for they know not what they do."[361]

But all those in the presence of the cross were not forgiven. In the second chapter of the book of Acts, Peter is preaching to the crowds on the day of Pentecost (fifty days after Jesus' crucifixion).

After speaking of how Jesus was killed "lawlessly" (i.e., in total violation of the legal principles of the day),[362] Peter called on his listeners to repent—in other words, to acknowledge that they shared in the guilt of Jesus' death.[363] His logic was sound, for the crowd with one voice had pressured the Roman governor, Pontius Pilate, to deliver the death sentence. Nearly 2000 years later, some may scoff at Peter's appeal. However, three thousand in the crowd didn't scoff; instead, they repented of their role in the crucifixion, and Jesus' prayer of forgiveness became effectual for them.

These dynamics of forgiveness were recently modeled in Charleston, South Carolina. Invoking the same prayer of Jesus from Calvary, *USA Today* published the words of John S. Dickerson in the aftermath of the brutal murder of nine members of Charleston, South Carolina's Emanuel African Methodist Episcopal Church. Pastor Dickerson commented on an event that captured the world's collective attention:

> Did you see the families of the shooting victims in Charleston, S.C., confront the accused killer at his bond hearing Friday?
>
> Did you see the video — them pleading with Dylann Roof through tears?
>
> They said they forgave him — the very soul who, days earlier police said, held the weight of the gun, pulled the trigger and, having seen the mess of blood spurting from one writhing victim, continued to another. And another. And another. Until nine lay dead on the seats and the floor of a Christian house of worship.[364]

Dickerson also noted that the murderer, in that initial confrontation, did not accept the gift of forgiveness: "Like the Boston bomber, the Charleston suspect stood unmoved by the words of mourning survivors, his eyes veiled by the evil of hatred. We have

340

witnessed concentrated, unthinkable evil — met by concentrated, undeserved forgiveness."[365]

In that practical vignette, Dickerson bore explicit testimony to the biblical world's understanding of mercy: There is a difference between extending forgiveness and it being relationally effectual through its acceptance.

Countercultural Forgiveness

"Stand up for your rights." "What's in it for me?" "You've got to look out for number one." Phrases like these encapsulate a pervasive worldview: *my personal interests trump all other considerations.* However, Christianity embraces a counterintuitive worldview. As the apostle Paul expressed it: "I am debtor." Listen to his words as he writes to the early Christian church in Rome: "I am debtor both to the Greeks, and to the Barbarians; both to the wise, and to the unwise."[366]

In other words, Paul's focus was on his obligations to others, not on what was in it for himself. Such a perspective helps illuminate this Beatitude and the remaining ones. If I see myself as a debtor, under obligation to bless others, then, when wronged, I will not focus on the injustice but rather on the opportunity to respond to another with undeserved kindness. From this perspective we can appreciate that forgiveness is about far more than forgetting or ignoring wrongs. If we are really interested in healed relationships, forgiveness requires confrontation. True, Dylann Roof appeared to be fully cognizant of the pain that he had inflicted. Many times, however, individuals are unaware that they have hurt us. Consequently, we need to lovingly confront them, and let them know how we feel wronged—and, then, offer forgiveness.

The "confrontation" should not be emotionally charged. The spirit should lend itself to something like the following: "I've already chosen to forgive you. You really hurt me by doing _____, but I want to let you know that I am choosing not to let that stand between the two of us. My offer of forgiveness, however, doesn't fully make amends until you accept it. That's why I am speaking to you now."

A wise Christian mother and writer commented on this aspect of forgiveness:

> Until the judgment you will never know the influence of a kind, considerate course toward the inconsistent, the unreasonable, the unworthy. When we meet with ingratitude and betrayal of sacred trusts, we are roused to show our contempt or indignation. This the guilty expect; they are prepared for it. But kind forbearance takes them by surprise and often awakens their better impulses and arouses a longing for a nobler life.[367]

Please note, however, that forgiveness is far different from going back into abusive or destructive relationships. You can forgive someone who cheated you in a business deal, but that doesn't mean that you give him another $10,000 to invest on your behalf. You can forgive an abusive spouse for the physical and emotional scars he caused, but that doesn't necessarily mean you will ever move in with him again.

There can be healing on some levels of a relationship without full trust being restored. Even for the most merciful, however, trusting a person who deeply wronged you involves a process that takes time—and evidence of trustworthiness demonstrated in the life of the one forgiven. As a pro football coach recently said when commenting on the lack of integrity in one of his players: "it will be a process ... to regain trust that was violated -- you lose it in buckets and regain it in drops."[368]

The Practical Significance of Forgiveness

Dr. Dick Tibbits and colleagues at Florida Hospital designed a controlled study to look at the effects of a forgiveness training program and how it impacted blood pressure. Over an eight-week time frame, the investigators found that those who began the program with elevated anger expression scores registered significant decreases in their blood pressure.[369] Other experimental data suggest that some of the benefits may have occurred through decreased stress levels.[370] Or, as expressed by yet another group of researchers, "these results demonstrate divergent cardiovascular effects of anger and forgiveness, such that anger is associated with a more cardiotoxic autonomic and hemodynamic profile, whereas TF [trait forgiveness] is associated with a more cardioprotective profile. These findings suggest that interventions aimed at decreasing anger while increasing forgiveness may be clinically relevant."[371]

Indeed, forgiveness has been garnering more and more interest in medical research, which has extended far beyond high blood pressure and stress, encompassing disease processes as diverse as fibromyalgia[372] and cancer.[373]

Finally, a fascinating aspect of the forgiveness literature brings us back to the biblical world—and to a few applications for each of us. Researchers talk about two different types of forgiveness: *decisional* forgiveness and *emotional* forgiveness. By the former, they're referring to "a behavioral intention to resist an unforgiving stance and to respond differently toward a transgressor." Emotional forgiveness, on the other hand, "is the replacement of negative unforgiving emotions with positive other-oriented emotions."[374] This latter emotional forgiveness appears to be the most powerful when it comes to effecting beneficial health outcomes.

Of interest, it is this emotional type of forgiveness that the Bible says Jesus manifested. Consider the words of the apostle Paul, "For while we were still weak, at the right time Christ died for the ungodly. For one will scarcely die for a righteous person—though perhaps for a good person one would dare even to die— but God shows his love for us in that while we were still sinners, Christ died for us."[375] Despite the abuse and enmity he received, Christ, in love for his transgressors, willingly gave up even his life.

This dialogue on forgiveness begs at least two important questions. First, to whom do I need to extend forgiveness? Second, who do I think I've forgiven, yet still feel emotionally cold toward? The answers to these questions can open doors to better health—and to lower blood pressure. Why not add at least one behavioral goal at the end of this chapter that deals with forgiveness?

Still stumped when it comes to practical directions to take? Let me suggest one more aspect highlighted in the medical literature: self-forgiveness. You may not think you are harboring ill will toward anyone else, but you may be blaming yourself. If you can relate to a Judeo-Christian illustration, look at it this way: if God can forgive you, why can't you forgive yourself?[376] If that spiritual perspective doesn't connect with you, try this: if the families of murder victims can forgive the murderer, why can't you forgive yourself? After all, no matter how you feel you've hurt yourself, you're still very much alive.

Timeless Prescription #6: Don't Compromise

Blessed are the pure in heart, for they shall see God. Matthew 5:8

Richard had fallen upon hard times: he had lost his job, his wife had left him, and he found himself out on the street with three children. Rachel, a friend from years back, was dealing with her own challenges. Although reeling from a bitter divorce, Rachel graciously invited Richard to stay in her home with her and her daughter. Without much thought, Richard accepted her offer. After all, he and his kids needed a place to stay. It also seemed like an emotionally safe environment; there was never anything romantic between him and Rachel.

Within a few days of his moving in, however, Rachel began a blatant process of seduction. Richard was determined to avoid a sexual relationship, and he soon was forced to move out. But more damage was done. Rachel resorted to social media to further sully his reputation, adding a mass of lies to his already difficult situation.

Modern dictionaries equate "purity" with freedom from contamination and, particularly, with freedom from immorality, especially in the sexual realm. Should we even be concerned about such notions when many are trying to tell us there really is no objective right or wrong? After all, if there are no moral absolutes, *then how can anything be immoral?*

In contrast to the sometimes questionable nature of morality, there was no question that Richard's situation had become more difficult and painful because he wouldn't compromise. Making his situation more complex was this: one easily could reason that Richard and his children would have been better off had he given in. To be out on the street is, generally, not a health-enhancing situation. But what does the medical literature reveal? Could compromise ultimately entail a greater cost than retaining purity? Before we go there, lets first look at the scriptural approach.

Moral Purity in the Biblical World

Even in biblical times, standing for right often appeared—at least on the surface—to be the wrong decision. Consider the classic story of Joseph. After being sold into slavery by his brothers, he found himself in the position of steward for a wealthy Egyptian named Potiphar.[377] Under Joseph's direction, all went very well in Potiphar's household, until Potiphar's wife decided she wanted to sleep with the handsome young Hebrew. However, Joseph refused her repeated overtures, ultimately declaring, "There is no one greater in this house than I, nor has he kept back anything from me but you, because you are his wife. How then can I do this great wickedness and sin against God?"[378]

His failure to compromise didn't earn Joseph a medal but a stiff prison sentence instead. Nonetheless, as events transpired, Joseph's time in prison remarkably became the pathway to him serving as the Egyptian prime minister.

This foundational story in the Bible's first book sets the stage for similar stories and teachings throughout Scripture. The counterintuitive message resonates today: refusing to compromise may bring short-term difficulties; however, in the long term, God blesses the lives of those who remain pure.

The Practical Significance of Moral Rectitude, Avoiding Compromise

Elsa came into my office concerned about depression. When I asked her about any precipitating factors, she hung her head low and described a sexual indiscretion. Whether or not you believe in "sexual sin," Elsa was clearly struggling with shame, guilt, and remorse.

Recent evidence suggests that shame may be related to high blood pressure. Researchers from Brandeis University and the University of Rhode Island have linked shame to higher stress hormone levels, a connection with clear implications for poorer blood pressure control.[379] Unfortunately, in this and many similar papers, researchers look at shame or shame-proneness as primarily individual character traits, as opposed to looking at shame as a response to specific life choices. This oversight may underestimate how the *causes* of shame impact high blood pressure. Even common dictionary definitions of shame highlight painful feelings like regret, sadness, humiliation, guilt or distress "caused by consciousness of guilt, shortcoming, or impropriety."[380]

Sure, some individuals are more prone to shame and guilt. However, it could be argued that at some point—at least on some level—everyone feels ashamed when caught doing something wrong. Furthermore, although shame can be linked to personal failures or compromise, it too often has its roots in the indiscretions of others. Victims typically feel shame—although they personally did nothing worthy of blame. For example, individuals who are the victims of sexual abuse often feel ashamed of their history, despite having no personal responsibility for being violated.

In some particularly provocative research, experts from three prestigious institutions, Columbia, Yale and Duke, analyzed data from New York City. They focused their attention on 247 HIV-infected adults who had been sexually abused as children. No attempt was made to determine whether the childhood abuse was related to their HIV infection. The investigators' goal was to see if shame affected quality of life. In order to make their analyses, the team honed in on two sources of shame: shame associated with their childhood sexual trauma and shame related to being HIV positive. Neither of these two historical characteristics inevitably causes shame or guilt. However, many affected individuals are at least somewhat ashamed of one or both. When all the data was in, only the HIV-related shame was linked to poor health outcomes, including decreased health-related quality of life, poorer social well-being and impaired cognitive functioning.[381]

Consider some important implications of this study:

1. Shame and guilt reflect individual experiences. We can't necessarily predict what life events will produce such feelings. Consequently, it is typically unwise to make assumptions about the presence of shame or its causes.

2. It is generally best to cultivate compassion toward those dealing with potentially shame-inducing life situations.

3. If you're dealing with a condition through no apparent fault of your own (such as childhood sexual abuse, or contracting HIV in a setting where you were violated), don't punish yourself. Even if you don't know who to blame, inappropriately blaming yourself only hurts you and your body.

4. If you wish to avoid experiencing shame from your own choices, realize that making choices contrary to your own values often lays the foundation for shame. Even a single

violation of your moral principles may set the stage for life-long feelings of shame or guilt. Such violations—and the weight of the resultant shame—can increase the risk of stress-related conditions like hypertension. (Don't despair, if you're speeding through this chapter and didn't make the connection, Timeless Prescription #2 already provided some antidotes to shame and guilt.)

5. Finally, healing is available, regardless of whether you are the victim of your own bad choices, the choices of others, or even have no idea where to place blame. In the New York City study, for example, the researchers concluded that HIV-positive individuals would likely gain significant benefit from stress management interventions as well as programs fostering better social support.

The investigators' observations are noteworthy. Although avoiding compromise is always the best personal choice, far too often we are victimized by the compromises of others. This is not the end of the road—despite the beatitude's call for purity. From a Christian perspective, as we have already observed, God offers forgiveness to everyone. However, even from a totally secular perspective, we can come to terms with our past and move on. Some of those resources involve just what the research literature highlights: greater investments in stress management and socially-connecting activities.

Although compromise involves many other areas of life beyond the sexual, sexuality is extremely important in these regards, not only because of the traditional connections with purity, but also because of the far-ranging physical and mental health implications of our sexual choices. Generations of health professional students have been vividly reminded of this reality when our teachers repeated the aphorism: "One night with Venus and the rest of your life with mercury." That saying hearkened back to the days when chronic syphilis was treated with mercury-laden pharmaceuticals.

Today, of course, chronic syphilis may seem like a disease of interest only to medical historians. Most people think that modern medicine has conquered most sexually transmitted diseases (STDs). Not true. STDs, even those that seem largely subjugated, are again rearing their heads, some in epidemic proportions. Even syphilis, as illustrated in Figure 14.5, is on the rise.[382] Of note, the rise in syphilis is largely a male epidemic, with 91% of the cases being among men, and 83% of those male cases occurring among men who have sex with men.

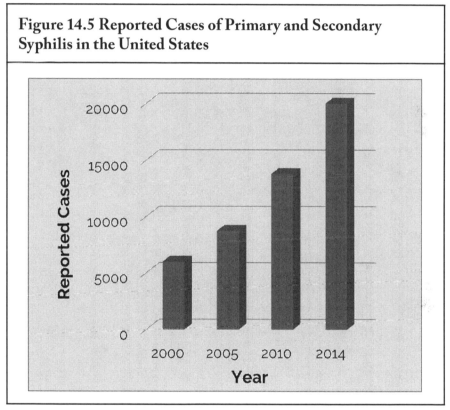

Figure 14.5 Reported Cases of Primary and Secondary Syphilis in the United States

Though presenting this data in a section dealing with moral choices, I'm not taking a position here on what your moral values should be. I'm merely making the observation that—regardless of your sexual orientation, regardless of whether you are married to a single partner or have multiple sexual partners—it is likely you have some sense of what is right and wrong when it comes to sexual practices.[383] For example, some heterosexual religionists may label all homosexual relations wrong; while others, equally religious, may be living in a committed gay or lesbian relationship. However, even gay couples who don't consider themselves religious still may feel (at least in certain circumstances) it is "wrong" for their partner to be sexually involved with another. Here's my point from a cross-cultural perspective: be true to your own values. Live a pure and moral life in your own eyes (regardless of how others label you). And interestingly, those values across cultural and sexual-orientation lines *generally* decrease your number of lifetime sexual partners, which yields health benefits. By all means, don't compromise your own morality just because you don't measure up to someone else's moral code, or desires. Be true to yourself, and don't compromise.

I could make the same appeal in dealing with any other aspect of morality. Clearly, these connections are not limited to sexuality. Investigators from UCLA's Department of Psychology[384] documented a number of negative outcomes when volunteers wrote about a variety of life events for which they blamed themselves. Among their results was an increase in shame and guilt, as well as a rise in markers of inflammation (recall that inflammation in the body contributes to higher blood pressure).

Sure, we can blame ourselves for honest mistakes and other human failings. These can never be totally avoided. However, valuing purity and moral rectitude can be a safeguard against one category of major stressors, blaming ourselves for our own moral failings. From the biblical worldview, God never asks us to do something he is not committed to help us accomplish. If that doesn't offer you encouragement, please remember the power of your own will. Making a choice to stop doing something you believe is wrong is extremely powerful.

If there are moral compromises in your life, why not, today, begin addressing them? If you can visualize some concrete steps in that direction, why not add them to your goals at the end of this chapter?

Timeless Prescription #7: Mediate

Blessed are the peacemakers, for they shall be called sons of God.
Matthew 5:9

I grew up in a nuclear family that was estranged from my mother's parents and siblings. Much of the tension stemmed from an event that occurred years before I was born: my mother's expulsion from a conservative Christian college on grounds that she deemed unjust. My mom's bitterness toward the college spilled over into her relationship with her parents (who had encouraged her to attend that particular school) and to the Christian church of her youth. Although I didn't realize it for many years, the estrangement—and the unresolved issues it represented—was a major stressor for my mother.

When I was a teenager, my grandparents began seeking reconciliation with my family. They sought to rebuild that relationship in an unusual way: they requested permission to park their motorhome outside our house and live in it during the summer. (Those dynamics may seem a bit more understandable when you realize we lived in Canada, and my grandfather was a university professor in the States.)

Although initially resisting, my mother did ultimately allow the motorhome to become a summer fixture at our place. Relationships were gradually rebuilt. I have fond memories of my grandparents visiting with the whole family in the evenings, as well as spending time with my teenage brother and me while my parents were at work.

I found my grandparents to be very loving and gentle. They taught me about a loving God who called us to love and to help each other. It took three full summers of visiting but my family, and most importantly, my mom, slowly began warming up to her siblings and parents again. We all began attending church, and a peace entered our family and my own heart that I had never experienced before. To this day I value my grandparents as peacemakers of the highest order.

Of course, I am not alone in appreciating the value of reconciliation. In a world filled with hostilities, we still value peace across cultural lines. So enshrined is peace in the world's consciousness that we collectively celebrate peace and mediation when the Nobel Foundation names its annual recipient of the Peace Prize.

In addition to the societal value of peace, the concept has broad medical implications. Perhaps this truth is most clearly seen in studies looking at the antithesis of peace: hostility. Earlier in this book, I presented data from the CARDIA Study (Coronary Artery Risk Development in Young Adults Study), which showed the connection between hostility and the development of high blood pressure (see Chapter 11). This provides only a glimpse into the broad health literature database showing the dangers of hostility. A quick look at the wealth of data on this subject is provided by a search of the National Library of Medicine's database. The term "hostility" pulls up over 8000 scientific references.

Consequently, in this section we look at the value of supporting peace, reconciliation, and harmony. However, in order to extend this gift to others, we must first accept it ourselves. We must be at peace with ourselves before we can most effectively mediate between others. Similarities between this beatitude and the fifth, highlighting the importance of mercy and forgiveness, abound. However, there are also important nuances, with special relevance in the blood pressure arena.

Peacemaking in the Biblical World

Making peace, restoring harmony into broken relationships, is the underlying theme of the Bible. Looked at structurally, the first two chapters of the Bible tell how God created a perfect world; the last two chapters tell how he will recreate such an idyllic state. What intervenes is, first, the story of humankind's sin, and then the work of God in mediating or making peace.

From a biblical perspective, sin—at its very heart—is rebellion against God's just and loving provisions. Unlike many religious codes (even those advocated by some Jews and Christians, who say they are advocating scriptural principles), the Bible's commandments were never arbitrary exactions.

As an example of the motive behind all God's counsel, consider the words of Deuteronomy 5, in the context of the second recitation of the Ten Commandments:

> You shall be careful therefore to do as the LORD your God has commanded you. You shall not turn aside to the right hand or to the left. You shall walk in all the way that the LORD your God has commanded you, that you may live, and that it may go well with you, and that you may live long in the land that you shall possess.[385]

Thus, God's law was always an expression of the *best,* most peaceful, and happiest way for mankind to live. This is likely one reason why Jesus taught that the entire law could be summarized by a single word: love.[386] On the other hand, sin—or violation of God's law[387]—could be crystalized in another single word: rebellion. Sin is, at its heart, rebellion against God's orderly universe. But it is more than that; in the biblical worldview, sin is that which breaks trusting, loving relationships with our heavenly father and our fellow humans.

God illustrated his desire—and commitment to reconciliation—to a nation who had been enslaved in Egypt for generations. Beginning with the Passover meal on the day that they were miraculously delivered from Egyptian bondage, God instituted a sanctuary service that was to serve as a model for what he wanted to do in every human heart.

So central was this service to the day-to-day life of his people that God instructed them to construct a portable tabernacle or temple in the midst of the Jewish encampment. This sanctuary was all about restoring right relations between a people prone to sin/rebel and a God even more determined to love, forgive and make whole. If there was any doubt that the whole service was focused on mediation, forgiveness and peace, one only has to look at the day when the most important service took place there. It was Yom Kippur, the Day of Atonement. At its heart, atonement is all about *at-one-ment*, bringing peace to estranged parties.

To a world today largely made up of urban dwellers, aspects of that sanctuary service may seem macabre and politically incorrect. Indeed, from our superficial vantage point, many of the services may seem to show disregard for animal life. However, understood from the agricultural context of the Jewish people, the services made perfect sense. Before the sanctuary system was formalized in the wilderness of Sinai, each family was slaying domesticated animals for food. In the sanctuary system, God connected this necessary taking of life with what he was going to do, which was give his own life for his people.

In fact, what happened at the wilderness sanctuary, also known as the tabernacle, was very different from the animal sacrifices of other indigenous peoples. Anthropologically, most cultures that engaged in animal sacrifices did so, hoping to please or placate their gods. In the biblical worldview, the situation was just the opposite. The only purpose of the sanctuary was for God's people to show their faith in the deliverance that He Himself would accomplish *for them*. When people forgot about this underlying meaning of the services, God spoke in no uncertain terms:

> I desire steadfast love and not sacrifice,
>   the knowledge of God rather than burnt offerings.[388]

The sanctuary and its message of reconciliation were not reserved for a single nationality. Throughout the New Testament, sanctuary terminology (language from the Old Testament sacrificial system) was used to refer to what Jesus' ministry accomplished for all of mankind. Although such comparisons abound in books like Hebrews and Romans, other books also embrace this theme. For example, Paul in this second letter to the Corinthian church wrote:

> God... through Christ reconciled us to himself and gave us the ministry of reconciliation; that is, in Christ God was reconciling the world to himself, not counting their trespasses against them, and entrusting to us the message of reconciliation. Therefore, we are ambassadors for Christ, God making his appeal through us. We implore you on behalf of Christ, be reconciled to God. For our sake he made him to be sin who knew no sin, so that in him we might become the righteousness of God.[389]

In the passage above we see evidence of the recurring connections between the ministry of Jesus and reconciliation (the latter providing implicit testimony to the underlying theme of the sanctuary services). That connection is strengthened when we realize that, in an earlier letter to the same Greek church, Paul made it clear that the Passover, in and of itself, was not the central issue. Although the service was commemorative, it also pointed forward to an ultimately greater reality. Of the Messiah, this Hebrew apostle wrote: "For Christ, our Passover lamb, has been sacrificed."[390]

Some might try to argue that Paul, although himself a Jew, was still involved in a type of cultural appropriation, trying to make the Hebrew services applicable to non-Jews. However, even a careful reading of the Hebrew Scriptures themselves makes it clear that from a biblical standpoint their religion was given them as a trust in order to be a benefit to all nations. Thus when the patriarch Abraham was called by God he was promised,

> I will make of you a great nation, and I will bless you and make

your name great, so that you will be a blessing. I will bless those who bless you, and him who dishonors you I will curse, and in you all the families of the earth shall be blessed.[391]

The idea that God called Abraham and his offspring to be a blessing to the whole world seems largely forgotten. After all, many of the world's conflicts have been fueled—or at least supported—by individuals who identified themselves as Abraham's descendants. But the truth is that the biblical vision of our existence is one primarily of promoting unity and harmony rather than conflict!

Don't read into my words an unthinking pacifism. In the biblical worldview there were "just wars." However, for those who criticize the religions that stem from Abraham's offspring (Judaism, Catholicism, Protestant Christianity, and Islam) for their role in human carnage, I suggest you think again. The fault is not with Abraham or the religion God instituted, but with humans superimposing their often perverse ideas on what God has called them to do and be.

The book of Isaiah provides another line of evidence that the Bible intended the sanctuary message of reconciliation to reach the whole planet, not merely a single race. Isaiah wrote:

> Let not the foreigner who has joined himself to the Lord say,
> "The Lord will surely separate me from his people..."
> For thus says the LORD...
> "the foreigners who join themselves to the Lord,
> to minister to him, to love the name of the Lord,
> and to be his servants,
> everyone who keeps the Sabbath and does not profane it,
> and holds fast my covenant—
> these I will bring to my holy mountain,
> and make them joyful in my house of prayer;
> their burnt offerings and their sacrifices
> will be accepted on my altar;
> for my house shall be called a house of prayer

for all peoples."
The Lord God,
who gathers the outcasts of Israel, declares,
"I will gather yet others to him
besides those already gathered."[392]

Certainly, even toward "outsiders," God was all about making peace. What I find particularly interesting about the words of Isaiah above is this: the sign of the covenant was keeping the Sabbath. The sanctuary connection here is profound, for special occasions in the sanctuary services were often marked by specially designated Sabbaths.[393] These Sabbaths, like the weekly Sabbath (kept biblically from sundown Friday to sundown Saturday), were times when God's people rested in what he was doing (or had done) on their behalf. At the heart of each of these Sabbath occasions—whether the Passover, Yom Kippur, or the weekly Sabbath—was a message about a God who reaches out to humanity, offering them healing and wholeness, and does so most often through reconciliation.

See it through the eyes of the Bible writers: the first Sabbath was given as a memorial of God's work in creating our planet.[394] No reconciliation was needed during that first Sabbath, for mankind was in harmony with God. However after the entrance of sin, the weekly Sabbath was infused with additional significance as a memorial of God's work of redemption.[395] From then on, the Sabbath observances, whether weekly or connected with the sanctuary's festivals, had a redemptive or reconciliatory purpose.

Consequently, Sabbath observance was a sign that a person accepted God's provision for his wholeness. Contrary to the critics of Sabbath observance today, Sabbath keeping was never a work that had merit in itself.

In summary, the biblical world saw mediation and harmony as central to its entire message. The sanctuary and the Sabbath both were intimately connected with this peacemaking purpose. God is the one who reaches out the hand of reconciliation. Our job is to accept it. We are first brought into harmony with God, and then we can extend the gift of reconciliation to the rest of the world.

The Practical Significance of Mediation and Harmony

Medical research indicates that one of the mechanisms by which religion and spirituality confer health benefits is by fostering stronger social relationships. One of the world's classic population health studies, the Alameda County Study, begun by Dr. Lester Breslow in the 1960s, sheds some fascinating light on this subject.[396]

In 2001, Breslow's successors, led by William J. Strawbridge, looked at thirty years' worth of data involving 2,676 participants. Those reporting weekly religious attendance tended to have more social relationships and greater marital stability. Those connections may not be all that surprising. However, what was remarkable in light of our *No Pressure* journey was this: those attending religious services regularly "were more likely to both improve poor health behaviors and maintain good ones"—over a period of three decades! Additionally, weekly religious attendance was associated with better mental health.

From this physician's vantage point, those results are striking. First, if you maintain a long-term connection with a group of people in a faith community, you can be sure that your "peacemaking" skills will be occasionally put to the test. Sure, anyone can disown their family, leave their job, or stop attending their church, synagogue, or temple. However, when we stay in those settings, we have opportunities to grow as we negotiate our way through life's conflicts. What is unique in the faith community setting is that attendance is voluntary. We may not feel at liberty to leave our place of employment. Even if we abandon our family, we'll still probably share a common surname. However, for most of us, few constraints bind us that closely to a specific congregation for worship. In other words, faith communities provide a voluntary arena where we are called to deal with social difficulties in a constructive way. Perhaps this very feature provides an aid to mental health and healthy behavior maintenance.

Second, faith communities historically present messages about the importance of reconciliation, often first on the vertical or spiritual dimension, but then also on a human level. What we saw in the biblical world is mirrored in the Orient by Buddhists who, like the Dalai Lama, preach a message of peace and compassion. It is reflected by Muslims worldwide who decry the brutal practices of some who have brought Islam into disrepute. It is seen in the lives of Native Americans, who, in spite of historical mistreatment by those of European stock, find meaning and encouragement in their traditional worship practices, yet also seek harmony with the descendants of their oppressors. I could give other examples.[397] But the bottom line is this: across denominational and cultural labels many congregations value peace, harmony and reconciliation. Sure, there are some glaring exceptions. However, many—if not most—places of worship are settings where mediation is valued and promoted.

If not part of a faith community, don't view these observations as a slight. You may be an even greater advocate for harmony in your village, town, or city than is the most devout churchgoer or temple worshipper. The values of peace and mediation can be embraced by secular humanists, and often are. However, my point is that if you are not in a committed social relationship with others—as occurs with faith community membership—you're missing a powerful source of reinforcement when it comes to your most noble values.

To summarize the seventh beatitude, consider how you can promote peace in all the social networks where you find yourself. As far as arriving at practical goals along these lines consider the following questions:

- Are there interpersonal problems in my nuclear or extended family that I can help address?

- Can I use my influence to make a difference as far as defusing tensions in my community?

- What can I do in my workplace to foster better collegiality and respect?

Timeless Prescription #8: Persist

Blessed are those who are persecuted for righteousness' sake, for theirs is the kingdom of heaven. Blessed are you when others revile you and persecute you and utter all kinds of evil against you falsely on my account. Rejoice and be glad, for your reward is great in heaven, for so they persecuted the prophets who were before you. Matthew 5:10-12

On-demand videos. Instant, on-line purchases. Remote control devices. No-waiting-in-line internet banking. We are a society accustomed to getting what we want when we want it. But is our instant-gratification culture exacting a hefty price? Could we be losing the virtue of patience?

One interesting dynamic of any given virtue is that its optimal development occurs only in settings that test or stress it. Patience is, perhaps, most tested in circumstances where we have every right to be impatient. Situations pervaded by injustice like unwarranted persecution surely fit that bill. Therefore, the final beatitude describes a context calculated to produce either optimal patience or its antithesis.

However, this beatitude speaks not merely of a stoical patience, but rather a persistence infused with rejoicing. It is this aspect of the prescription that connects us with today's positive psychology movement, a movement that declares we have the power to cultivate optimism in spite of persecution or other difficulties.[398] Such optimism, in turn, offers significant physical—as well as mental—health benefits.

Persistence in the Biblical World

In this chapter we have been looking at the power of virtues to change health outcomes. However, our last beatitude brings us to a strange conclusion. The very things that help our health and increase our capacity for blessing others may be turned against us.

Dr. Gary Namie and colleagues at the Workplace Bullying Institute recently conducted a survey to ascertain the qualities of those most likely to attract a bully's ire. Many lay people likely found the results surprising. Although a third of the victims met the stereotypes of appearing vulnerable and unlikely to defend themselves, 61% of the victims were defined primarily as kind, giving, altruistic, or agreeable.[399] In other words, developing the very characteristics described in the first seven beatitudes is likely (in the right—or wrong—context) to result in persecution.

From the biblical worldview, Jesus and his followers also acknowledged this same dynamic. Paul said unequivocally, "all who desire to live a godly life in Christ Jesus will be persecuted."[400] Jesus himself told his disciples:

> Behold, I am sending you out as sheep in the midst of wolves, so be wise as serpents and innocent as doves. Beware of men, for they will deliver you over to courts and flog you in their synagogues, and you will be dragged before governors and kings for my sake, to bear witness before them... do not fear those who kill the body but cannot kill the soul. Rather fear him who can destroy both soul and body in hell. Are not two sparrows sold for a penny? And not one of them will fall to the ground apart from your Father. But even the hairs of your head are all numbered. Fear not, therefore; you are of more value than many sparrows.[401]

How could Christ's followers remain free of worry, and even go so far as to rejoice? The secret was distilled by one Christian author: "It is easy living after we are dead."[402] However, for those not familiar with a biblical worldview such a declaration sounds oxymoronic.

The death being referred to hearkens back to the third beatitude, for it refers to submission. *Death* in this biblical setting indicates a total surrender, giving up our own desires to submit fully to God's will for our lives.

In the biblical worldview, the true believer surrenders herself fully to God, so that her highest desire is to follow the directions of her Creator and Redeemer. The Bible speaks of this experience as dying to self or the crucifixion of self (which could be more precisely defined as dying to selfishness and sin).

However, the analogy with death has another dimension. As we have already observed in this chapter, the Bible teaches that eternal death—not an immortal roasting in hell fire—is the natural consequence of sin. For example, Adam and Eve were banished from the Garden of Eden after sin, in order to ensure there would never be an immortal sinner.[403] That's right, if sinners are suffering in a hell for eternity, then they are by definition *immortal* sinners, something that God took pains to prevent from the beginning. Furthermore, the idea of sinners burning for eternity is not consistent with the Bible's messages either of a loving God, or of a God who will ultimately have a universe free of sin and evil. Instead, the Bible focuses on God's redemption and reconciliation of his wayward children, not their destruction. Even Jesus endorsed such a view. As one example, did you catch the words I recently cited from the *Gospel of Matthew*, Chapter 10: "do not fear those who kill the body but cannot kill the soul; rather fear him who can destroy both soul and body in hell"?[404] But Jesus doesn't stop with a message of doom and gloom. Luke adds these words of the master teacher: "Fear not, little flock, for it is your Father's good pleasure to give you the kingdom."[405]

So here's how the other dimension to the death analogy comes into the picture: the believer considers herself dead to the world (surrendering her selfishness and sin), but also accepts by faith the death of Jesus on her behalf. In other words, she believes that, somehow, in God's system of justice, Jesus was dying on that cross some 2000 years ago to pay the penalty for her sins. This concept of the substitutionary atonement is unique in the biblical world, and it has its foundations in the sanctuary services.

How could someone suffer the penalty for someone else's crime, especially when that penalty was death, and when the one dying allegedly rose from the grave a few days later? That's a good question. However, I'm not writing a theological treatise; rather, I'm trying to give you some unique health principles in their original cultural context. So for now, just take my summary of God's legal system at face value. See if the following doesn't follow logically and, also, shed light on dealing with some of life's most difficult situations.

This aspect of the biblical worldview (the concept of the substitutionary atonement) informs another practice that seems strange to the uninitiated: that of baptism by immersion. Although it has become fashionable to baptize by sprinkling, dipping, or other means, Bible baptism was always by full immersion. (Jesus himself was so baptized.[406]) Why? Baptism was a sign that a consenting individual was choosing to accept the death (or crucifixion) of Christ on his behalf. It was a public proclamation he was dying to self and sin. Going fully under the water represented death, emerging from the water represented the "born again" or "new life" experience.[407]

When writing to the church in Colossae, Paul again makes the connection between baptism and death to self and sin. However, he doesn't stop there. He gives some amazing insights into living the principles of all *The Beatitudes* and being joyful, even in the face of persecution. Listen to his logic:

> ...having been buried with him [Christ] in baptism, in which you were also raised with him through faith in the powerful working of God, who raised him from the dead. And you, who were dead in your trespasses... God made alive together with him, having forgiven us all our trespasses,

by canceling the record of debt that stood against us with its legal demands. This he set aside, nailing it to the cross...

If then you have been raised with Christ, seek the things that are above, where Christ is, seated at the right hand of God. Set your minds on things that are above, not on things that are on earth. For you have died, and your life is hidden with Christ in God...

Put to death therefore what is earthly in you: sexual immorality, impurity, passion, evil desire, and covetousness, which is idolatry... In these you too once walked, when you were living in them. But now you must put them all away: anger, wrath, malice, slander, and obscene talk from your mouth. Do not lie to one another, seeing that you have put off the old self with its practices and have put on the new self...

Put on then, as God's chosen ones, holy and beloved, compassionate hearts, kindness, humility, meekness, and patience, bearing with one another and, if one has a complaint against another, forgiving each other; as the Lord has forgiven you, so you also must forgive. And above all these put on love, which binds everything together in perfect harmony. And let the peace of Christ rule in your hearts, to which indeed you were called in one body. And be thankful. Let the word of Christ dwell in you richly, teaching and admonishing one another in all wisdom, singing psalms and hymns and spiritual songs, with thankfulness in your hearts to God. And whatever you do, in word or deed, do everything in the name of the Lord Jesus, giving thanks to God the Father through him.[408]

Have you written Christianity off because of the sexual immorality of professed Christians—or their anger, loss of patience, unkindness, etc.? If so, you haven't been rightly judging Christianity—just those who are either false professors or those who have not fully allowed Christ to bear sway in their lives. Yes, one of the best arguments against Christianity is the shortcomings of its professors. It's a humbling admission, for years ago I left the agnostic camp to become a Christian—and I still fall short. This doesn't leave me depressed or despondent, just longing for a closer relationship with the risen Christ, the only one who can help me live a life worthy of his name.

But there are other implications to that passage in Colossians that speak to us regardless of our religious persuasion. And it's this: perhaps Jesus spent the longest time articulating the eighth and final beatitude because, in a sense, that which tries our patience most is what we desperately need, in order to fully embrace—and practice—all the virtues. For many of us, only when we go through difficulties like persecution do we really look heavenward in full dependence. One aged Christian gentleman put it this way, "The worse the outlook, the better the up-look." Indeed, it's only during the storms of life that many of us finally realize our need to fully surrender to the God of the universe.

To summarize, the biblical world tells us to be prepared for persecution when we follow *The Beatitudes*. However, it assures us we can stand fearless and even rejoice in the midst of such onslaughts. The secret to such a stance is realizing God wants to live his life in me, giving me the strength to stand, representing his loving and just character.[409]

The Practical Significance of Persistence

If you've been following the *No Pressure* program to this point, you probably already have been facing some persecution. This is true whether or not anything resonated with you regarding the biblical world's perspective on the eighth beatitude.

Think about it. You've embarked on a new lifestyle. Many of your friends and family likely have been threatened by some of your new good habits. (Perhaps they too have hypertension and don't want to believe they have to change their lives to get the best blood pressure results.) Although some may respect you for your resolve, others—often just as well meaning—will engage in overt (or perhaps covert) persecution. It may be frank mocking or overt disdain. You may have heard things like, "So you think you're better than us?" or, "So now our food isn't good enough for you?"

Others will assail your new lifestyle in subtler ways. They'll send you a link to a website that says salt and obesity are really good for your blood pressure. Or they'll leave a news clipping on your desk that alleges you can have great blood pressure, and follow any lifestyle you want, as long as you take some proprietary over-the-counter pill.

Don't succumb to any of these forms of "persecution." Instead, be patient. The full impact of lifestyle changes takes time and persistence. And, interestingly, the patience you exercise will be providing you with additional tools to help keep your blood pressure in check.

Consider a fascinating study that comes from a Muslim population. Researchers in Tehran, Iran assessed 252 Iranian college students (123 males and 129 females). They found those with greater levels of patience (measured in any one of three different realms: interpersonal, life hardship, and daily hassles) had better health. Specifically, students who were more patient had greater life satisfaction and less depression, as well as lower levels of anxiety and psychological dysfunction.[410]

The benefits of patience are not confined to the Muslim world. Sarah Schnitker, PhD, Associate Professor of Psychology at Fuller Theological Seminary's School of Psychology, has looked at patience in other populations. She too has found that this virtue has far-reaching benefits. Of particular interest, Dr. Schnitker demonstrated that patience aids in goal pursuit—especially when faced with obstacles.[411]

This is of great importance when it comes to developing new habits. Think about it: if you want to make lasting changes that will help normalize your blood pressure for the rest of your life, then you want to keep your eyes on that goal. Patience will aid you in so doing—especially when you hit those bumps along life's road. But let's not stop here. The last of the eight divine prescriptions provides a secret to building patience: rejoicing in the face of persecution.

There's probably no better note on which to close this chapter, and the main didactic portion of this book. You're on the path to success. Persist. Stick with it. The greatest benefits typically come to those who are patient and don't deviate from their goals.

A Final Question

For three decades I've been helping people change their lifestyles.[412] Some people see results within days (or even hours) of making lifestyle changes; others see few improvements until they stick with their new behaviors for weeks or months.

I've often asked myself the question: "Who is better off, the person who sees results quickly or the one who notches positive changes only after a long time?" Well, honestly, I don't know. There are dangers in both camps.

Those who see quick improvements are in danger of minimizing the importance of long-lasting lifestyle changes. It's easy for them to reason: "Wow, it's really easy to control blood pressure. Just walk a little bit, watch my diet for a few days, and shed a few pounds. I can do that any time I want." The very ease of improvement belies how critical it is to not deviate from the healthy lifestyle that you've been following for the better part of a month. If you're in this camp, congratulations. However, don't rest on your laurels. Adhere to the good changes you've made. Stick with your new *No Pressure* lifestyle.

On the other hand, if you've not yet seen much improvement, you're likely in the second group, the ones who only see progress after what can seem like an inordinate time.

Years ago, at the Lifestyle Center of America, we had a patient, "Juan," who came to our facility with only one goal in mind: lowering his staggering triglyceride level. (Marked elevations of triglycerides, a type of blood fat, increases the risk not only of cardiovascular problems but also of pancreatitis, a serious digestive disorder.) After two weeks at our residential facility, we ran a second set of blood tests on Juan, and all his fellow participants. Imagine Juan's excitement as he heard rumblings of remarkable drops in cholesterol, blood sugar and triglycerides from other patients who had seen their physicians before him.

When Juan's physician entered the exam room, an expectant Juan was not prepared for what would soon follow. "So Doc, how did my triglycerides fare?" were the first words out of his mouth. Rather than answering his query, his doctor simply placed a copy of his lab work in front of him. Juan's eyes scanned the paper, then stopped in disbelief. All he could manage was a feeble, "What?"

"Yes, Juan, I'm sorry but your triglycerides went up." Before his physician could say anything more, an enraged Juan stormed out of his office. Although he was determined to pack his bags, leave the facility and never come back, the staff prevailed upon Juan to be patient. His physician reinforced the same message.

Six months later Juan came back to the Lifestyle Center of America a very happy man; he had stuck with a lifestyle that seemed to make no difference at first, but now his triglycerides where literally a fraction of what they had been before coming to our facility.

If you're in that second group with Juan, you see the danger, don't you? If you haven't had impressive results on your *No Pressure* journey, you may be tempted to throw in the towel. But follow Juan's example, and don't give up. In the long run, the Juans in life may be more fortunate than the rapid responders. After all, there's much less danger that they will slip back into their old ways, knowing what an arduous task it was to normalize their numbers in the first place.

So, whether your journey has been easy or hard to this point I encourage you with that single word: Persist.

Chapter 14 Spirituality – Draft Worksheet

	Week 1							Week 2						
Day #	1	2	3	4	5	6	7	8	9	10	11	12	13	14
Behavioral Goals														
Example 1: Cultivate altruism, humility and selflessness by performing at least one daily random act of kindness (i.e., an unplanned act where you spontaneously help someone without any expectation of personal gain).														
Example 2: Attempt to get connected or reconnected with a faith community by attending worship services once a week (visiting one or more congregations)														
Example 3: Take steps to restoring a broken relationship with a family member or coworker (make this goal SMART with your own specifics, etc.)														
My Goal 14:1														
My Goal 14:2														
My Goal 14:3														
My Goal 14:4														
My Goal 14:5														

15

PUTTING IT ALL TOGETHER

IF YOU'VE BEEN "WORKING the *No Pressure* program" on your way to this concluding chapter, then odds are that you've already noted some significant benefits. If you're like many of the patients who have even followed a portion of the elements we've covered, you've seen not only physical benefits, but there's a good chance your mind is clearer and your sense of well-being has improved.

I promised this was a 30-day journey. By this time you should be approaching that terminus. However, where do you go from here? I would suggest you take a few days to seriously consider which elements of this program you will commit to long term.

The amazing thing about lifestyle change is that we can develop new habits, and enjoy them as much or more than our old practices. We just have to be persistent.

Some years ago I was leading out in a group session at one of the several residential health centers I've worked at over the years. One of the participants, who I'll call Brenda, made a startling announcement to the whole group: "I didn't come here with any intention of following all the elements of this program when I went home. However, after seeing my results, I'd be a fool not to."

Granted, Brenda had an advantage over some of you. You see, shortly after Brenda arrived for our 18-day residential program she had extensive blood testing. She had the same blood work repeated at the end of the program. Marked improvement on those tests apparently contributed to her bold proclamation.

Even if you didn't have a blood test immediately preceding your 30-day journey, you can still follow Brenda's example. Why not ask your physician to have a blood panel drawn this week? You can then compare your results with tests you had before. You might be surprised by the progress.

Even if you never part with a drop of blood, I hope you've taken some time to gauge your actual blood pressure progress. Has your doctor been able to eliminate or reduce any of your medications? What has happened with your average blood pressure readings? Why not spend some time analyzing Appendix A. Calculate your average blood pressure for week one, then compare it with your blood pressure during the most recent week.

One other measurement is even easier to access: your weight. Unless you began this journey already quite thin or on a lifestyle very much like I've recommended, you should have lost at least a few pounds over the 30 days. Eating better, drinking more water and less caloric beverages, exercising regularly, and even getting more sleep, all help effect modest weight loss—even if you're not consciously cutting back on your calories. (If you have a lot to lose, 3-5 pounds may not seem like much, but think of it this way: if you keep up that rate of loss, you're on a trajectory to lose some 50 pounds in the next year.)

Blood tests and other standard measurements aside, have you made other quantifiable improvements? Can you walk farther without shortness of breath? Are you waking up more refreshed? Have you dropped a dress size; can you tighten your belt an extra notch?

As you reflect on this program, I want to give you an assignment:

take at least 30 minutes to write down all the benefits that you've reaped. These may include direct benefits, like the ones I've just mentioned, or even indirect benefits, which might include:

- Saving money by eating on a lower salt diet (you're making more food from scratch and eating out less)
- Getting more compliments about your appearance
- Cutting your commuting budget by walking or riding your bike to work (or to the train station for the daily commute)
- Sleeping better

Once you've made a gratitude journal, listing the benefits of this program, then you're prepared to answer the question about what will be different from here on out. I hope you'll conclude that you want to follow all ten facets of the *No Pressure* Program. And I hope—even if you're not there yet—those ten program elements will ensure we never bump into each other waiting in line for blood pressure meds at the pharmacy.

Continued success is my earnest wish and prayer.

Appendix A. Blood Pressure Chart

As mentioned in the text, we recommend you start checking and charting your blood pressure three or four times per day at least one week before beginning your thirty-day journey. (That's what the "Week 0" column is all about.) Then continue to check your BPs at that frequency over the 30 days when applying this book's principles. Note: if you're on BP meds, check with your doctor if your blood pressure is consistently running below 130 systolic or 80 diastolic. However, ask your doctor personally what thresholds she wants you to use, both high and low, before calling her office. (Note: to make calculations easier we have separate columns for systolic [S] and diastolic [D] readings.)

Day of the Week	Week 0		Week 1		Week 2		Week 3		Week 4		Week 5	
	S	D	S	D	S	D	S	D	S	D	S	D
Sun												
Mon												
Tues												
Wed												

Day of the Week	Week 0		Week 1		Week 2		Week 3		Week 4		Week 5	
	S	D	S	D	S	D	S	D	S	D	S	D
Thurs												
Fri												
Sat												
Weekly Ave												

Appendix B

Note: Ch = Chapter

	Week 1							Week 2							Week 3							Week 4							Wk 5	
	1	2	3	4	5	6	7	8	9	10	11	12	13	14	15	16	17	18	19	20	21	22	23	24	25	26	27	28	29	30
Ch 5																														
Ch 6																														
Ch 7																														
Ch 8																														
Ch 9																														
Ch 10																														
Ch 11																														

Appendix B (continued)

	Week 1							Week 2							Week 3							Week 4							Wk 5	
	1	2	3	4	5	6	7	8	9	10	11	12	13	14	15	16	17	18	19	20	21	22	23	24	25	26	27	28	29	30
Ch 12																														
Ch 13																														
Ch 14																														

ENDNOTES

[1] World Health Organization. *A Global Brief on Hypertension: Silent Killer, Global Public Health Crisis.* Geneva, Switzerland: WHO Press; 2013.

[2] CRED (Centre for Research on the Epidemiology of Disasters). Disaster Data: A Balanced Perspective. *CRED Crunch.* 2016 February; 41:1-3. Accessed 25 April 2016 at http://www.cred.be/publications.

[3] Centers for Disease Control and Prevention (CDC). High blood pressure fact sheet. http://www.cdc.gov/DHDSP/data_statistics/fact_sheets/fs_bloodpressure.htm. Updated 3 January 2014. Accessed 15 December 2014.

[4] The common statistical term, *prevalence*, refers to the percentage of a population affected by a given condition at a specific point in time.

[5] World Health Organization. *A Global Brief on Hypertension: Silent Killer, Global Public Health Crisis.* Geneva, Switzerland: WHO Press; 2013.

[6] Egan BM, Zhao Y, Axon RN. US trends in prevalence, awareness, treatment, and control of hypertension, 1988-2008. *JAMA.* 2010 May 26; 303(20):2043-50.

[7] Fields LE, Burt VL, Cutler JA, et al. The burden of adult hypertension in the United States 1999 to 2000: a rising tide. *Hypertension.* 2004; 44:398-404.

[8] Bengtsson H, Bergqvist D. Ruptured abdominal aortic aneurysm: a population-based study. *J Vasc Surg.* 1993 Jul;18(1):74-80. See also Schermerhorn ML, Bensley RP, Giles KA, et al. *Ann Surg.* 2012 Oct; 256(4): 651–658.

[9] Michel MC, Heemann U, Schumacher H, et al. Association of hypertension with symptoms of benign prostatic hyperplasia. *J Urol.* 2004 Oct;172(4 Pt 1):1390-3.

[10] Raz N, Rodrigue KM, Haacke EM. Brain aging and its modifiers: insights from in vivo neuromorphometry and susceptibility weighted imaging. *Ann N Y Acad Sci.* 2007 Feb;1097:84-93.

[11] Gąsecki D, Kwarciany M, Nyka W, Narkiewicz K. Hypertension, brain damage and cognitive decline. *Curr Hypertens Rep.* 2013 Dec;15(6):547-58.

[12] Smith PJ, Blumenthal JA, Babyak MA, et al. Effects of the dietary approaches to stop hypertension diet, exercise, and caloric restriction on neurocognition in overweight adults with high blood pressure. *Hypertension*. 2010 Jun;55(6):1331-8.

[13] Goldstein FC, Levey AI, Steenland NK. High blood pressure and cognitive decline in mild cognitive impairment. *J Am Geriatr* Soc. 2013;61(1):67–73.

[14] Lenfant C, Chobanian AV, Jones DW, Roccella EJ. Seventh report of the Joint National Committee on the Prevention, Detection, Evaluation, and Treatment of High Blood Pressure (JNC 7): resetting the hypertension sails. *Hypertension*. 2003 Jun;41(6):1178-9.

[15] Sheridan S, Pignone M, Donahue, K. Screening for high blood pressure: review of the evidence. *Am J Prev Med* 2003;25:151-8.

[16] Adapted from (a) Chobanian AV, Bakris GL, Black HR, et al. The seventh report of the Joint National Committee on Prevention, Detection, Evaluation, and Treatment of High Blood Pressure: the JNC 7 report. *JAMA*. 2003 May 21;289(19):2560-72; and (b) Egan BM, Zhao Y, Axon RN. US trends in prevalence, awareness, treatment, and control of hypertension, 1988-2008. *JAMA*. 2010 May 26;303(20):2043-50.

[17] Heart diagram. Wikipedia Commons website. Created by Wapcaplet in Sodipodi, CC BY-SA 3.0, https://commons.wikimedia.org/w/index.php?curid=830253.

[18] Lenfant C, Chobanian AV, Jones DW, et al. Seventh report of the Joint National Committee on the Prevention, Detection, Evaluation, and Treatment of High Blood Pressure (JNC 7): resetting the hypertension sails. *Hypertension*. 2003 Jun;41(6):1178-9.

[19] Lenfant C, Chobanian AV, Jones DW, et al. Seventh report of the Joint National Committee on the Prevention, Detection, Evaluation, and Treatment of High Blood Pressure (JNC 7): resetting the hypertension sails. *Hypertension*. 2003 Jun;41(6):1178-9.

[20] Thomas G, Shishehbor M, Brill D, Nally JV Jr. New hypertension guidelines: one size fits most? *Cleve Clin J Med*. 2014 Mar;81(3):178-88.

[21] Sleight P, Redon J, Verdecchia P, et al. Prognostic value of blood pressure in patients with high vascular risk in the Ongoing Telmisartan Alone and in combination with Ramipril Global Endpoint Trial study. *J Hypertens*. 2009 Jul;27(7):1360-9.

[22] Cushman WC, Whelton PK, Fine LJ, et al. SPRINT Trial results: latest news in hypertension management. *Hypertension.* 2016 Feb; 67(2):263-5.

[23] SPRINT Research Group, Wright JT Jr, Williamson JD, et al. A randomized trial of intensive versus standard blood-pressure control. *N Engl J Med.* 2015 Nov 26;373(22):2103-16.

[24] Carter BL, Chrischilles EA, Rosenthal G, et al. Efficacy and safety of nighttime dosing of antihypertensives: review of the literature and design of a pragmatic clinical trial. *J Clin Hypertens (Greenwich).* 2014 Feb;16(2):115-21.

[25] Perkovic V, Rodgers A. Redefining blood-pressure targets--SPRINT starts the marathon. *N Engl J Med.* 2015 Nov 26;373(22):2175-8.

[26] Stamler J, Stamler R, Neaton JD. Blood pressure, systolic and diastolic, and cardiovascular risks. US population data. *Arch Intern Med.* 1993 Mar 8;153(5):598-615.

[27] Kronish IM, Woodward M, Sergie Z, et al. Meta-analysis: impact of drug class on adherence to antihypertensives. *Circulation.* 2011 Apr 19;123(15):1611-21.

[28] Kronish IM, Woodward M, Sergie Z, et al. Meta-analysis: impact of drug class on adherence to antihypertensives. *Circulation.* 2011 Apr 19;123(15):1611-21.

[29] Keller G, Zimmer G, Mall G, et al. Nephron number in patients with primary hypertension. *N Engl J Med.* 2003 Jan 9;348(2):101-8.

[30] Zohdi V, Sutherland MR, Lim K, et al. Low birth weight due to intrauterine growth restriction and/or preterm birth: Effects on nephron number and long-term renal health. *Int J Nephrol.* 2012;2012:136942.

[31] Jones JE, Jurgens JA, Evans SA, et al. Mechanisms of fetal programming in hypertension. *Int J Pediatr.* 2012;2012:584831.

[32] Just a reminder: the accounts in this book are generally based on real patients who have been cared for by one or more of us. Except for rare cases where individuals have authorized us to use their exact story, personal details have been changed to ensure confidentiality.

[33] Morton DP, Rankin P, Morey P, et al. The effectiveness of the Complete Health Improvement Program (CHIP) in Australasia for reducing selected chronic disease risk factors: a feasibility study. *N Z Med J.* 2013 Mar 1;126(1370):43-54.

[34] Rankin P, Morton DP, Diehl H, et al. Effectiveness of a volunteer-delivered lifestyle modification program for reducing cardiovascular disease risk factors. *Am J Cardiol*. 2012 Jan 1;109(1):82-6.

[35] Adapted from Allen D. *Getting Things Done: the Art of Stress-Free Productivity*. New York: Penguin Books; 2002. See also: http://gettingthings-done.com/fivesteps/.

[36] Myers MG, Kaczorowski J, Dawes M, Godwin M. Automated office blood pressure measurement in primary care. *Can Fam Physician*. 2014 Feb;60(2):127-32.

[37] Ward AM, Takahashi O, Stevens R, Heneghan C. Home measurement of blood pressure and cardiovascular disease: systematic review and meta-analysis of prospective studies. *J Hypertens*. 2012 Mar;30(3):449-56.

[38] Mancia G, Bertinieri G, Grassi G, et al. Effects of blood-pressure measurement by the doctor on patient's blood pressure and heart rate. *Lancet*. 1983 Sep 24;2(8352):695-8.

[39] Clark CE, Horvath IA, Taylor RS, Campbell JL. Doctors record higher blood pressures than nurses: systematic review and meta-analysis. *The British Journal of General Practice*. 2014;64(621):e223-e232.

[40] Franklin SS, Thijs L, Hansen TW, et al. White-coat hypertension: new insights from recent studies. *Hypertension*. 2013 Dec;62(6):982-7.

[41] Ward AM, Takahashi O, Stevens R, Heneghan C. Home measurement of blood pressure and cardiovascular disease: systematic review and meta-analysis of prospective studies. *J Hypertens*. 2012 Mar;30(3):449-56.

[42] Cuspidi C, Sala C, Tadic M, et al. Is white-coat hypertension a risk factor for carotid atherosclerosis? A review and meta-analysis. *Blood Press Monit*. 2015 Apr;20(2):57-63.

[43] Cuspidi C, Rescaldani M, Tadic M, et al. White-coat hypertension, as defined by ambulatory blood pressure monitoring, and subclinical cardiac organ damage: a meta-analysis. *J Hypertens*. 2015 Jan;33(1):24-32.

[44] Newer studies show manual BP methods to be less accurate than automatic BP methods. See: Myers MG, Kaczorowski J, Dawes M, Godwin M. Automated office blood pressure measurement in primary care. *Can Fam Physician*. 2014 Feb;60(2):127-32.

[45] Landgraf J, Wishner SH, Kloner RA. Comparison of automated oscillometric

versus auscultatory blood pressure measurement. *Am J Cardiol.* 2010 Aug 1;106(3):386-8.

[46] Myers MG, Kaczorowski J, Dawes M, Godwin M. Automated office blood pressure measurement in primary care. *Can Fam Physician.* 2014 Feb;60(2):127-32.

[47] Mort JR, Kruse HR. Timing of blood pressure measurement related to caffeine consumption. *Ann Pharmacother.* 2008 Jan;42(1):105-10.

[48] Dr. DeRose's DVD resources can be purchased at www.compasshealth.net/purchase.

[49] Melby CL, Goldflies DG, Hyner GC, Lyle RM. Relation between vegetarian/nonvegetarian diets and blood pressure in black and white adults. *Am J Public Health.* 1989 Sep;79(9):1283-8.

[50] Fraser GE. Vegetarian diets: what do we know of their effects on common chronic diseases? *Am J Clin Nutr.* 2009 May;89(5):1607S-1612S.

[51] Berkow SE, Barnard ND. Blood pressure regulation and vegetarian diets. *Nutr Rev.* 2005 Jan;63(1):1-8.

[52] For an example of a study that connects dietary heart disease risk factors to high blood pressure see: Stamler J, Caggiula A, Grandits GA, et al. Relationship to blood pressure of combinations of dietary macronutrients. Findings of the Multiple Risk Factor Intervention Trial (MRFIT). *Circulation.* 1996 Nov 15;94(10):2417-23.

[53] Michaëlsson K, Wolk A, Langenskiöld S, et al. Milk intake and risk of mortality and fractures in women and men: cohort studies. *BMJ.* 2014 Oct 28;349:g6015.

[54] Feskanich D, Bischoff-Ferrari HA, Frazier AL, Willett WC. Milk consumption during teenage years and risk of hip fractures in older adults. *JAMA Pediatr.* 2014 Jan;168(1):54-60.

[55] Byberg L, Bellavia A, Orsini N, et al. Fruit and vegetable intake and risk of hip fracture: A cohort study of Swedish men and women. *J Bone Miner Res.* 2015 Jun;30(6):976-84.

[56] United States Department of Agriculture. National Nutrient Database for Standard Reference, Release 27. Agricultural Research Service, National Agricultural Library. http://ndb.nal.usda.gov/ndb/nutrients/index. Accessed 1 January 2015.

[57] Guang C, Phillips RD. Plant food-derived Angiotensin I converting enzyme inhibitory peptides. *J Agric Food Chem*. 2009 Jun 24;57(12):5113-20.

[58] Melby CL, Dunn PJ, Hyner GC, et al. Correlates of blood pressure in elementary schoolchildren. *J Sch Health*. 1987 Nov;57(9):375-8.

[59] Whelton PK, Appel L, Charleston J, et al. The effects of nonpharmacologic interventions on blood pressure of persons with high normal levels. Results of the Trials of Hypertension Prevention, Phase I. *JAMA*. 1992 Mar 4;267(9):1213-20.

[60] Leonard AD, Brey RL. Patient page. Blood pressure control and stroke: an ounce of prevention is worth a pound of cure. *Neurology*. 2002 Jul 9;59(1):E1-2.

[61] Mozaffarian D, Hao T, Rimm EB, et al. Changes in diet and lifestyle and long-term weight gain in women and men. *N Engl J Med*. 2011 Jun 23;364(25):2392-404. Note: The graph shows pooled, multivariable-adjusted results based on 20 years of follow-up in the Nurses Health Study, 12 years of follow-up in the Nurses Health Study II, and 20 years of follow-up in the Health Professionals Follow-up Study. All data is highly statistically significant, $p < .001$.

[62] See for example: Armstrong S, Shahbaz C, Singer G. Inclusion of meal-reversal in a behaviour modification program for obesity. *Appetite*. 1981 Mar;2(1):1-5.

[63] CDC. Controlling blood pressure. http://www.cdc.gov/bloodpressure/control. htm. Published 7 July 2014. Accessed 24 April 2016.

[64] World Health Organization. *Guideline: Sodium Intake for Adults and Children*. Geneva: World Health Organization; 2012. http://www.ncbi.nlm.nih.gov/books/NBK133290/. Accessed 24 April 2016.

[65] He FJ, Li J, Macgregor GA. Effect of longer term modest salt reduction on blood pressure: Cochrane systematic review and meta-analysis of randomised trials. *BMJ*. 2013 Apr 3;346:f1325.

[66] Bibbins-Domingo K, Chertow GM, Coxson PG, et al. Projected effect of dietary salt reductions on future cardiovascular disease. *N Engl J Med*. 2010 Feb 18;362(7):590-9.

[67] CDC. Sodium reduction toolkit: A global opportunity to reduce population-level sodium intake. http://www.cdc.gov/salt/sodium_toolkit.htm. Updated 4 Sept 2013. Accessed 1 May 2016.

[68] CDC. Sodium: the facts. http://www.cdc.gov/salt/pdfs/Sodium_Fact_Sheet.pdf. Published April 2016. Accessed 1 May 2016.

[69] Jackson SL, King SM, Zhao L, Cogswell ME. Prevalence of Excess Sodium Intake in the United States - NHANES, 2009-2012. *MMWR Morb Mortal Wkly Rep.* 2016 Jan 8;64(52):1393-7.

[70] O'Donnell M, Mente A, Rangarajan S, et al. Urinary sodium and potassium excretion, mortality, and cardiovascular events. *N Engl J Med.* 2014 Aug 14;371(7):612-23.

[71] Felder RA, White MJ, Williams SM, Jose PA. Diagnostic tools for hypertension and salt sensitivity testing. *Curr Opin Nephrol Hypertens.* 2013 Jan; 22(1): 65–76.

[72] Logan, AG. Dietary sodium intake and its relation to human health: a summary of the evidence. *J Am Coll Nutr.* 2006 Jun;25(3):165-9.

[73] O'Donnell M, Mente A, Rangarajan S, et al. Urinary sodium and potassium excretion, mortality, and cardiovascular events. *N Engl J Med.* 2014 Aug 14;371(7):612-23.

[74] For example see: Colin-Ramirez E, McAlister FA, Zheng Y, et al. The long-term effects of dietary sodium restriction on clinical outcomes in patients with heart failure. The SODIUM-HF (Study of Dietary Intervention Under 100 mmol in Heart Failure): a pilot study. *Am Heart J.* 2015 Feb;169(2):274-281.

[75] Rothberg MB, Sivalingam SK. The new heart failure diet: less salt restriction, more micronutrients. *J Gen Intern Med.* 2010 Oct;25(10):1136-7.

[76] Doukky R, Avery E, Mangla A, et al. Impact of dietary sodium restriction on heart failure outcomes. *JACC Heart Fail.* 2016 Jan;4(1):24-35.

[77] See for example: Graudal N, Jürgens G, Baslund B, Alderman MH. Compared with usual sodium intake, low- and excessive- sodium diets are associated with increased mortality: a meta-analysis. *Am J of Hypertension.* 2014 Apr 26;27(9):1129-1137.

[78] CDC. Sodium and food sources. http://www.cdc.gov/salt/food.htm. Updated 29 February 2016. Accessed 8 May 2016.

[79] Blais CA, Pangborn RM, Borhani NO, et al. Effect of dietary sodium restriction on taste responses to sodium chloride: a longitudinal study. *Am J Clin Nutr.* 1986 Aug;44(2):232-43.

[80] See for example: Schütze M, Boeing H, Pischon T, et al. Alcohol attributable burden of incidence of cancer in eight European countries based on results from prospective cohort study. *BMJ*. 2011 Apr 7;342:d1584.

[81] Stokowski LA. No amount of alcohol is safe. *Medscape*. April 30, 2014. http://www.medscape.com/viewarticle/824237_1. Published 30 April 2014. Accessed 5 January 2015.

[82] Beilin LJ, Puddey IB. Alcohol and hypertension: an update. *Hypertension*. 2006 Jun;47(6):1035-8.

[83] Husain K, Ansari RA, Ferder L. Alcohol-induced hypertension: Mechanism and prevention. *World J Cardiol*. 2014 May 26;6(5):245-52.

[84] Marchi KC, Muniz JJ, Tirapelli CR. Hypertension and chronic ethanol consumption: What do we know after a century of study? *World J Cardiol*. 2014 May 26;6(5):283-94.

[85] Malik VS, Schulze MB, Hu FB. Intake of sugar-sweetened beverages and weight gain: a systematic review. *Am J Clin Nutr* 2006 Aug;84(2):274-88.

[86] Gardener H, Rundek T, Markert M, et al. Diet soft drink consumption is associated with an increased risk of vascular events in the Northern Manhattan Study. *J Gen Intern Med*. 2012 Sep;27(9):1120-6.

[87] Mort JR, Kruse HR. Timing of blood pressure measurement related to caffeine consumption. *Ann Pharmacother*. 2008 Jan;42(1):105-10.

[88] James JE. Critical review of dietary caffeine and blood pressure: a relationship that should be taken more seriously. *Psychosom Med*. 2004 Jan-Feb;66(1):63-71.

[89] Chan J, Knutsen SF, Blix GG, et al. Water, other fluids, and fatal coronary heart disease: the Adventist Health Study. *Am J Epidemiol*. 2002 May 1;155(9):827-33.

[90] Letcher RL, Chien S, Pickering TG, et al. Direct relationship between blood pressure and blood viscosity in normal and hypertensive subjects. Role of fibrinogen and concentration. *Am J Med*. 1981 Jun;70(6):1195-1202.

[91] Ciuffetti G, Schillaci G, Lombardini R, et al. Plasma viscosity in isolated systolic hypertension: the role of pulse pressure. *Am J Hypertens*. 2005 Jul;18(7):1005-8.

[92] Lamarre Y, Lalanne-Mistrih ML, Romana M, et al. Male gender, increased blood viscosity, body mass index and triglyceride levels are independently

associated with systemic relative hypertension in sickle cell anemia. *PLoS One.* 2013 Jun 13;8(6):e66004.

[93] Rylander R, Arnaud MJ. Mineral water intake reduces blood pressure among subjects with low urinary magnesium and calcium levels. *BMC Public Health.* 2004; 4: 56.

[94] May M, Jordan J. The osmopressor response to water drinking. *Am J Physiol Regul Integr Comp Physiol.* 2011 Jan;300(1):R40-6.

[95] McHugh J, Keller NR, Appalsamy M, et al. Portal osmopressor mechanism linked to transient receptor potential vanilloid 4 and blood pressure control. *Hypertension.* 2010 Jun;55(6):1438-43.

[96] Goldhamer A, Lisle D, Parpia B, et al. Medically supervised water-only fasting in the treatment of hypertension. *J Manipulative Physiol Ther.* 2001 Jun;24(5):335-9.

[97] Kamhieh-Milz S, Kamhieh-Milz J, Tauchmann Y, et al. Regular blood donation may help in the management of hypertension: an observational study on 292 blood donors. *Transfusion.* 2016 Mar;56(3):637-44.

[98] Boschmann M, Steiniger J, Franke G, et al. Water drinking induces thermogenesis through osmosensitive mechanisms. *J Clin Endocrinol Metab.* 2007 Aug;92(8):3334-7.

[99] Wirtz PH, von Känel R, Mohiyeddini C, et al. Low social support and poor emotional regulation are associated with increased stress hormone reactivity to mental stress in systemic hypertension. *J Clin Endocrinol Metab.* 2006 Oct;91(10):3857-65.

[100] Bell CN, Thorpe RJ Jr, Laveist TA. Race/Ethnicity and hypertension: the role of social support. *Am J Hypertens.* 2010 May;23(5):534-40.

[101] Gallos LK, Barttfeld P, Havlin S, et al. Collective behavior in the spatial spreading of obesity. *Sci Rep.* 2012;2:454.

[102] Paiva PC, de Paiva HN, de Oliveira Filho PM, et al. Development and validation of a social capital questionnaire for adolescent students (SCQ-AS). *PLoS One.* 2014 Aug 5;9(8):e103785.

[103] Chen X, Stanton B, Gong J, et al. Personal Social Capital Scale: an instrument for health and behavioral research. *Health Educ Res.* 2009 Apr;24(2):306-17.

[104] The Greater Good Science Center. Social Capital Quiz. Accessed 15 April 2016 at http://greatergood.berkeley.edu/quizzes/take_quiz/13.

[105] The Quiz in Figure 7.1 was adapted from several instruments including: (a) Chen X, Stanton B, Gong J, et al. Personal Social Capital Scale: an instrument for health and behavioral research. *Health Educ Res*. 2009 Apr;24(2):306-17; (b) The Greater Good Science Center. Social capital quiz. http://greatergood.berkeley.edu/quizzes/take_quiz/13. Accessed 15 April 2016; (c) Paiva PC, de Paiva HN, de Oliveira Filho PM, et al. Development and validation of a social capital questionnaire for adolescent students (SCQ-AS). *PLoS One*. 2014 Aug5;9(8):e103785; and (d) the Social Capital Community Benchmark Survey. http://www.ksg.harvard.edu/saguaro/communitysurvey/index.html. Accessed 17 April 2016.

[106] Kamiya Y, Whelan B, Timonen V, Kenny RA. The differential impact of subjective and objective aspects of social engagement on cardiovascular risk factors. *BMC Geriatr*. 2010 Nov 2;10:81.

[107] Hagberg JM for the American College of Sports Medicine. *Exercising Your Way to Lower Blood Pressure* [brochure]. 2011. http://www.acsm.org/docs/brochures/exercising-your-way-to-lower-blood-pressure.pdf. Accessed 1 May 2015.

[108] Ishikawa-Takata K, Ohta T, Tanaka H. How much exercise is required to reduce blood pressure in essential hypertensives: a dose-response study. *Am J Hypertens*. 2003 Aug;16(8):629-33.

[109] Hagberg JM for the American College of Sports Medicine. *Exercising Your Way to Lower Blood Pressure* [brochure]. 2011. Accessed 1 May 2015 at http://www.acsm.org/docs/brochures/exercising-your-way-to-lower-blood-pressure.pdf.

[110] Even if it doesn't seem so on the surface, the math really does add up. There are only nine three-minute increases over the course of ten weeks, so the exercise subjects never quite reached 50-minute sessions during the 10-week program.

[111] If you're interested in the technical research details: both IT and CT group members had their target heart rate initially set at 40% of their measured V02max heart rate reserve (HRR). Training intensity increased 5% each week to a maximum of 85% V02max HRR.

[112] Beddhu S, Wei G, Marcus RL, et al. Light-intensity physical activities and mortality in the United States general population and CKD subpopulation. *Clin J Am Soc Nephrol*. 2015 Jul 7;10(7):1145-53.

[113] Fagard RH, Cornelissen VA. Effect of exercise on blood pressure control in hypertensive patients. *Eur J Cardiovasc Prev Rehabil*. 2007 Feb;14(1):12-7.

[114] Cornelissen VA, Fagard RH, Coeckelberghs E, Vanhees L. Impact of resistance training on blood pressure and other cardiovascular risk factors: a meta-analysis of randomized, controlled trials. *Hypertension*. 2011 Nov;58(5):950-8.

[115] Bowen R. The Migrating Motor Complex. In: *Pathophysiology of the Digestive System*. Colorado State University Hypertextbook; 1995. http://www.vivo. colostate.edu/hbooks/pathphys/digestion/stomach/mmcomplex.html. Accessed 2 May 2015.

[116] Dalenbäck J, Abrahamson H, Björnson E, et al. Human duodenogastric reflux, retroperistalsis, and MMC. *Am J Physiol*. 1998 Sep;275(3 Pt 2):R762-9.

[117] Nagai M, Hoshide S, Kario K. Sleep duration as a risk factor for cardiovascular disease- a review of the recent literature. *Curr Cardiol Rev*. 2010 Feb;6(1):54-61.

[118] Marin JM, Agusti A, Villar I, et al. Association between treated and untreated obstructive sleep apnea and risk of hypertension. *JAMA*. 2012 May 23;307(20):2169-76.

[119] Grebenev AL, Sheptulin AA, Saltykov BB. Analysis of association of peptic ulcer and essential hypertension from the standpoint of the problem of concomitant pathology. A possible role of vascular factor in the genesis of ulcer formation. *Mater Med Pol*. 1992 Jan-Mar;24(1):9-13.

[120] Thollander M, Gazelius B, Hellström PM. Adrenergic modulation of small bowel haemodynamics in interdigestive motility state of man. *Eur J Gastroenterol Hepatol*. 1999 Mar;11(3):257-65.

[121] Thor PJ, Krolczyk G, Gil K, et al. Melatonin and serotonin effects on gastrointestinal motility. *J Physiol Pharmacol*. 2007 Dec;58 Suppl 6:97-103.

[122] Chen CQ, Fichna J, Bashashati M, et al. Distribution, function and physiological role of melatonin in the lower gut. *World J Gastroenterol*. 2011 Sep 14;17(34):3888-98.

[123] Grossman E, Laudon M, Zisapel N. Effect of melatonin on nocturnal blood pressure: meta-analysis of randomized controlled trials. *Vasc Health Risk Manag*. 2011;7:577-84.

[124] Nedley N. Proof Positive: *How to Reliably Combat Disease and Achieve*

Optimal Health Through Nutrition and Lifestyle. Ardmore, OK: Nedley Publishing; 1998..

[125] See for example: Mozaffari S, Rahimi R, Abdollahi M. Implications of melatonin therapy in irritable bowel syndrome: a systematic review. *Curr Pharm Des.* 2010;16(33):3646-55; and Chen CQ, Fichna J, Bashashati M, et al. Distribution, function and physiological role of melatonin in the lower gut. *World J Gastroenterol.* 2011 Sep 14;17(34):3888-98.

[126] Niigaki M, Adachi K, Hirakawa K, et al. Association between metabolic syndrome and prevalence of gastroesophageal reflux disease in a health screening facility in Japan. *J Gastroenterol.* 2013 Apr;48(4):463-72.

[127] See for example: Dang Y, Reinhardt JD, Zhou X, Zhang G. The effect of probiotics supplementation on Helicobacter pylori eradication rates and side effects during eradication therapy: a meta-analysis. *PLoS One.* 2014 Nov 3;9(11):e111030.

[128] Husain K, Ansari RA, Ferder L. Alcohol-induced hypertension: Mechanism and prevention. *World J Cardiol.* 2014 May 26;6(5):245-52.

[129] Sagawa Y, Kondo H, Matsubuchi N, et al. Alcohol has a dose-related effect on parasympathetic nerve activity during sleep. *Alcohol Clin Exp Res.* 2011 Nov;35(11):2093-100.

[130] European Society of Cardiology. Midday naps associated with reduced blood pressure and fewer medications. http://www.escardio.org/The-ESC/Press-Office/Press-releases/Last-5-years/Midday-naps-associated-with-reduced-blood-pressure-and-fewer-medications. Public Release: 29 August 2015. Accessed 20 September 2015.

[131] Cao Z, Shen L, Wu J, et al. The effects of midday nap duration on the risk of hypertension in a middle-aged and older Chinese population: a preliminary evidence from the Tongji-Dongfeng Cohort Study, China. *J Hypertens.* 2014 Oct;32(10):1993-8.

[132] Dhand R, Sohal H. Good sleep, bad sleep! The role of daytime naps in healthy adults. *Curr Opin Pulm Med.* 2006 Nov;12(6):379-82.

[133] Takahashi M. The role of prescribed napping in sleep medicine. *Sleep Med Rev.* 2003 Jun;7(3):227-35.

[134] These include: Duffy JF, Czeisler CA. Effect of light on human circadian physiology. *Sleep Med Clin.* 2009 Jun;4(2):165-177; Western Australia Department of Health Centre for Clinical Interventions. Sleep hygiene.

http://www.cci.health.wa.gov.au/docs/Info-sleep%20hygiene.pdf. Accessed 20 September 2015; Bonnet MH, Arand DL. Treatment of insomnia. *UpToDate*. Accessed 18-20 September 2015; Thorpy M. Sleep hygiene. National Sleep Foundation. https://sleepfoundation.org/ask-the-expert/sleep-hygiene. Accessed 20 September 2015; Nedley N. Sleep. http://nedleyhealthsolutions. com/index.php/solutions/sleep.html. Accessed 20 September 2015.

[135] Anson J, Anson O. Death rests a while: holy day and Sabbath effects on Jewish mortality in Israel. *Soc Sci Med*. 2001 Jan;52(1):83-97.

[136] Jews who observe the biblical principles spelled out in the Torah (the first five books of the Judeo-Christian Old Testament) keep a weekly Sabbath from sundown Friday to sundown Saturday. See for example Exodus 20:8-11 and Exodus 31:13.

[137] See for example: Levi F, Halberg F. Circaseptan (about-7-day) bioperiodicity--spontaneous and reactive--and the search for pacemakers. *Ric Clin Lab*. 1982 Apr-Jun;12(2):323-70.

[138] Lee MS, Lee JS, Lee JY, et al. About 7-day (circaseptan) and circadian changes in cold pressor test (CPT). *Biomed Pharmacother*. 2003 Oct;57 Suppl 1:39s-44s.

[139] Lee JS, Lee MS, Lee JY, et al. Effects of diaphragmatic breathing on ambulatory blood pressure and heart rate. *Biomed Pharmacother*. 2003 Oct;57 Suppl 1:87s-91s.

[140] Zhao P, Xu P, Wan C, Wang Z. Evening versus morning dosing regimen drug therapy for hypertension. *Cochrane Database Syst Rev*. 2011 Oct 5;(10):CD004184.

[141] Ndrepepa A, Twardella D. Relationship between noise annoyance from road traffic noise and cardiovascular diseases: a meta-analysis. *Noise Health*. 2011 May-Jun;13(52):251-9.

[142] Kelishadi R, Poursafa P, Keramatian K. Overweight, air and noise pollution: Universal risk factors for pediatric pre-hypertension. *J Res Med Sci*. 2011 Sep;16(9):1234-50.

[143] Hu RF, Jiang XY, Zeng YM, et al. Effects of earplugs and eye masks on nocturnal sleep, melatonin and cortisol in a simulated intensive care unit environment. *Crit Care*. 2010;14(2):R66.

[144] Huang HW, Zheng BL, Jiang L, et al. Effect of oral melatonin and wearing earplugs and eye masks on nocturnal sleep in healthy subjects in a simulated

intensive care unit environment: which might be a more promising strategy for ICU sleep deprivation? *Crit Care.* 2015 Mar 19;19:124.

[145] Zhang L, Gong JT, Zhang HQ, et al. Melatonin attenuates noise stress-induced gastrointestinal motility disorder and gastric stress ulcer: Role of gastrointestinal hormones and oxidative stress in rats. *J Neurogastroenterol Motil.* 2015 Mar 30;21(2):189-99.

[146] Nahas R. Complementary and alternative medicine approaches to blood pressure reduction: An evidence-based review. *Can Fam Physician.* 2008 Nov;54(11):1529-33.

[147] Dowdy JC, Sayre RM, Holick MF. Holick's rule and vitamin D from sunlight. *J Steroid Biochem Mol Biol.* 2010 Jul;121(1-2):328-30.

[148] Holick MF. Vitamin D deficiency. *N Engl J Med.* 2007 Jul 19;357(3):266-81.

[149] Groppelli A, Giorgi DM, Omboni S, et al. Persistent blood pressure increase induced by heavy smoking. *J Hypertens.* 1992 May;10(5):495-9.

[150] Burhansstipanov L, Harjo LD. Native American tobacco education fact sheets: Ceremonial use. http://natamcancer.org/nnacc_dwnlds/ SHEETS/02-18-07_Tob-ceremony_04-12-09.pdf Accessed 18 April 2016.

[151] Kaplan NM. Smoking and hypertension. *UpToDate.* Updated 4 February 2015. Accessed 4 May 2015.

[152] Virdis A, Giannarelli C, Neves MF, et al. Cigarette smoking and hypertension. *Curr Pharm Des.* 2010;16(23):2518-25.

[153] Cymerys M, Bogdański P, Pupek-Musialik D, et al. Influence of hypertension, obesity and nicotine abuse on quantitative and qualitative changes in acute-phase proteins in patients with essential hypertension. *Med Sci Monit.* 2012 May;18(5):CR330-6.

[154] See for example: Almarshad HA, Hassan FM. Alterations in blood coagulation and viscosity among young male cigarette smokers of Al-Jouf Region in Saudi Arabia. *Clin Appl Thromb Hemost.* 2016 May;22(4):386-9.

[155] Czoli CD, Hammond D. TSNA Exposure: Levels of NNAL Among Canadian Tobacco Users. *Nicotine Tob Res.* 2015 Jul;17(7):825-30.

[156] Westman EC. Does smokeless tobacco cause hypertension? *South Med J.* 1995 Jul;88(7):716-20.

[157] See for example: Nascimento LF, Francisco JB. Particulate matter and hospital admission due to arterial hypertension in a medium-sized Brazilian city. *Cad Saude Publica*. 2013 Aug;29(8):1565-71. Pedersen M, Stayner L, Slama R, et al. Ambient air pollution and pregnancy-induced hypertensive disorders: a systematic review and meta-analysis. *Hypertension*. 2014 Sep;64(3):494-500.

[158] See, for example, Lee JS, Lee MS, Lee JY, et al. Effects of diaphragmatic breathing on ambulatory blood pressure and heart rate. *Biomed Pharmacother*. 2003 Oct;57 Suppl 1:87s-91s.

[159] Cernes R, Zimlichman R. RESPeRATE: the role of paced breathing in hypertension treatment. *J Am Soc Hypertens*. 2015 Jan;9(1):38-47.

[160] Landman GW, van Hateren KJ, van Dijk PR, et al. Efficacy of device-guided breathing for hypertension in blinded, randomized, active-controlled trials: a meta-analysis of individual patient data. *JAMA Intern Med*. 2014 Nov;174(11):1815-21.

[161] Schuwald AM, Nöldner M, Wilmes T, et al. Lavender oil-potent anxiolytic properties via modulating voltage dependent calcium channels. Skoulakis EMC, ed. *PLoS ONE*. 2013;8(4):e59998.

[162] Cha JH, Lee SH, Yoo YS. Effects of aromatherapy on changes in the autonomic nervous system, aortic pulse wave velocity and aortic augmentation index in patients with essential hypertension [Korean language article]. *J Korean Acad Nurs*. 2010 Oct;40(5):705-13.

[163] Sayorwan W, Siripornpanich V, Piriyapunyaporn T, et al. The effects of lavender oil inhalation on emotional states, autonomic nervous system, and brain electrical activity. *J Med Assoc Thai*. 2012 Apr;95(4):598-606.

[164] Hur MH, Lee MS, Kim C, Ernst E. Aromatherapy for treatment of hypertension: a systematic review. *J Eval Clin Pract*. 2012 Feb;18(1):37-41.

[165] Park BJ, Tsunetsugu Y, Kasetani T, et al. The physiological effects of Shinrin-yoku (taking in the forest atmosphere or forest bathing): evidence from field experiments in 24 forests across Japan. *Environ Health Prev Med*. 2010 Jan;15(1):18-26.

[166] Anderson WP, Reid CM, Jennings GL. Pet ownership and risk factors for cardiovascular disease. *Med J Aust*. 1992 Sep 7;157(5):298-301.

[167] For example, see Headey B, Grabka M, Kelley J, et al. Pet ownership is good for your health and saves public expenditure too: Australian and German longitudinal evidence. *Aust Social Monitor* 2002 Nov 4;5(4): 93-99.

[168] Friedmann E, Thomas SA. Pet ownership, social support and one year survival after acute myocardial infarction in the Cardiac Arrhythmic Suppression Trial (CAST). *Am J Cardiol* 1995; 76: 1213-1217.

[169] Parslow RA, Jorm AF. Pet ownership and risk factors for cardiovascular disease: another look. *Med J Aust.* 2003 Nov 3;179(9):466-8.

[170] See for example: Grassi G, Seravalle G, Quarti-Trevano F. The "neuroadrenergic hypothesis" in hypertension: current evidence. *Exp Physiol.* 2010 May;95(5):581-6.

[171] Schnall PL, Schwartz JE, Landsbergis PA, et al. Relation between job strain, alcohol, and ambulatory blood pressure. *Hypertension.* 1992 May;19(5):488-94.

[172] Alcoholics Anonymous. The origin of our serenity prayer. www.aahistory. com/prayer.html. Published August 1992. Accessed 1 May 2015.

[173] Markovitz JH, Matthews KA, Kannel WB, et al. Psychological predictors of hypertension in the Framingham Study. Is there tension in hypertension? *JAMA.* 1993 Nov 24;270(20):2439-43.

[174] Jayakody K, Gunadasa S, Hosker C. Exercise for anxiety disorders: systematic review. *Br J Sports Med.* 2014 Feb;48(3):187-96.

[175] Anxiety and Depression Association of America. Exercise for stress and anxiety. http://www.adaa.org/living-with-anxiety/managing-anxiety/exercise-stress-and-anxiety. Updated July 2014. Accessed 17 September 2015.

[176] Helmes E, Wiancko DC. Effects of music in reducing disruptive behavior in a general hospital. *J Amer Psych Nurses Assoc.* 2006 Feb;12(1):37-44.

[177] See, for example: Carlson E, Saarikallio S, Toiviainen P, et al. Maladaptive and adaptive emotion regulation through music: a behavioral and neuroimaging study of males and females. *Front Hum Neurosci.* 2015 Aug 26;9:466; Watkins GR. Music therapy: proposed physiological mechanisms and clinical implications. *Clin Nurse Spec.* 1997 Mar;11(2):43-50.

[178] See, for example: Eerola T. Are the emotions expressed in music genre-specific? An audio-based evaluation of datasets spanning classical, film, pop and mixed genres. *J New Music Research.* 2011 Nov 25; 40(4):349-366.

[179] Nedley N. *The Lost Art of Thinking: How to Improve Emotional Intelligence and Achieve Peak Mental Performance.* Ardmore, Oklahoma: Nedley Publishing; 2011.

[180] Kunikullaya KU, Goturu J, Muradi V, et al. Music versus lifestyle on the autonomic nervous system of prehypertensives and hypertensives-a randomized control trial. *Complement Ther Med*. 2015 Oct;23(5):733-40.

[181] Eerola T, Vuoskoski JK. A comparison of the discrete and dimensional models of emotion in music. *Psychology of Music*. 2011 January; 39(1): 18–49.

[182] See, for example: Crippa JA, Derenusson GN, Ferrari TB, et al. Neural basis of anxiolytic effects of cannabidiol (CBD) in generalized social anxiety disorder: a preliminary report. *J Psychopharmacol*. 2011 Jan;25(1):121-30.

[183] Ghosh A, Basu D. Cannabis and psychopathology: The meandering journey of the last decade. *Indian J Psychiatry*. 2015 Apr-Jun;57(2):140-9.

[184] Ghosh A, Basu D. Cannabis and psychopathology: The meandering journey of the last decade. *Indian J Psychiatry*. 2015 Apr-Jun;57(2):140-9.

[185] Schmits E, Quertemont E. So called "soft" drugs: cannabis and the amotivational syndrome. [Article in French] *Rev Med Liege*. 2013 May-Jun;68(5-6):281-6.

[186] Jones RT. Cardiovascular system effects of marijuana. *J Clin Pharmacol*. 2002 Nov;42(11 Suppl):58S-63S.

[187] Vandrey R, Umbricht A, Strain EC. Increased blood pressure after abrupt cessation of daily cannabis use. *J Addict Med*. 2011 Mar;5(1):16-20.

[188] Ghosh A, Basu D. Cannabis and psychopathology: The meandering journey of the last decade. *Indian J Psychiatry*. 2015 Apr-Jun;57(2):140-9.

[189] American Psychological Association. Controlling anger before it controls you. http://www.apa.org/topics/anger/control.aspx?item=2. Accessed 18 September 2015.

[190] Yan LL, Liu K, Matthews KA, et al. Psychosocial factors and risk of hypertension: the Coronary Artery Risk Development in Young Adults (CARDIA) study. *JAMA*. 2003 Oct 22;290(16):2138-48.

[191] Yan LL, Liu K, Matthews KA, et al. Psychosocial factors and risk of hypertension: the Coronary Artery Risk Development in Young Adults (CARDIA) study. *JAMA*. 2003 Oct 22;290(16):2138-48.

[192] Izzo AA, Ernst E. Interactions between herbal medicines and prescribed drugs: a systematic review. *Drugs*. 2001;61(15):2163-75.

[193] Bradley R, Kozura E, Kaltunas J, et al. Observed changes in risk during naturopathic treatment of hypertension. *Evid Based Complement Alternat Med*. 2011;2011:826751.

[194] Nahas R. Complementary and alternative medicine approaches to blood pressure reduction: An evidence-based review. *Can Fam Physician*. 2008 Nov;54(11):1529-33.

[195] Sirtori CR, Arnoldi A, Cicero AF. Nutraceuticals for blood pressure control. *Ann Med*. 2015; 47(6):447-56.

[196] Rosenfeldt F, Haas SJ, Krum H, et al. Coenzyme Q10 in the treatment of hypertension: a meta-analysis of the clinical trials. *J Hum Hypertens*. 2007 Apr;21(4):297-306.

[197] Natural Medicines Comprehensive Database. Coenzyme Q-10. http://naturaldatabase.therapeuticresearch.com/nd/PrintVersion.aspx?id=938. Updated 20 October 2014. Accessed 21 September 2015.

[198] Office of Dietary Supplements (U.S. Department of Health & Human Services). Magnesium: Fact sheet for health professionals. https://ods.od.nih.gov/factsheets/Magnesium-HealthProfessional/#h7. Updated 2013 November. Accessed 29 September 2015.

[199] Kass L, Weekes J, Carpenter L. Effect of magnesium supplementation on blood pressure: a meta-analysis. *Eur J Clin Nutr*. 2012 Apr;66(4):411-8.

[200] Kass LS, Poeira F. The effect of acute vs chronic magnesium supplementation on exercise and recovery on resistance exercise, blood pressure and total peripheral resistance on normotensive adults. *J Int Soc Sports Nutr*. 2015 Apr 24;12:19.

[201] Office of Dietary Supplements (U.S. Department of Health & Human Services). Magnesium: Fact sheet for health professionals. https://ods.od.nih.gov/factsheets/Magnesium-HealthProfessional/#h7. Updated 2013 November. Accessed 29 September 2015.

[202] See for example: Haag M. Essential fatty acids and the brain. *Can J Psychiatry*. 2003 Apr;48(3):195-203.

[203] Office of Dietary Supplements (U.S. Department of Health & Human Services). Omega-3 fatty acids and health: Fact sheet for health professionals. https://ods.od.nih.gov/factsheets/Omega3FattyAcidsandHealth-HealthProfessional/. Updated 28 October 2005. Accessed 29 Sept 2015.

[204] Cole GM, Ma QL, Frautschy SA. Omega-3 fatty acids and dementia.

Prostaglandins Leukot Essent Fatty Acids. 2009 Aug-Sep;81(2-3):213-21.

[205] Tagetti A, Ericson U, Montagnana M, et al. Intakes of omega-3 polyunsaturated fatty acids and blood pressure change over time: Possible interaction with genes involved in 20-HETE and EETs metabolism. *Prostaglandins Other Lipid Mediat.* 2015 Jul;120:126-33.

[206] National Center for Complementary and Integrative Health (US Department of Health and Human Services; National Institutes of Health). Omega-3 supplements: An introduction. https://nccih.nih.gov/health/omega3/introduction.htm. Updated August 2015. Accessed 4 October 2015.

[207] Natural Resources Defense Council. Mercury contamination in fish: A guide to staying healthy and fighting back. http://www.nrdc.org/health/effects/mercury/sources.asp. Accessed 4 October 2015.

[208] US Environmental Protection Agency (EPA). Polychlorinated biphenyls (PCBs)(Arochlors): Hazard Summary. http://www3.epa.gov/ttn/atw/hlthef/polychlo.html. Revised January 2000. Accessed 4 October 2015.

[209] Connor WE, Connor, SL. Omega-3 Fatty Acids from Fish. In: Bendich A, Deckelbaum RJ, ed. *Preventive Nutrition: The Comprehensive Guide for Health Professionals.* New York, NY: Humana Press; 1997: 225-243.

[210] United States Department of Agriculture. National Nutrient Database for Standard Reference Release 27 Agricultural Research Service National Agricultural Library. http://ndb.nal.usda.gov. Accessed 6 October 2015.

[211] Gerster H. Can adults adequately convert alpha-linolenic acid (18:3n-3) to eicosapentaenoic acid (20:5n-3) and docosahexaenoic acid (22:6n-3)? *Int J Vitam Nutr Res.* 1998;68(3):159-73.

[212] de Goede J, Verschuren WM, Boer JM, et al. Alpha-linolenic acid intake and 10-year incidence of coronary heart disease and stroke in 20,000 middle-aged men and women in the Netherlands. *PLoS One.* 2011 Mar 25;6(3):e17967.

[213] Fleming JA, Kris-Etherton PM. The evidence for alpha-linolenic acid and cardiovascular disease benefits: Comparisons with eicosapentaenoic acid and docosahexaenoic acid. *Adv Nutr.* 2014 Nov 14;5(6):863S-76S.

[214] FAO (Food and Agriculture Organization of the United Nations). The state of world fisheries and aquaculture. http://www.fao.org/3/a-i3720e.pdf. Published 2014:37. Accessed 24 October 2015.

[215] FAO (Food and Agriculture Organization of the United Nations). General

situation of world fish stocks. http://www.fao.org/newsroom/common/ecg/1000505/en/stocks.pdf. Accessed 24 October 2015.

[216] American Heart Association. Fish and Omega-3 Fatty Acids. http://www.heart.org/HEARTORG/GettingHealthy/NutritionCenter/HealthyDietGoals/Fish-and-Omega-3-Fatty-Acids_UCM_303248_Article.jsp#.Vi0oIcsvlNM. Updated 15 June 2015. Accessed 25 October 2015.

[217] Gerster H. Can adults adequately convert alpha-linolenic acid (18:3n-3) to eicosapentaenoic acid (20:5n-3) and docosahexaenoic acid (22:6n-3)? *Int J Vitam Nutr Res.* 1998;68(3):159-73.

[218] Talahalli RR, Vallikannan B, Sambaiah K, Lokesh BR. Lower efficacy in the utilization of dietary ALA as compared to preformed EPA + DHA on long chain n-3 PUFA levels in rats. *Lipids.* 2010 Sep;45(9):799-808.

[219] University of Maryland Medical Center. Omega-3 fatty acids. http://umm.edu/health/medical/altmed/supplement/omega3-fatty-acids. Updated 5 August 2015. Accessed 6 October 2015.

[220] Martek Biosciences Corporation. The *life's DHA* Advantage. http://www.lifesdha.com/what-is-dha/lifesdha-advantage.aspx. Accessed 25 October 2015.

[221] University of Maryland Medical Center. Omega-3 fatty acids. http://umm.edu/health/medical/altmed/supplement/omega3-fatty-acids. Updated 5 August 2015. Accessed 6 October 2015.

[222] Seely D, Kanji S, Yazdi F, et al. Dietary supplements in adults taking cardiovascular drugs. *Agency for Healthcare Research and Quality.* https://effective-healthcare.ahrq.gov/ehc/products/223/1038/CER51_DietarySupplements_execsumm.pdf. Published April 2012. Accessed 25 October 2015.

[223] See for example: Bixquert Jiménez M. Treatment of irritable bowel syndrome with probiotics. An etiopathogenic approach at last? *Rev Esp Enferm Dig.* 2009 Aug;101(8):553-64; Dang Y, Reinhardt JD, Zhou X, Zhang G. The effect of probiotics supplementation on Helicobacter pylori eradication rates and side effects during eradication therapy: a meta-analysis. *PLoS One.* 2014 Nov 3;9(11):e111030; Didari T, Mozaffari S, Nikfar S, Abdollahi M. Effectiveness of probiotics in irritable bowel syndrome: Updated systematic review with meta-analysis. *World J Gastroenterol.* 2015 Mar 14;21(10):3072-84.

[224] Khalesi S, Sun J, Buys N, Jayasinghe R. Effect of probiotics on blood pressure: a systematic review and meta-analysis of randomized, controlled trials. *Hypertension.* 2014 Oct;64(4):897-903.

[225] Dong JY, Szeto IM, Makinen K, et al. Effect of probiotic fermented milk on blood pressure: a meta-analysis of randomised controlled trials. *Br J Nutr*. 2013 Oct;110(7):1188-94 citing: Research Group of Gamma-Aminobutyric Acid in Tokyo (1960) Clinical aspects on the use of gamma-aminobutyric acid. In *Inhibition in the Nervous System and Gamma-aminobutyric Acid: Proceedings of an International Symposium*, 22–24 May 1959, City of Hope Medical Center, Duarte, CA, pp. 579–581. Oxford: Pergamon Press.

[226] See for example: Sawada H, Furushiro M, Hirai K, et al. Purification and characterization of an antihypertensive compound from Lactobacillus casei. *Agric Biol Chem*. 1990 Dec;54(12):3211-9.

[227] Tabuchi M, Ozaki M, Tamura A, et al. Antidiabetic effect of Lactobacillus GG in streptozotocin-induced diabetic rats. *Biosci Biotechnol Biochem*. 2003 Jun;67(6):1421-4.

[228] Xu JY, Qin LQ, Wang PY, et al. Effect of milk tripeptides on blood pressure: a meta-analysis of randomized controlled trials. *Nutrition*. 2008 Oct;24(10):933-40.

[229] Schecter A, Cramer P, Boggess K, et al. Intake of dioxins and related compounds from food in the U.S. population. *J Toxicol Environ Health A*. 2001 May 11;63(1):1-18.

[230] Reddy BS, Simi B, Patel N, et al. Effect of amount and types of dietary fat on intestinal bacterial 7 alpha-dehydroxylase and phosphatidylinositol-specific phospholipase C and colonic mucosal diacylglycerol kinase and PKC activities during stages of colon tumor promotion. *Cancer Res*. 1996 May 15;56(10):2314-20.

[231] Conlon MA, Bird AR. The impact of diet and lifestyle on gut microbiota and human health. *Nutrients*. 2014 Dec 24;7(1):17-44.

[232] Roberfroid M, Gibson GR, Hoyles L, et al. Prebiotic effects: metabolic and health benefits. *Br J Nutr*. 2010 Aug;104 Suppl 2:S1-63.

[233] Peng M, Bitsko E, Biswas D. Functional properties of peanut fractions on the growth of probiotics and foodborne bacterial pathogens. *J Food Sci*. 2015 Mar;80(3):M635-41.

[234] Lacombe A, Wu VC, White J, et al. The antimicrobial properties of the lowbush blueberry (Vaccinium angustifolium) fractional components against foodborne pathogens and the conservation of probiotic Lactobacillus rhamnosus. *Food Microbiol*. 2012 May;30(1):124-31.

[235] Koutsos A, Tuohy KM, Lovegrove JA. Apples and cardiovascular health--is the gut microbiota a core consideration? *Nutrients*. 2015 May 26;7(6):3959-98.

[236] Reddy BS. Possible mechanisms by which pro- and prebiotics influence colon carcinogenesis and tumor growth. *J Nutr*. 1999 Jul;129(7 Suppl):1478S-82S.

[237] Roberfroid MB. Prebiotics and synbiotics: concepts and nutritional properties. *Br J Nutr*. 1998 Oct;80(4):S197-202.

[238] Chow J. Probiotics and prebiotics: A brief overview. *J Ren Nutr*. 2002 Apr;12(2):76-86.

[239] Flores AC, Morlett JA, Rodriguez R. Inulin potential for enzymatic obtaining of prebiotic oligosaccharide. *Crit Rev Food Sci Nutr*. 2015 Mar 6:0.

[240] See for example: Endres M, Laufs U. Discontinuation of statin treatment in stroke patients. *Stroke*. 2006 Oct;37(10):2640-3.

[241] Dashtabi A, Mazloom Z, Fararouei M, Hejazi N. Oral L-arginine administration improves anthropometric and biochemical indices associated with cardiovascular diseases in obese patients: a randomized, single blind placebo controlled clinical trial. *Res Cardiovasc Med*. 2015 Dec 29;5(1):e29419.

[242] Böger RH. L-arginine therapy in cardiovascular pathologies: beneficial or dangerous? *Curr Opin Clin Nutr Metab Care*. 2008 Jan;11(1):55-61.

[243] Willeit P, Freitag DF, Laukkanen JA, et al. Asymmetric dimethylarginine and cardiovascular risk: systematic review and meta-analysis of 22 prospective studies. *J Am Heart Assoc*. 2015 May 28;4(6):e001833.

[244] Böger RH. Asymmetric dimethylarginine, an endogenous inhibitor of nitric oxide synthase, explains the "L-arginine paradox" and acts as a novel cardiovascular risk factor. *J Nutr*. 2004 Oct;134(10 Suppl):2842S-2847S.

[245] Serban C, Sahebkar A, Ursoniu S, et al. Effect of sour tea (Hibiscus sabdariffa L.) on arterial hypertension: a systematic review and meta-analysis of randomized controlled trials. *J Hypertens*. 2015 Jun;33(6):1119-27.

[246] Nwachukwu DC, Aneke EI, Obika LF, Nwachukwu NZ. Effects of aqueous extract of Hibiscus sabdariffa on the renin-angiotensin-aldosterone system of Nigerians with mild to moderate essential hypertension: A comparative study with lisinopril. *Indian J Pharmacol*. 2015 Sep-Oct;47(5):540-5.

[247] National Woman's Christian Temperance Union. Early history. http://www. wctu.org/history.html. Accessed 15 November 2015.

[248] National Woman's Christian Temperance Union. Home page. http://www.wctu.org/. Accessed 15 November 2015.

[249] U.S. Food and Drug Administration (FDA). Non-aspirin nonsteroidal anti-inflammatory drugs (NSAIDs): Drug safety communication - FDA strengthens warning of increased chance of heart attack or stroke. http://www.fda.gov/Safety/MedWatch/SafetyInformation/SafetyAlertsforHumanMedicalProducts/ucm454141.htm. Published 9 July 2015. Accessed 14 November 2015.

[250] Snowden S, Nelson R. The effects of nonsteroidal anti-inflammatory drugs on blood pressure in hypertensive patients. *Cardiol Rev*. 2011 Jul-Aug;19(4):184-91.

[251] Bautista LE, Vera LM. Antihypertensive effects of aspirin: what is the evidence? *Curr Hypertens Rep*. 2010 Aug;12(4):282-9.

[252] Wall R, Ross RP, Fitzgerald GF, Stanton C. Fatty acids from fish: the anti-inflammatory potential of long-chain omega-3 fatty acids. *Nutr Rev*. 2010 May;68(5):280-9.

[253] Zhou H, Beevers CS, Huang S. The targets of curcumin. *Curr Drug Targets*. 2011 Mar 1;12(3):332-47.

[254] Sahbaie P, Sun Y, Liang DY, et al. Curcumin treatment attenuates pain and enhances functional recovery after incision. *Anesth Analg*. 2014 Jun;118(6):1336-44.

[255] Lorente-Cebrián S, Costa AG, Navas-Carretero S, et al. An update on the role of omega-3 fatty acids on inflammatory and degenerative diseases. *J Physiol Biochem*. 2015 Jun;71(2):341-9.

[256] Souza PR, Norling LV. Implications for eicosapentaenoic acid- and docosahexaenoic acid-derived resolvins as therapeutics for arthritis. *Eur J Pharmacol*. 2015 Jul 9. pii: S0014-2999(15)30148-5.

[257] National Institutes of Health National Center for Complementary and Integrative Health. Turmeric at a glance. https://nccih.nih.gov/health/turmeric/ataglance.htm. Updated April 2012. Accessed 20 June 2016.

[258] Adaramoye OA, Anjos RM, Almeida MM, et al. Hypotensive and endothelium-independent vasorelaxant effects of methanolic extract from Curcuma longa L. in rats. *J Ethnopharmacol*. 2009 Jul 30;124(3):457-62.

[259] Boonla O, Kukongviriyapan U, Pakdeechote P, et al. Curcumin improves

endothelial dysfunction and vascular remodeling in 2K-1C hypertensive rats by raising nitric oxide availability and reducing oxidative stress. *Nitric Oxide.* 2014 Nov 15;42:44-53.

[260] Kimmatkar N, Thawani V, Hingorani L, Khiyani R. Efficacy and tolerability of Boswellia serrata extract in treatment of osteoarthritis of knee--a randomized double blind placebo controlled trial. *Phytomedicine.* 2003 Jan;10(1):3-7.

[261] Pickering, TG. Pain and blood pressure. *Medscape Family Medicine.* http://www.medscape.com/viewarticle/465355. Accessed 20 June 2016.

[262] Bruehl S, Chung OY, Ward P, et al. The relationship between resting blood pressure and acute pain sensitivity in healthy normotensives and chronic back pain sufferers: the effects of opioid blockade. *Pain.* 2002 Nov;100(1-2):191-201.

[263] Mayo Clinic. Medications and supplements that can raise your blood pressure. http://www.mayoclinic.org/diseases-conditions/high-blood-pressure/in-depth/blood-pressure/art-20045245?pg=1. Published 13 March 2013. Accessed 25 October 2015.

[264] Weber F, Anlauf M. Treatment resistant hypertension--investigation and conservative management. *Dtsch Arztebl Int.* 2014 Jun 20;111(25):425-31.

[265] Grossman A, Messerli FH, Grossman E. Drug induced hypertension - An unappreciated cause of secondary hypertension. *Eur J Pharmacol.* 2015 Sep 15;763(Pt A):15-22.

[266] Sudano I, Flammer AJ, Périat D, et al. Acetaminophen increases blood pressure in patients with coronary artery disease. *Circulation.* 2010 Nov 2;122(18):1789-96.

[267] Glasser SP, Khodneva Y. Should acetaminophen be added to the list of anti-inflammatory agents that are associated with cardiovascular events? *Hypertension.* 2015 May;65(5):991-2.

[268] Burstein R, Noseda R, Borsook D. Migraine: multiple processes, complex pathophysiology. *J Neurosci.* 2015 Apr 29;35(17):6619-29.

[269] Mayo Clinic . Medications and supplements that can raise your blood pressure. http://www.mayoclinic.org/diseases-conditions/high-blood-pressure/in-depth/blood-pressure/art-20045245?pg=2. Published 13 March 2013. Accessed 25 October 2015.

[270] Torres AD, Rai AN, Hardiek ML. Mercury intoxication and arterial hypertension: report of two patients and review of the literature. *Pediatrics.* 2000 Mar;105(3):E34.

[271] Clarkson TW, Magos L, Myers GJ. The toxicology of mercury -- Current exposures and clinical manifestations. *N Engl J Med.* 2003; 349:1731-1737.

[272] Alissa EM, Ferns GA. Heavy metal poisoning and cardiovascular disease. *J Toxicol.* 2011;2011:870125.

[273] Agency for Toxic Substances and Disease Registry (ATSDR). ToxFAQsTM for cadmium. *Centers for Disease Control.* http://www.atsdr.cdc.gov/toxfaqs/ TF.asp?id=47&tid=15. Updated 12 March 2015. Accessed 15 November 2015.

[274] Vogt R, Bennett D, Cassady D, et al. Cancer and non-cancer health effects from food contaminant exposures for children and adults in California: a risk assessment. *Environ Health.* 2012 Nov 9;11:83.

[275] See for example: Mastin JP. Environmental cardiovascular disease. *Cardiovasc Toxicol.* 2005;5(2):91-4; O'Toole TE, Conklin DJ, Bhatnagar A. Environmental risk factors for heart disease. *Rev Environ Health.* 2008 Jul-Sep;23(3):167-202.

[276] Rancière F, Lyons JG, Loh VH, et al. Bisphenol A and the risk of cardiometabolic disorders: a systematic review with meta-analysis of the epidemiological evidence. *Environ Health.* 2015 May 31;14:46.

[277] Ha MH, Lee DH, Son HK, et al. Association between serum concentrations of persistent organic pollutants and prevalence of newly diagnosed hypertension: results from the National Health and Nutrition Examination Survey 1999-2002. *J Hum Hypertens.* 2009 Apr;23(4):274-86. See also: Huang X, Lessner L, Carpenter DO. Exposure to persistent organic pollutants and hypertensive disease. *Environ Res.* 2006 Sep;102(1):101-6.

[278] Boada LD, Sangil M, Alvarez-León EE, et al. Consumption of foods of animal origin as determinant of contamination by organochlorine pesticides and polychlorobiphenyls: results from a population-based study in Spain. *Chemosphere.* 2014 Nov;114:121-8.

[279] Zhang L, Li J, Zhao Y, et al. Polybrominated diphenyl ethers (PBDEs) and indicator polychlorinated biphenyls (PCBs) in foods from China: levels, dietary intake, and risk assessment. *J Agric Food Chem.* 2013 Jul 3;61(26):6544-51.

[280] Hennig B, Ormsbee L, McClain CJ, et al. Nutrition can modulate the toxicity of environmental pollutants: implications in risk assessment and human health. *Environ Health Perspect.* 2012 Jun;120(6):771-4.

[281] Petriello MC, Newsome B, Hennig B. Influence of nutrition in PCB-induced vascular inflammation. *Environ Sci Pollut Res Int.* 2014 May;21(10):6410-8.

282 Oishi K, Sato T, Yokoi W, et al. Effect of probiotics, Bifidobacterium breve and Lactobacillus casei, on bisphenol A exposure in rats. *Biosci Biotechnol Biochem*. 2008 Jun;72(6):1409-15.

283 Kukongviriyapan U, Pannangpetch P, Kukongviriyapan V, et al. Curcumin protects against cadmium-induced vascular dysfunction, hypertension and tissue cadmium accumulation in mice. *Nutrients*. 2014 Mar 21;6(3):1194-208.

284 For example see: Newberg A, Waldman MR. *Born to Believe: God, Science, and the Origin of Ordinary and Extraordinary Beliefs*. New York, NY: Simon & Schuster Inc; 2007. Newberg,A, Waldman MR. *How God Changes Your Brain: Breakthrough Findings from a Leading Neuroscientist*. New York: Ballantine Books; 2010.

285 Oken, BS. *Complementary Therapies in Neurology: An Evidence-Based Approach*. New York, NY: The Parthenon Publishing Group; 2004:225.

286 Graham TW, Kaplan BH, Cornoni-Huntley JC, et al. Frequency of church attendance and blood pressure elevation. *J Behav Med*. 1978 Mar;1(1):37-43.

287 Larson DB, Koenig HG, Kaplan BH, et al. The impact of religion on men's blood pressure. *J Relig Health*. 1989 Dec;28(4):265-78.

288 Koenig HG, George LK, Hays JC, et al. The relationship between religious activities and blood pressure in older adults. *Int J Psychiatry Med*. 1998;28(2):189-213.

289 Lucchese FA, Koenig HG. Religion, spirituality and cardiovascular disease: research, clinical implications, and opportunities in Brazil. *Rev Bras Cir Cardiovasc*. 2013 Mar;28(1):103-28.

290 Pargament KI, Koenig HG, Tarakeshwar N, Hahn J. Religious struggle as a predictor of mortality among medically ill elderly patients: a 2-year longitudinal study. *Arch Intern Med*. 2001 Aug 13-27;161(15):1881-5.

291 Pargament KI, Koenig HG, Tarakeshwar N, Hahn J. Religious coping methods as predictors of psychological, physical and spiritual outcomes among medically ill elderly patients: a two-year longitudinal study. *J Health Psychol*. 2004 Nov;9(6):713-30.

292 Some Christians may be uncomfortable with Jesus' call to embrace a virtuous life. Let me reassure you, I also believe the foundation of true Christianity rests on our freely accepting Christ's love and forgiveness—we can do nothing to merit God's favor. Nevertheless, the Holy Scriptures repeatedly call Christians to holy living. This does not constitute "a religion of works" since God's Spirit

works to change our life and habits in response to His love. Paul's prison epistles, Ephesians and Colossians, provide examples of this balance. They begin with statements of God's free forgiveness but end with moral imperatives.

[293] Howard R, Lash J. *This Was Your Life! Preparing to Meet God Face to Face.* Grand Rapids, MI: Chosen Books; 1998:85.

[294] Stein T. Humility: The art of self-forgetfulness. http://blogs.bible.org/engage/tiffany_stein/humility_the_art_of_self-forgetfulness. Published 18 March 2015. Accessed 29 February 2016.

[295] Coulehan J. On humility. *Ann Intern Med.* 2010 Aug 3;153(3):200-1.

[296] Micah 6:8. *The Holy Bible: English Standard Version.* Wheaton, IL: Standard Bible Society; 2001.

[297] Luke 18:9–14. *The Holy Bible: English Standard Version.* Wheaton, IL: Standard Bible Society; 2001.

[298] Your authors collectively have a significant international presence. As a single point of contact you can reach any of us through the "Contact Us" link at www.compasshealth.net.

[299] Picard RW. Intellectual assurance Christianity is sound. Talk presented at: the Massachusetts Institute of Technology (MIT); 19 April 1995. http://web.media.mit.edu/~picard/personal/ccc-talk.php. Accessed 29 November 2015.

[300] Isaiah 6:5. *The Holy Bible: English Standard Version.* Wheaton, IL: Standard Bible Society; 2001.

[301] Luke 5:8. *The Holy Bible: English Standard Version.* Wheaton, IL: Standard Bible Society; 2001.

[302] Philippians 2:6–8. *The Holy Bible: English Standard Version.* Wheaton, IL: Standard Bible Society; 2001.

[303] Proverbs 15:1. *The Holy Bible: English Standard Version.* Wheaton, IL: Standard Bible Society; 2001.

[304] Coulehan J. "A gentle and humane temper": humility in medicine. *Perspect Biol Med.* 2011 Spring;54(2):206-16.

[305] Crape BL, Latkin CA, Laris AS, Knowlton AR. The effects of sponsorship in 12-step treatment of injection drug users. *Drug Alcohol Depend.* 2002 Feb 1;65(3):291-301.

[306] Mark 1:4. *The Holy Bible: English Standard Version*. Wheaton, IL: Standard Bible Society; 2001.

[307] Mark 1:15. *The Holy Bible: English Standard Version*. Wheaton, IL: Standard Bible Society; 2001.

[308] John 6:37. *The Holy Bible: English Standard Version*. Wheaton, IL: Standard Bible Society; 2001.

[309] 1 John 1:9. *The Holy Bible: English Standard Version*. Wheaton, IL: Standard Bible Society; 2001.

[310] Job 5:17–18. *The Holy Bible: English Standard Version*. Wheaton, IL: Standard Bible Society; 2001.

[311] For example, see: Zemore SE, Subbaraman M, Tonigan JS. Involvement in 12-step activities and treatment outcomes. *Subst Abus*. 2013;34(1):60-9.

[312] For example, see: Weiss RD, Griffin ML, Gallop RJ, et al. The effect of 12-step self-help group attendance and participation on drug use outcomes among cocaine-dependent patients. *Drug Alcohol Depend*. 2005 Feb 14;77(2):177-84.

[313] Alcoholics Anonymous Australia. The twelve steps of AA. www.aa.org.au/members/twelve-steps.php. Accessed 21 November 2015.

[314] Kretzer K, Davis J, Easa D, et al. Self identity through Ho'oponopono as adjunctive therapy for hypertension management. *Ethn Dis*. 2007 Autumn;17(4):624-8.

[315] Kretzer K, Evelo AJ, Durham RL. Lessons learned from a study of a complementary therapy for self-managing hypertension and stress in women. *Holist Nurs Pract*. 2013 Nov-Dec;27(6):336-43.

[316] See John 1:1-3, 14; Colossians 1:12-17; Genesis 1: 1-2; note also, in Genesis 1:26-28, the word "us," indicating a plurality of persons referred to as "God."

[317] Philippians 2:5-10.

[318] Ezekiel 18:20; Romans 6:23.

[319] See John 14:15; 15:10.

[320] Proverbs 20:1. *The Holy Bible: English Standard Version*. Wheaton, IL: Standard Bible Society; 2001.

[321] Pompili M, Serafini G, Innamorati M, et al. Suicidal behavior and alcohol abuse. *Int J Environ Res Public Health*. 2010 April; 7(4): 1392–1431.

[322] Driscoll T, Harrison J, Steenkamp M. Review of the role of alcohol in drowning associated with recreational aquatic activity. *Inj Prev*. 2004 April; 10(2): 107–113.

[323] *Alcohol and Violence*. Volume 25, Number 1, 2001.

[324] Carroll AE. Alcohol or marijuana? A pediatrician faces the question. *New York Times*. 6 March 2015.

[325] CDC. Alcohol and public health: Fact sheets - Binge drinking. http://www.cdc.gov/alcohol/fact-sheets/binge-drinking.htm. Published 7 November 2012. Accessed 7 June 2013.

[326] See Exodus 20 for the Bible's famed "ten commandments" or Jesus' summary of them as "love God and love your neighbor" in Matthew 22:36-40.

[327] See Genesis 1:29.

[328] Animal fat is saturated fat. See Leviticus 7:23 and 3:17. Recall also our discussions about saturated fat earlier in this book.

[329] See Leviticus 15. Bathing lowers blood pressure for at least 60 minutes. Kawabe H, Saito I. Influence of nighttime bathing on evening home blood pressure measurements: how long should the interval be after bathing? *Hypertens Res*. 2006 Mar;29(3):129-33.

[330] See Leviticus 14:8-9,47; 15:5-13,21-22,27; 16:26-28; 17:15-16.

[331] See Leviticus 13. Although there is no direct connection to biblical infectious disease control practices, infection may play a role in blood pressure. Haarala and associates found that a more potent chronic infection with cytomegalovirus is associated with higher blood pressures. Haarala A, Kähönen M, Lehtimäki T, et al. Relation of high cytomegalovirus antibody titres to blood pressure and brachial artery flow-mediated dilation in young men: the Cardiovascular Risk in Young Finns Study. *Clin Exp Immunol*. 2012 Feb; 167(2):309–316.

[332] See Deuteronomy 23:13.

[333] See Leviticus 18. For example, note that inbreeding was responsible for 36% of all hypertension cases on three Croatian Islands. Rudan I, Smolej-Narancic N, Campbell H, et al. Inbreeding and the Genetic Complexity of Human Hypertension. *Genetics*. 2003 March 1; 163(3):1011-1021.

[334] See Leviticus 13. Although there is no direct connection to biblical infectious disease control practices, infection may play a role in blood pressure. Haarala and associates found that a more potent chronic infection with cytomegalovirus is associated with higher blood pressures. Haarala A. et al. Relation of high cytomegalovirus antibody titres to blood pressure and brachial artery flow-mediated dilation in young men: the Cardiovascular Risk in Young Finns Study. *Clin Exp Immunol*. 2012 Feb; 167(2):309–316.

[335] Matthew 27:46. *The Holy Bible: English Standard Version*. Wheaton, IL: Standard Bible Society; 2001.

[336] See, for example, Luke 3:22; John 12:27-33.

[337] See Galatians 3:13; 2 Corinthians 5:21.

[338] See Colossians 2:20-23.

[339] See Hebrews 1:1-3.

[340] See 1 Peter 2:21-25.

[341] See John 10:17.

[342] Compare Romans 6:6-7,12.

[343] See Proverbs 16:9; Isaiah 40:28-31; 2 Corinthians 5:17, 21; 1 Thessalonians 5:24; Romans 6:17-18, 22.

[344] Also called the second death in Revelation 20:6,14 and 21:8.

[345] Revelation 20:11-15.

[346] See John 5:21-30.

[347] Matthew 26:39. *The Holy Bible: English Standard Version*. Wheaton, IL: Standard Bible Society; 2001.

[348] Habakkuk 1:2. *The Holy Bible: English Standard Version*. Wheaton, IL: Standard Bible Society; 2001.

[349] Habakkuk 3:17–18. *The Holy Bible: English Standard Version*. Wheaton, IL: Standard Bible Society; 2001.

[350] Koenig HG, George LK, Hays JC, et al. The relationship between religious activities and blood pressure in older adults. *Int J Psychiatry Med*. 1998;28(2):189-213.

351 Shin J. Great is thy faithfulness: My journey into medicine [audio recording]. https://www.audioverse.org/english/sermons/recordings/13570/great-is-thy-faithfulness-my-journey-into-medicine.html. Published 31 October 2015. Accessed 22 November 2015.

352 Dossey L. Biography. http://www.dosseydossey.com/larry/default.html. Accessed 22 November 2015.

353 Matthew 6:25–34. *The Holy Bible: English Standard Version*. Wheaton, IL: Standard Bible Society; 2001.

354 Philippians 4:11–12. *The Holy Bible: English Standard Version*. Wheaton, IL: Standard Bible Society; 2001.

355 Matthew 5:16. *The Holy Bible: English Standard Version*. Wheaton, IL: Standard Bible Society; 2001.

356 Matthew 6:1–8. *The Holy Bible: English Standard Version*. Wheaton, IL: Standard Bible Society; 2001.

357 See for example: Duéñez-Guzmán EA, Sadedin S. Evolving righteousness in a corrupt world. *PLoS One*. 2012; 7(9): e44432.

358 Fønnebø V. The Tromsø Heart Study: diet, religion, and risk factors for coronary heart disease. *Am J Clin Nutr*. 1988 Sep;48(3 Suppl):826-9.

359 Zak PJ. Why inspiring stories make us react: the neuroscience of narrative. *Cerebrum*. 2015 Feb 2;2015:2.

360 Zak PJ, Stanton AA, Ahmadi S. Oxytocin increases generosity in humans. *PLoS One*. 2007; 2(11): e1128.

361 Luke 23:34. *The Holy Bible: English Standard Version*. Wheaton, IL: Standard Bible Society; 2001.

362 Acts 2:23, ESV.

363 Acts 2:38-39.

364 Dickerson JS. Charleston victims wield power of forgiveness: Column. *USA Today*. http://www.usatoday.com/story/opinion/2015/06/21/charleston-church-shooting-families-forgiveness-column/29069731/. Published 22 June 2015. Accessed 22 November 2015.

365 Dickerson JS. Charleston victims wield power of forgiveness: Column. *USA Today*. http://www.usatoday.com/story/opinion/2015/06/21/

charleston-church-shooting-families-forgiveness-column/29069731/. Published 22 June 2015. Accessed 22 November 2015.

366 Romans 1:14. *The Holy Bible: King James Version* (electronic ed. of the 1769 edition of the 1611 Authorized Version). Bellingham, WA: Logos Research Systems, Inc.

367 White EG. *The Ministry of Healing.* Nampa, ID: Pacific Press Publishing; 1905:495.

368 Wilson R. Mike Pettine: No discussion of cutting Manziel, QB can regain trust. http://www.cbssports.com/nfl/news/mike-pettine-no-discussion-of-cutting-manziel-qb-can-regain-trust/. Published 25 November 2015. Accessed 29 November 2015.

369 Tibbits D, Ellis G, Piramelli C, et al. Hypertension reduction through forgiveness training. *J Pastoral Care Counsel.* 2006 Spring-Summer;60(1-2):27-34.

370 Harris AH, Luskin F, Norman SB, et al. Effects of a group forgiveness intervention on forgiveness, perceived stress, and trait-anger. *J Clin Psychol.* 2006 Jun;62(6):715-33.

371 May RW, Sanchez-Gonzalez MA, Hawkins KA, et al. Effect of anger and trait forgiveness on cardiovascular risk in young adult females. *Am J Cardiol.* 2014 Jul 1;114(1):47-52.

372 Lee YR, Enright RD. A forgiveness intervention for women with fibromyalgia who were abused in childhood: A pilot study. *Spiritual Clin Pract* (Wash DC). 2014 Sep;1(3):203-217.

373 Toussaint L, Barry M, Bornfriend L, Markman M. Restore: the journey toward self-forgiveness: a randomized trial of patient education on self-forgiveness in cancer patients and caregivers. *J Health Care Chaplain.* 2014;20(2):54-74.

374 Worthington EL Jr, Witvliet CV, Pietrini P, Miller AJ. Forgiveness, health, and well-being: a review of evidence for emotional versus decisional forgiveness, dispositional forgivingness, and reduced unforgiveness. *J Behav Med.* 2007 Aug;30(4):291-302.

375 Romans 5:6–8. *The Holy Bible: English Standard Version.* Wheaton, IL: Standard Bible Society; 2001.

376 Don't minimize the far-reaching forgiveness Jesus offers. After all he said: "every sin and blasphemy will be forgiven people" Matthew 12:31 (ESV).

[377] Genesis 39:1.

[378] Genesis 39:9. *The Holy Bible: English Standard Version*. Wheaton, IL: Standard Bible Society; 2001.

[379] Lupis SB, Sabik NJ, Wolf JM. Role of shame and body esteem in cortisol stress responses. *J Behav Med*. 2016 Apr;39(2):262-75.

[380] Merriam-Webster On-line Dictionary. Shame. http://www.merriam-webster.com/dictionary/shame. Accessed 29 November 2015.

[381] Persons E, Kershaw T, Sikkema KJ, Hansen NB. The impact of shame on health-related quality of life among HIV-positive adults with a history of childhood sexual abuse. *AIDS Patient Care and STDs*. 2010;24(9):571-580.

[382] CDC. 2014 Sexually transmitted diseases surveillance. http://www.cdc.gov/std/stats14/default.htm. Updated 17 November 2015. Accessed 29 November 2015.

[383] Some may judge gay men based on Figure 14.5. However, public health consequences don't discriminate based on sexual preferences. Regardless of sexual orientation, wide-spread sexual expression without a moral basis is problematic from several standpoints including that of infectious diseases, reproductive health, and social and family stability—apart from any concerns derived from Judeo-Christian spiritual traditions (e.g., see Leviticus 18). Furthermore, research suggests that among some men, testosterone may have failed to fully androgenize or masculinize their brains between 14 and 17 weeks gestation, a critical time period in development. (See, for example, Rice WR, Friberg U, Gavrilets S . Homosexuality as a consequence of epigenetically canalized sexual development. *Q Rev Biol*. 2012 Dec;87(4):343-68). This theoretically could lead to an individual who has a male appearing body but a more feminine brain. An analogous situation may occur in women who develop with a more masculinized brain. For those of us without this experience, compassion rather than condemnation is of utmost importance. Condemnation itself can produce guilt and affect our stress response, ultimately influencing our health and blood pressure.

[384] Dickerson SS, Kemeny ME, Aziz N, et al. Immunological effects of induced shame and guilt. *Psychosom Med*. 2004 Jan-Feb;66(1):124-31.

[385] Deuteronomy 5:32–33. *The Holy Bible: English Standard Version*. Wheaton, IL: Standard Bible Society; 2001.

[386] See Matthew 22:36-40.

[387] See 1 John 3:4.

[388] Hosea 6:6. *The Holy Bible: English Standard Version*. Wheaton, IL: Standard Bible Society; 2001.

[389] 2 Corinthians 5:18–21. *The Holy Bible: English Standard Version*. Wheaton, IL: Standard Bible Society; 2001.

[390] 1 Corinthians 5:7. *The Holy Bible: English Standard Version*. Wheaton, IL: Standard Bible Society; 2001.

[391] Genesis 12:2–3. *The Holy Bible: English Standard Version*. Wheaton, IL: Standard Bible Society; 2001.

[392] Isaiah 56:3–8. *The Holy Bible: English Standard Version*. Wheaton, IL: Standard Bible Society; 2001.

[393] See, for example, the Sabbath connection with the Day of Atonement/Yom Kippur as described in Leviticus 16:29-34.

[394] Genesis 2:1-3; Exodus 20:8-11.

[395] Deuteronomy 5:12-15.

[396] Strawbridge WJ, Shema SJ, Cohen RD, Kaplan GA. Religious attendance increases survival by improving and maintaining good health behaviors, mental health, and social relationships. *Ann Behav Med*. 2001 Winter;23(1):68-74.

[397] For an excellent, and detailed, example of this from a Judeo-Christian perspective, consider the work of attorney Ken Sande and his associates at www.peacemaker.net.

[398] See, for example, Seligman MEP. *Learned Optimism: How to Change Your Mind and Your Life*. New York: Vintage Books; 2006.

[399] Workplace Bullying Institute. WBI survey: Personal attributes of bullied targets at work. http://www.workplacebullying.org/wbi-2014-ip-a/. Published 25 September 2014. Accessed 27 November 2015.

[400] 2 Timothy 3:12. *The Holy Bible: English Standard Version*. Wheaton, IL: Standard Bible Society; 2001.

[401] Matthew 10:16–31. *The Holy Bible: English Standard Version*. Wheaton, IL: Standard Bible Society; 2001.

[402] White EG. *Messages to Young People*. Nampa, ID: Pacific Press Publishing Association; 1930:127.

[403] Genesis 3:22-24.

[404] Matthew 10:28. *The Holy Bible: English Standard Version*. Wheaton, IL: Standard Bible Society; 2001.

[405] Luke 12:32. *The Holy Bible: English Standard Version*. Wheaton, IL: Standard Bible Society; 2001.

[406] For example, see John 3:23 (why would you need *much water* if people were just being ritually sprinkled?) and Mark 1:10 (if Jesus came *up out of the water* he must have gone down into it).

[407] See Romans 6:4–11. *The Holy Bible: English Standard Version*. Wheaton, IL: Standard Bible Society; 2001.

[408] Colossians 2:12-3:17. *The Holy Bible: English Standard Version*. Wheaton, IL: Standard Bible Society; 2001.

[409] See also Galatians 2:20.

[410] Aghababaei N, Tabik MT. Patience and mental health in Iranian students. *Iran J Psychiatry Behav Sci*. 2015 Sep;9(3):e1252.

[411] Schnitker SA. An examination of patience and well-being. *J Positive Psychol*. 2012 Jun;7(4):263–80.

[412] Actually, between your three co-authors we've collectively been helping people with lifestyle changes for some six decades.

CONTACT US

Thank you for taking the time to invest in your health. Your authors value your feedback. Feel free to contact any of us at the following addresses:

Dr. DeRose – drderose@compasshealth.net

Dr. Steinke – drgreg@programsforhealth.com

Nurse Practitioner Li – trullurn@yahoo.com

KEEP ON LEARNING

If you enjoyed *30 Days to Natural Blood Pressure Control,* you'll love the other educational resources produced by Dr. DeRose and his colleagues at CompassHealth Consulting, Inc. CompassHealth produces free materials as well as inexpensive educational resources like Dr. DeRose's popular DVD programs. **Why not continue to learn from some of Dr. DeRose's best seminars as described on the following pages?**

Take special note: if you're still struggling with some of the lifestyle changes recommended in this book, check out Dr. DeRose's motivational mini-series, *Changing Bad Habits for Good.*

All of the resources depicted on the pages that follow are available at http://www.compasshealth.net/purchase/.

Reversing Hypertension Naturally

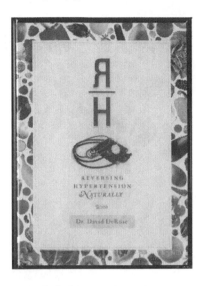

JOIN DR. DAVID DeROSE in this three-part series that complements the material in *30 Days to Natural Blood Pressure Control*!

(Three presentations, approximately 1-hour each; i.e., approx. 3 hours total run time.)

Reversing Diabetes Naturally

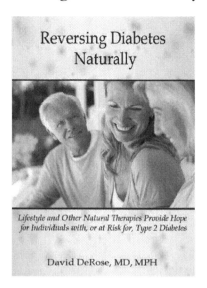

THIS LIFE-CHANGING SERIES unlocks the power of a non-drug approach for type 2 diabetes. Viewers will learn how to address diabetes' root cause known as "insulin resistance" and much, much more.

(Four presentations, approximately 1-hour each; i.e., approx. 4 hours total run time.)

Longevity Plus

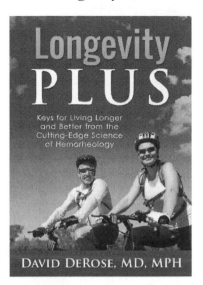

IN THIS DVD SERIES, Dr. DeRose unlocks the fascinating science of hemorheology, showing how we can increase our likelihood of living longer and better by following simple lifestyle practices that enhance blood fluidity.

(Two presentations, approximately 60-min each; i.e., approx. 2 hours total run time.)

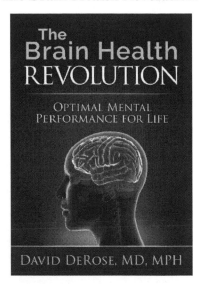

MODERN NEUROSCIENCE HAS UNLEASHED nothing short of a revolution when it comes to naturally optimizing brain health. In this two-part, approximately 2-hour long mini-series, Dr. DeRose walks you through some of the keys to enhancing brain performance without relying on drugs or expensive therapies.

Listening to the Buffalo

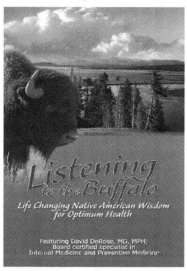

STARTING WITH THE TRUE STORY of an American Indian-raised homesteader who survived a buffalo stampede, Dr. DeRose takes a scientific look at the Native Americans who held bison in high esteem. You'll gain amazing insights into how modern science validates simple lifestyle strategies that can help prevent or treat diabetes and other lifestyle-related metabolic conditions.

(Two presentations, approximately 30-min each; i.e., approx. 1 hour total run time.)

Healing Insights from the Gospel of Mark

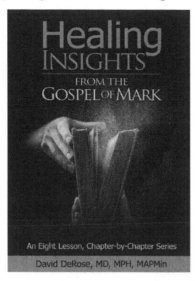

IF CHAPTER 14 DEALING WITH SPIRITUALITY left you longing for more of Dr. DeRose's health insights from the ancient scriptures, this series is perfect for you. *Healing Insights from the Gospel of Mark* offers a great way to learn and reinforce the health principles of *30 Days to Natural Blood Pressure Control*. Suitable for individual or group use, this series is designed to be viewed once weekly for eight weeks. Begin each session with Dr. DeRose's 30-minute video and then conclude with a 30-minute group health-focused Bible study (aided by Dr. DeRose's free study guides). Participants go through the entire 16 chapters of *The Gospel of Mark* over the course of the eight weeks.

(Eight presentations, approximately 30-min each; i.e., approx. 4 hours total run time.)

Changing Bad Habits for Good

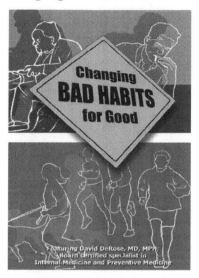

IF YOU KNOW WHAT YOU should be doing for your health but are having trouble translating that into practice, this DVD is for you. Finally master the dynamics of health behavior change in an engaging, practical way. You'll learn to develop new enjoyments and experience high quality living at the same time you shed unwanted habits.

(Two presentations, approximately 30-min each; i.e., approx. 1 hour total run time.)

Natural Strategies for Infectious Diseases

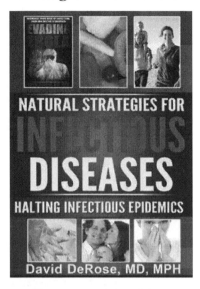

DR. DEROSE PROVIDES STRATEGIES TO HELP you keep well–even when it seems all those around you are getting sick. Whether dealing with the common cold, influenza, or more frightening infectious illnesses like Ebola or equine encephalitis, Dr. DeRose's simple strategies can truly spell the difference between sickness and health. DeRose shares insights into a variety of relevant, cutting-edge topics including fitness, dietary practices, vaccinations, beverage choices, and hygiene.

(Two presentations, approximately 60-min each; i.e., approx. 2 hours total run time.)

And don't forget the companion book to

the *Natural Strategies for Infectious Disease* DVD mini-series...

Evading Ebola

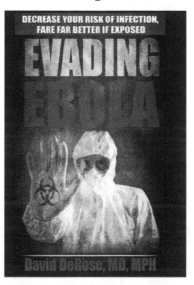

ALTHOUGH EBOLA MAY NO LONGER SEEM to be a threat, the untold story behind Ebola provides keys that could save your life from other infectious diseases. In *Evading Ebola*, physician and public health expert, David DeRose, MD, MPH, provides some of the most encouraging, yet untold, information to date. Drawn from research on "inapparent" Ebola infection (Africans who got the virus but never got sick), DeRose outlines simple practical steps to help you avoid ever getting sick with Ebola (and a host of other infections)—even if exposed. The book details research from infectious diseases as diverse as Ebola, food poisoning, colds and influenza. Don't miss the practical importance of this book to your overall health and well-being because you thought it merely dealt with Ebola.